D1394406

OXFORD MEDICAL PUBLICATIONS
Addiction
Medicine

Oxford Specialist Handbooks published and forthcoming

General Oxford Specialist Handbooks
A Resuscitation Room Guide
Addiction Medicine
Perioperative Medicine,
Second Edition
Post-Operative Complications,
Second edition

Oxford Specialist Handbooks in Anaesthesia
Cardiac Anaesthesia
General Thoracic Anaesthesia
Neuroanaesthesia
Obstetric Anaesthesia
Paediatric Anaesthesia
Regional Anaesthesia, Stimulation
and Ultrasound Techniques

Oxford Specialist Handbooks in Cardiology
Adult Congenital Heart Disease
Cardiac Catheterization and
Coronary Intervention
Echocardiography
Fetal Cardiology
Heart Failure
Hypertension
Nuclear Cardiology
Pacemakers and ICDs

Oxford Specialist Handbooks in Critical Care
Advanced Respiratory Critical Care

Oxford Specialist Handbooks in End of Life Care
End of Life Care in Cardiology
End of Life Care in Dementia
End of Life Care in Nephrology
End of Life Care in Respiratory
Disease
End of Life Care in the Intensive
Care Unit

Oxford Specialist Handbooks in Neurology
Epilepsy
Parkinson's Disease and Other
Movement Disorders
Stroke Medicine

Oxford Specialist Handbooks in Paediatrics
Paediatric Endocrinology and Diabetes
Paediatric Dermatology
Paediatric Gastroenterology,
Hepatology, and Nutrition
Paediatric Haematology and
Oncology
Paediatric Nephrology
Paediatric Neurology
Paediatric Radiology
Paediatric Respiratory Medicine

Oxford Specialist Handbooks in Psychiatry
Child and Adolescent Psychiatry
Old Age Psychiatry

Oxford Specialist Handbooks in Radiology
Interventional Radiology
Musculoskeletal Imaging

Oxford Specialist Handbooks in Surgery
Cardiothoracic Surgery
Hand Surgery
Hepato-pancreatobiliary Surgery
Oral Maxillo Facial Surgery
Neurosurgery
Operative Surgery, Second Edition
Otolaryngology and Head and Neck
Surgery
Plastic and Reconstructive Surgery
Surgical Oncology
Urological Surgery
Vascular Surgery

Oxford Specialist Handbooks

Addiction Medicine

Noeline Latt
Drug and Alcohol Department, Royal North Shore
Hospital and Faculty of Medicine, University of Sydney,
Australia

Katherine Conigrave
Drug Health Service, Royal Prince
Alfred Hospital, Faculty of Medicine,
University of Sydney, Australia

John B. Saunders
Faculty of Medicine
University of Sydney, Australia

E. Jane Marshall
South London and Maudsley
NHS Foundation Trust, and Institute of Psychiatry,
King's College London, London, UK

David Nutt
Psychopharmacology Unit
University of Bristol, UK

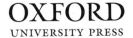

OXFORD
UNIVERSITY PRESS

OXFORD
UNIVERSITY PRESS

Great Clarendon Street, Oxford OX2 6DP

Oxford University Press is a department of the University of Oxford.
It furthers the University's objective of excellence in research, scholarship,
and education by publishing worldwide in

Oxford New York

Auckland Cape Town Dar es Salaam Hong Kong Karachi
Kuala Lumpur Madrid Melbourne Mexico City Nairobi
New Delhi Shanghai Taipei Toronto

With offices in

Argentina Austria Brazil Chile Czech Republic France Greece
Guatemala Hungary Italy Japan Poland Portugal Singapore
South Korea Switzerland Thailand Turkey Ukraine Vietnam

Oxford is a registered trade mark of Oxford University Press
in the UK and in certain other countries

Published in the United States
by Oxford University Press Inc., New York

© Oxford University Press, 2009

British Library Cataloguing in Publication Data
Data available

Library of Congress Cataloging in Publication Data
Data available

Typeset by Newgen Imaging Systems (P) Ltd., Chennai, India
Printed in China
on acid-free paper through
Asia Pacific Offset

ISBN 978–0–19–953933–8

10 9 8 7 6 5 4 3 2

Foreword

The appearance of this major work is a fortunate event for the student and practitioner of addictions treatment. There is a need for people who work in this field to be conversant with both the social and also the biological aspects of substance dependence.

A by-product of the ease with which today both materials and cultures can travel across continents has been that the human species has access to an ever widening range of psychoactive substances. The brain's mosaic of mood pathways can be titillated in myriad subtle ways and our bodies seem able to metabolise many potentially toxic substances. Indeed, the breakdown catalyst of ethanol, ethanol dehydrogenase, has been evolutionarily important in our transition from fruit eating primate to homo erectus. Our forebears could eat the fermenting fruit lying on the ground, and not have to rely on scaling the heights of the trees. Fermenting fruit became a sophisticated industry—it can sometimes even charge a higher price for its ageing products, which is an ingenious marketing device.

For alcoholic beverages, multinational business ensures that the breadth of choice is getting ever wider. World Trade Agreements indirectly aid availability. There are limits however. The radio-astronomical discovery 6 years ago of a galaxy several light years away, whose atmosphere is made up principally of ethanol vapour, does not announce the extension of Trade Agreements to outer space.

As long as societies wish to care for those who become ill, whether or not through their recreation or lifestyle or diet, there will be a growing need for health and social carers to understand addictions. They will find this magnificent scholarly textbook, representing huge dedication by many writers, a boon and a blessing to their studies and their labours.

Jonathan Chick
University of Edinburgh, Scotland

Preface

Origin of the handbook
This Handbook of Addiction Medicine is the result of many years preparation by a group of us who have been clinicians, teachers and researchers in the alcohol and drug field in Australia and the United Kingdom. It has its origins in a series of clinical protocols that were originally developed by one of us (JBS) in the mid-1970s, which then formed the basis of lecture courses in the University of London. The protocols and lecture notes have been developed progressively since then, and have been made available to successive groups of students and practitioner colleagues in Australia and the UK. In preparing the *Handbook of Addiction Medicine* we sought the contributions of fellow specialists in several countries to produce a contemporary, clinically-grounded text that summarizes the theory and the practice of addiction medicine.

Evidence and practice
The material in this handbook is informed by the evidence base—the clinical trials and systematic reviews of study findings, and the underpinning science. It also draws upon our clinical practice and experience, as it has been shaped over the years to respond to changing patterns of substance use and various interventions that have been developed. All the approaches described have been thoroughly tested in practice and are what we employ in our daily work.

Who is this book for?
The handbook is intended as a concise and practical guide for students and practitioners of medicine and other health professions who come into contact with people with substance use disorders. This means just about every student and practitioner! More specifically, it is designed for medical students, postgraduate trainees in internal medicine, psychiatry and general (family) practice, trainees in addiction medicine, and established practitioners and specialists in these areas. We believe it will also be useful and relevant to nurses, psychologists, counsellors, and other clinicians, and for specialist multi-disciplinary agencies providing treatment for people with substance use disorders.

Why is this book important?
Substance use rates amongst the top four risk factors contributing to the global burden of disease. Substance use disorders can cause, mimic, underlie, or complicate a large number of common medical and psychiatric disorders. They contribute immense personal suffering, as well as cost to society, which is often not well recognized. Patients may be reticent about revealing their substance use and may not see its relevance. The fact that

many patients use more than one substance, adds to the complexity of the problem. Making a correct diagnosis of the substance use disorder can facilitate clinical diagnosis, avoid unnecessary tests, shorten hospital stay and make the clinician and patient's life easier—and safer! Increasingly, the ability to diagnose and initiate management of substance use disorders is the responsibility of all medical and health professionals. Traditionally, however, they have not been confident in managing alcohol and drug problems. The knowledge base and the skill set required for good professional practice in this field has been increasingly defined. Addiction Medicine now has a range of treatments that compare in their effectiveness to those in other areas of medicine.

What is covered?

The handbook provides a practical and easy reference guide to the management of people with substance use disorders. As the text is confined to disorders relating to psychoactive substances, it does not cover gambling or electronic addiction. The first chapter outlines important background information and summarizes the principles of addiction medicine. It encompasses the epidemiology of psychoactive substance use, the pharmacology and neurobiology of the major substances, and the natural history of the main clinical disorders. The following two chapters summarize the principles of assessment and diagnosis and management that inform the practice of addiction medicine.

Following this there are seven chapters on specific types of psychoactive substance, in which the main clinical syndromes associated with that particular substance type and aspects of management that are specific to that substance are described. The remainder of the handbook is devoted to management of specific groups and in specific circumstances and places addiction medicine within the broad professional and legal context. The needs and relevant treatments for particular age and socio-economic groups are described, together with the more complex clinical situations, such as pain and dependence and psychiatric co-morbidity. Following the main text there are a series of appendices which provide summaries of concepts and practical tools to aid management.

The handbook provides detailed guidelines on how to obtain a history of alcohol and other drug use, as well as assessment and diagnosis of the core clinical syndromes and related medical and psychosocial problems. In it you will also find practical guides to the range of treatments available, including early intervention, management of withdrawal syndromes ('detoxification'), pharmacotherapies for relapse prevention, and other management approaches, such as psychological therapies, supportive approaches, and group programmes.

Contents

Acknowledgements

In presenting this handbook to our colleagues and students, we would in turn like to thank our own teachers. We accordingly wish to dedicate this handbook to those who helped influence and shape our own professional careers, including Griffith Edwards, Alex Paton, David Graham-Smith, Markku Linnoila, Boris Tabakoff, Harding Burns, Edith Collins, Norman Sartorius and Harold Kalant.

Thanks are also due to:

Dr Elizabeth Proude, University of Sydney, for her careful editing and formatting of the text and co-ordination of the final stages.

New South Wales Department of Health, Centre for Drug and Alcohol and Mental Health who provided funds for the compiling and editing of the text.

Our colleagues who reviewed various sections of the manuscript, and in particular, Professor Robert Batey who reviewed the entire text relating to physical disorders and Dr Glenys Dore who contributed to and reviewed all the mental health aspects of the handbook.

Authors and editors

Dr Noeline Latt MBBS, MPhil, MRCP (UK), FAChAM is an Addiction Medicine Specialist with a background in clinical pharmacology. She is a Senior Staff Specialist in Addiction Medicine at Royal North Shore Hospital in Sydney, Clinical Lecturer at the University of Sydney, Consultant to the NSW Drug and Alcohol Specialist Advisory Service and a Foundation Fellow of the Chapter of Addiction Medicine, Royal Australasian College of Physicians. She has more than 15 years experience in clinical treatment and teaching of alcohol and substance use disorders. Her research has focused on treatment of alcohol dependence, hepatitis C in pregnant injecting drug users and substance induced psychosis.

Associate Professor Kate Conigrave MBBS (Hons), FAFPHM, FAChAM, PhD is an Addiction Medicine Specialist and a Public Health Physician. As well as her clinical practice as a Staff Specialist in Addiction Medicine at Royal Prince Alfred Hospital she has extensive research experience in alcohol and drug use disorders. Associate Professor Conigrave has conjoint appointments at the Faculty of Medicine, University of Sydney, The National Drug and Alcohol Research Centre, University of New South Wales, and Menzies School of Population Health Research, Darwin. Her research has a focus on detection and early intervention for alcohol problems, and how to better implement evidence-based practice into the clinical routine. In recent years she has also worked with Aboriginal communities on addressing substance use disorders. She has acted as short-term consultant to the World Health Organization on brief intervention. She is on the Editorial Advisory Board for *Alcohol and Alcoholism*.

Professor John Saunders MA, MB BChir, MD, FRCP, FRACP, FAChAM, FAFPHM is a Professor of Medicine and addiction studies with appointments at the Universities of Queensland and Sydney, Australia, and a Consultant Physician in internal medicine and addiction medicine, and medical director in the Healthscope, St John of God Health Care and Wesley Health Services groups. He qualified in pharmacology and then medicine from the University of Cambridge, UK, and undertook specialist medical training in acute general medicine, gastroenterology and liver disease, and addiction medicine in Birmingham and London. His career as a clinician, service director, researcher and academic in the alcohol and drug field extends back over 30 years. His research over this time has included screening and early diagnosis, brief interventions, assessment instruments, susceptibility to alcohol- and drug-related disorders, treatment of alcohol, opioid, and psychostimulant dependence, and medical education in addiction studies. He has worked with the World Health Organization for many years and was responsible for developing the AUDIT questionnaire. He is Editor-in-Chief of the Drug and Alcohol

Review, Vice-President of the International Society of Addiction Medicine, a member of WHO's Expert Advisory Panel on Mental Health and Substance Abuse, and Co-Chair of the DSM V Substance Use Disorders Workgroup. He has been a member of many state and federal Australian government committees, and was a member of the Australian National Council on Drugs from 2001 to 2007. He has published two books and over 300 scientific papers, reviews and book chapters.

Dr Jane Marshall MB BCh BAO MRCP(Ireland) FRCPsych is a Consultant Psychiatrist in Alcohol Studies at the South London and Maudsley NHS Foundation Trust and Senior Lecturer in the Addictions at the National Addiction Centre, Institute of Psychiatry, Kings College London. She trained in Psychiatry at St Patrick's Hospital, Dublin, and St Bartholomew's and the Maudsley Hospitals in London. Her clinical work is currently focused on a specialist out-patient and in-patient alcohol service, also a service for addicted healthcare professionals. Education and training commitments include being lead clinician for an MSc programme in the Clinical and Public Health Aspects of Addiction, based at the Institute of Psychiatry. This involves curriculum development, teaching, student supervision and assessment, also programme monitoring. Research interests include the evaluation of treatment for alcohol problems in specialist and generalist settings and, in particular, treatment for addicted healthcare professionals. Dr Marshall acts as a Medical Supervisor, Examiner and expert witness for the General Medical Council and as a Medical Advisor for the General Dental Council. Since 2003 she has been Joint Co-Director of Flexible Training at the Royal College of Psychiatrists. She also sits on the executive committee of the College's Faculty of the Addictions and is a member of the College's Psychiatrists' Support Service Committee. She is on the executive committee of the Society for the Study of Addiction. Dr Marshall has contributed to national guidelines, and has been a member of a number of Working Parties, including the Royal College of Physicians Working Party on Alcohol in the General Hospital (2001); an Alcohol Concern Research Forum (2002); and a Department of Health Working Group on Alcohol-related Brain Damage (2007).

Professor David Nutt MB BChir, MA DM FRCP FRCPsych FMedSci is currently Professor of Psychopharmacology and Head of the Department of Community Based Medicine at the University of Bristol. He received his undergraduate training in medicine at Cambridge and Guy's Hospital, and continued training in neurology to MRCP. After completing his psychiatric training in Oxford, he continued there as a lecturer and then later as a Wellcome Senior Fellow in Psychiatry. He then spent 2 years as Chief of the Section of Clinical Science in the National Institute of Alcohol Abuse and Alcoholism in NIH, Bethesda, USA. On returning to England in 1988 he set up the Psychopharmacology Unit in Bristol, an interdisciplinary research grouping spanning the departments of Psychiatry and Pharmacology. Their main research interests are in the brain mechanisms underlying anxiety, depression, and addiction and the mode of action of therapeutic drugs. He is currently chair-elect of the Advisory Council on the Misuse of Drugs (ACMD), and Chair of its Technical

Committee, President of the European College of Neuropsychopharmacology (ECNP) and a Director of the 'European Certificate in Anxiety and Mood Disorders' and the 'Masters in Affective Disorders' courses jointly administered by the Universities of Maastricht, Bristol and Florence. In addition, he is the Editor of the *Journal of Psychopharmacology*, advisor to the British National Formulary and a Past-President of the British Association of Psychopharmacology (BAP). He was also a member of the Independent Inquiry into the Misuse of Drugs Act 1971, chaired by Viscountess Runciman, that reported in 2000 and a member of the Committee on Safety of Medicines (CSM) from 2000 to 2005. In 2006 he was Director of Bristol Neuroscience.

Contributors

Dr Peter Anderson
Consultant in Public Health,
Apartat de Correus 352, 17230
Palamos, Girona, Spain
*Chapter 1: Epidemiology
of alcohol*

**Associate Professor Sawitri
Assanangkornchai**
Faculty of Medicine, Prince
of Songkla University,
Hat Yai, Songkla 90110,
Thailand
*Chapter 12: Substance use in
different cultural contexts*

Professor Robert Batey
Professor of Medicine,
University of New South Wales,
Department of Gastroenterology,
Bankstown Hospital,
Eldridge Road, Bankstown,
New South Wales 2200,
Australia
*Chapter 4: Alcohol-related liver
disease; Chapter 8: Hepatitis B
and Hepatitis C in injecting
drug users*

Prof James Bell
Drug and Alcohol Clinical Director
of South Eastern Sydney Illawarra
Area Health Service, Director,
Langton Clinic, 591
South Dowling Street,
Surry Hills, NSW 2210
*Chapter 13: Pain and opioid
dependence*

**Associate Professor Renee
Bittoun**
Brain and Mind Research Unit,
University of Sydney, 100 Mallett
St Camperdown, New South Wales
2050, Australia
Chapter 5: Tobacco

Dr Yvonne Bonomo
Addiction Medicine, St Vincents
Hospital Melbourne, and Departments
of Medicine and Paediatrics,
University of Melbourne. PO Box
2900, Fitzroy, Victoria 3065, Australia
Chapter 12: Adolescents

Dr Adam Brodie
Locum Consultant Addiction
Psychiatrist, Stobhill Hospital,
Glasgow G21 3UT, United Kingdom
Chapter 10: Volatile solvent misuse

**Associate Professor Alan
Clough**
School of Public Health, Tropical
Medicine & Rehabilitation Science
and School of Indigenous Australian
Studies, James Cook University
(Cairns Campus), PO Box 6811
Cairns, Queensland 4870, Australia
Chapter 10: Kava

Professor Louisa Degenhardt
Professor of Epidemiology, National
Drug and Alcohol Research Centre,
University of New South Wales,
New South Wales 2052,
Australia
*Chapter 1: Epidemiology of illicit
drugs*

Dr Glenys Dore

Medical Director, Northern Sydney Area Drug & Alcohol Services, Herbert Street Drug and Alcohol Clinic, Royal North Shore Hospital, Pacific Highway, St Leonards NSW 2065, Australia
Chapter 9: Psychostimulants; Chapter 11: Psychiatric co-morbidity Chapter 12: Special populations; Chapter 14: Difficult and urgent situations; and mental health aspects in all other chapters throughout the handbook.

Dr Emily Finch

Consultant Psychiatrist in the Addictions, South London and Maudsley NHS Foundation Trust Blackfriars Road Community Drug and Alcohol Team
151 Blackfairs Road, London SE1 8EL
Chapter 15: Drugs and driving

Dr Stephen Jurd

Director of Postgraduate Training in Psychiatry, Northern Sydney & Central Coast Health. Academic Unit, Macquarie Hospital, PO Box 169 North Ryde, New South Wales 1670, Australia
Chapter 12: Addicted physicians

Prof Edwina Kidd

Emerita Professor of Cariology, Dental School, Kings College London, Floor 18 Guys Tower, London Bridge SE1 9RT, United Kingdom.
Chapter 13: The oral complications of drug and alcohol misuse

Associate Professor Michael Levy

Director, Corrections Health Program ACT Health
GPO Box 825
Canberra ACT 2601, Australia
Chapter 12: Special populations: prisons

Associate Professor Harry Minas

Director, Centre for International Mental Health, School of Population Health, University of Melbourne, 207 Bouverie St, Carlton, Victoria 3053, Australia
Chapter 12: Special populations: mental health and substance use disorders in refugees and migrants

Dr Tim Neumann

Department of Anesthesiology and Intensive Care Medicine, Campus Virchow-Klinikum and Campus Charité Mitte, Charité—Universitätsmedizin Berlin, 10117 Berlin, Germany
Chapter 14: Dealing with alcohol within the emergency department

Dr Sally Porter

Addiction Psychiatry, South London and Maudsley NHS Trust, Crosfield House, Mint Walk, Croydon CR9 3JS, United Kingdom
Chapter 15: Child protection issues

Dr Janie Sheridan
School of Pharmacy, Faculty of
Medical and Health Sciences,
University of Auckland, Private
Bag 92019, Auckland Mail Centre,
Auckland 1142, New Zealand
*Chapter 10: Proprietary and
pharmacy drugs*

Dr Iain D. Smith
Consultant Addiction
Psychiatrist, Gartnavel Royal
Hospital, Glasgow G12 0XH,
United Kingdom
Chapter 10: Volatile solvent misuse

Professor Claudia Spies
Department of Anesthesiology
and Intensive Care Medicine,
Campus Virchow-Klinikum and
Campus Charité Mitte, Charité—
Universitätsmedizin Berlin,
10117 Berlin, Germany
*Chapter 14: Dealing with alcohol
in the Emergency Department*

Ms Georgina Spilsbury
A/Statewide Clinical Coordinator
"At Risk" Programs, Chief
Psychologist, NSW Department of
Corrective Services, 56 Clinton
Street, Goulburn, New South
Wales 2580, Australia.
Chapter 3: Motivational interviewing

Prof David Taylor,
Chief Pharmacist, South London
and Maudsley NHS Foundation
Trust, Pharmacy Department.
Maudsley Hospital, Denmark Hill,
London SE5 8AZ United Kingdom
Chapter 10: Anabolic steroids

Dr Peter K Thompson,
Director Emergency Medicine,
Rockhampton Base Hospital,
Queensland 4700, Australia;
Consultant Emergency Physician,
King's College Hospital,
Denmark Hill, London,
SE5 9RS, United Kingdom
*Chapter 14: Illicit drug users in
the Emergency Department*

Dr Sue Wilson
University of Bristol,
Psychopharmacology Unit,
Dorothy Hodgkin Building,
Whitson St, Bristol BS1 3NY
United Kingdom
*Chapter 13: The sleepless
patient*

Dr Adam R Winstock
Senior Staff Specialist Drug
Health Services SSWAHS-DHS
and Conjoint Senior Lecturer,
National Drug and Alcohol
Research Centre, University
of New South Wales,
New South Wales 2052
Australia
*Chapters 10: Party drugs,
Areca nut (Betel/pan), khat, and
clinical photographs*

Dr Kim Wolff
Addictions Head of Graduate
Studies, Institute of Psychiatry,
King's College London.
Windsor Walk, London SE5 8AF,
United Kingdom
Chapter 12: Pregnancy

Glossary

Addiction An umbrella term that encompasses a variety of substance dependence syndromes and also behavioural disorders, such as pathological gambling where no substance use is implicated, but where the features of the disorder are similar to those of substance dependence.

Misuse An umbrella term used to embrace a range of substance use disorders of different severity where the characteristic feature is the single or repetitive use of a psychoactive substance.

Abuse The use of this term is confined to its use as a diagnostic term according to DSM-IV criteria, examples being 'alcohol abuse' and 'cannabis abuse'. Occasionally, it is used to indicate physical, sexual, or other abuse, but this will be clear from the context.

Dependence This refers to a dependence syndrome as described in ICD-10 or DSM-IV. Occasionally, the term 'pharmacological dependence' is used specifically to indicate neuro-adaptation to a psychoactive substance and, again, the context will be clear.

Detailed contents

Symbols and abbreviations

5HIAA5	Hydroxy indoleacetic acid
5HT	5 hydroxytryptamine (serotonin)
AA	Alcoholics anonymous
Ab	Antibody
ACE	Angiotensin converting enzyme
ADH	Antidiuretic hormone
ADHD	Attention deficit hyperactivity disorder
ADIS	Alcohol and Drug Information Service, Australia
AFP	Alpha-foeto protein
Ag	Antigen
AIDS	Acquired immune deficiency syndrome
ALP	Alkaline phosphatase
ALT	Alanine aminotransferase
Anti HCV	Hepatitis C antibody
APTT	Activated partial thromboplastin time
ARND	Alcohol-related neurodevelopment disorder
ASPD	Antisocial personality disorder
ASSIST	The Alcohol, Smoking and Substance Involvement Screening Test
ASI	Addiction severity index
AST	Aspartate aminotransferase
ATS	Amphetamine-type stimulants
AUD	Alcohol use disorder
AUDIT	Alcohol use disorders identification test
AWS	Alcohol withdrawal scale
BAC	Blood alcohol concentration
BAP	British Association of Psychopharmacology
bd	Twice daily
BP	Blood pressure
BWS	Benzodiazepine withdrawal scale
CAGE	An acronym for four alcoholism screening questions described by Mayfield 1974
CAL	Chronic airways limitation (also known as COPD)
CB1, CB2	Cannabis receptors 1 & 2
CBT	Cognitive behavioural therapy
CCF	Congestive cardiac failure
CDT	Carbohydrate deficient transferrin
CIDI	Composite international diagnostic interview

CIWA-AR	Clinical Institute Withdrawal Assessment for Alcohol-revised
CIWA-B	Clinical Institute Withdrawal Assessment for Benzodiazepines
C-L	Consultation liaison
CNS	Central nervous system
COMT	Catechol-O-methyltransferase
COPD	Chronic obstructive pulmonary disease
CK-MB	Creatine kinase isoenzyme for diagnosis of myocardial infarction
CPK	Creatine phosphokinase
CRP	C-reactive protein
CT	Computed tomography
CVS	Cardiovascular system
CXR	Chest X-ray
DALYs	Disability adjusted life years
DA	Dopamine
DD	Differential diagnosis
DDS	Delirium detection scale
DIS	Diagnostic Interview Schedule, National Institutes of Mental Health
DNA	Deoxyribonucleic acid
DSM IV	Diagnostic and Statistical Manual, 4th Edition
DT	Delirium tremens
DVLA	Driver and Vehicle Licensing Agency (UK)
ECG	Electrocardiogram
ECHO	Echocardiogram
ED	Emergency department
EDOU	Emergency department observation unit
EEG	Electroencephalogram
EMR	Eastern mediterranean region
ERCP	Endoscopic retrograde cholangiopancreatography
ESR	Erythrocyte sedimentation rate
EUC	Electrolytes, urea and creatinine
FAE	Foetal alcohol effects
FAS	Foetal alcohol syndrome
FASD	Foetal alcohol spectrum disorder
FBC	Full blood count
FLAGS	Feedback, Listen, Advice, Goals, Strategies (Acronym for core elements of brief intervention)
fMRI	Functional magnetic resonance imaging
FTC	Framework of Tobacco Control
FTQ	Fagerström tolerance questionnaire

GABA	Gamma aminobutyric acid
GAD	Generalized anxiety disorder
GCS	Glasgow coma scale
GDP	Gross domestic product
GGT	Gamma glutamyltransferase
GHB	Gamma hydroxybutyrate
GI	Gastrointestinal
GIT	Gastrointestinal tract
GP	General practitioner
HADS	Hospital Anxiety and Depression Scale
Hb	Haemoglobin
HBV	Hepatitis B virus
HBcAb	Hepatitis B core antibody
HBeAg	Hepatitis B e antigen
HbsAg	Hepatitis B surface antigen
Hct	Haematocrit
HCV	Hepatitis C virus
HDL	High density lipoprotein
HIV	Human immunodeficiency virus
HoNOS	Health of the Nation Outcome Scales
hr	Hours
I$	International dollars
ICD	International Classification of Diseases
IM	Intramuscular
INR	International normalized ratio
IV	Intravenous
IU	International units
IUGR	Intra-uterine growth retardation
K or Special K	Ketamine
Kg	Kilograms
L	Litre(s)
LDL	Low density lipoprotein
LFT	Liver function tests
LSD	Lysergic acid
MAOI	Monoamine oxidase inhibitors
MCV	Mean corpuscular volume
MDMA	Methylenedioxymethamphetamine
MEOS	Microsomal ethanol oxidizing system
μg	Micrograms
mins	Minutes
mL	Millilitre(s)
mmHg	Millimetres of mercury
MRI	Magnetic resonance imaging
MRSA	Methicillin resistant staphylococcus aureus

MSE	Mental state examination
NA	Narcotics anonymous
NAD	Nicotinamide adenine dinucleotide (oxidized form)
NADH	Nicotinamide adenine dinucleotide (reduced form)
NARS	Nicotine Assisted Reduction to Stop
NaSSA	Noradrenaline and specific serotonergic agent
ng	Nanograms
NMDA	N-methyl-d-aspartate
NMS	Neuroleptic malignant syndrome
nocte	At night
NRT	Nicotine replacement therapy
NSAIDs	Non-steroidal anti-inflammatory drugs
OCD	Obsessive compulsive disorder
OTC	Over-the-counter
PAT	Paddington alcohol test
PCP	Phencyclidine
PCR	Polymerase chain reaction
PET	Positron emission tomography
PFC	Prefrontal cortex;
PMA	Para-methoxyamphetamine
po	Per oral
PPP	Purchasing power parity
prn	Pro re nata (as required)
PTSD	Post-traumatic stress disorder
qid	Four times daily
RASS	Richmond Agitation-Sedation Scale
RIMA	Reversible inhibitor of monoamine oxidase A
RNA	Ribonucleic acid
RTA	Road traffic accidents
SAD	Social anxiety disorder
SADQ	Severity of Alcohol Dependence Questionnaire
SAM	Substance abuse module
SC	Subcutaneous
SCAN	WHO Schedules for Clinical Assessment in Neuropsychiatry
SDS	Severity of Dependence Scale
secs	Seconds
SF14, SF36, SF96	Quality of life questionnaires
SIDS	Sudden infant death syndrome
SE	Side effects
SL	Sublingual
SNRI	Serotonin and noradrenaline reuptake inhibitor
SODQ	Severity of Opiate Dependence Questionnaire

SSRIs	Selective serotonin reuptake inhibitors
STI	Sexually transmitted infection
t$_{1/2}$	Half life
TB	Tuberculosis
TCA	Tricyclic antidepressant
tds	Three times daily
TFT	Thyroid function test
THC	Tetrahydrocannabinol
TIA	Transient ischaemic attacks
TSH	Thyroid-stimulating hormone
TTFC	Time to first cigarette
TWEAK	An acronym for screening questions for excess drinking—Tolerance, Worried, Eye-opener, Amnesia, K/Cut-down
UN	United nations
UNODC	United Nations Office on Drugs and Crime
VDRL	Venereal diseases research laboratory test for syphilis
VTA	Ventral tegmental area
VSM	Volatile solvent misuse
WE	Wernicke's encephalopathy
WBC	White blood cell count
WHO	World health organization
WPR	Western pacific region

The scope of addiction medicine

The use of psychoactive substances has formed an integral part of human society for millennia, but there are considerable differences in the nature of substances used and the reasons for their use. Thousands of naturally occurring substances exist and these have been supplemented over the past 200 years by synthetic compounds produced in the search for medications or simply for hedonic purposes. Worldwide 48% of the total adult population (approx 2 billion people), consume alcohol at least occasionally, 33% (approx 1.3 billion people) smoke tobacco, principally in the form of cigarettes, and 5% of adults (approx 200 million people) use illicit drugs. Increasingly, the pattern of substance use involves the use of multiple substances, often with different pharmacological effects.

Cigarette smoking, which peaked in many western countries in 1940s and 50s, when 75% of men and 30% of women smoked, has declined greatly in response to concerted public health campaigns and legislation, for example, in Australia and some Scandinavian countries the prevalence is 16–20% of both men and women. Elsewhere in Europe the prevalence of cigarette smoking reaches approx 50%, and in Southeast Asia and East Asia the prevalence has risen hugely over the past 2–3 decades.

The pattern of illicit drug use varies widely across the world. In part, it reflects traditional use of certain drugs, and elsewhere the effects of trafficking and the creation of markets for these substances. The most commonly used illicit drug is cannabis, the use of which involves up to 10–15% of the adult population in many countries of Africa and the Middle East, Europe, Australasia, and North America. Illicit opioid use affects approx 1% of the adult population in several countries in Europe, Southeast Asia, and North America, but there has been a downturn in use in some Southeast Asian countries and Australia since 2000. The geographical pattern of psychostimulant use varies between cocaine and amphetamine-type stimulants. Traditional use of coca leaf in the northern countries of South America continues, and there has been high-level importation of cocaine into the USA, Canada, and several Western European countries. In contrast, in Southeast Asia and the Middle East, Japan, and Australia, amphetamine-type stimulants are more commonly used. Recently, there has been an upsurge in the use of amphetamines in the West Coast of the United States of America and this form of use is presently spreading eastwards across the country.

Substance use contributes substantially to the global burden of disease. Tobacco is the fourth commonest risk factor causing disease burden and measured by disability adjusted life years (DALYs). Alcohol consumption is the 5th commonest disease burden and illicit drugs are also in the top 20 causes of disease. Substance use disorders expend 4–5% of global gross domestic product (GDP), with alcohol causing 1–2%, tobacco 1%, and illicit drugs 0.5%.

Epidemiology of substance use

Alcohol

Alcohol consumption per head of population has been substantially higher in western countries, such as Europe, North America, and Australasia than elsewhere. In most of these countries alcohol consumption has plateaued or declined in recent years and ranges from 6 to 15 L of absolute alcohol per annum. Consumption has greatly increased in many countries where historically alcohol intake was low, notably in countries of East and Southeast Asia. By contrast, countries in the Middle East where Islam is the predominant religion and forbids the use of alcohol, have overall low levels of alcohol consumption, which are below 1 L per year and in some countries are essentially zero.

Globally, just over half the adult population does not drink alcohol, with abstention rates being higher in poorer countries (Table 1.1). Much of the variation in *per capita* alcohol consumption between countries and regions of the world reflects variations in abstention rates; amongst drinkers there is less variation in alcohol consumption. The majority of people who drink have a detrimental drinking pattern and a considerable proportion of alcohol is consumed in potentially harmful ways. Detrimental drinking patterns seem to be more common amongst poorer than amongst richer drinking populations.

Across regions of the world, the rank-ordering of the percentage of the population who drink alcohol generally follows the rank ordering in terms of *per capita* purchasing power parity (PPP), with there being more drinkers in richer regions than in poorer. This does not hold true for the two lowest income groups in Table 1.1, which were separated on the basis of their rates of abstention. Generally, the gender differences in abstention are much greater in the three developing country regional groups than in the two developed regional groups. In the absence of strong cultural or religious bars, it is likely that abstention rates are likely to decline as affluence increases.

At the level of the individual country, the relationship between economic level and alcohol abstention rate is relatively close up to a PPP level of (International Dollars) I\$7000. Beyond a PPP of I\$7000, there is little relation between the degree of affluence of a country and the adult rate of abstention. Within countries, when categorizing the population by three daily income categories (<US\$1/day, US\$1–2/day, and >US\$2/day), people with higher incomes are more likely to use alcohol than people with lower incomes. Below a PPP of I\$10,000, adult *per capita* consumption increases by 1.2 L of pure alcohol per year for each increase in I\$1000 PPP, with the relationship flattening after I\$10,000.

Analysis of trends in alcohol consumption for the WHO regions finds that the European, African, and the Americas all reached their highest consumption about the same time, in the early 1980s, although the level of alcohol consumption is much higher in the European Region than in the other regions. The Eastern Mediterranean Region displays a steady low consumption. The two regions showing recent and continuing increases in alcohol consumption are the Southeast Asian Region (although still very low) and the Western Pacific Region. Based on recent trends in alcohol consumption, it is reasonable to assume that in most regions of the world, alcohol consumption is likely to remain reasonably stable over the next 10–20 years. The exceptions to this are the countries of the Southeast Asian Region and the low to middle income countries of the Western Pacific Region (constituting nearly half of the world's population), where alcohol consumption is likely to increase.

Alcohol-related harm

The World Health Organization's global burden of disease study has estimated the impact of alcohol consumption on the burden of disease for the year 2002 (Table 1.2). The disability adjusted life year (DALY) estimates the number of healthy years of life lost due to alcohol. For example, while a year of perfect health will count as 1 and a year of death will be 0, a year of damaged health that significantly affects quality of life will be somewhere in between. DALYs measure a gap in health between the current position and what could be achieved.

Overall, alcohol is estimated to cause a net harm of 4.4% of the global burden of disease, indicating that the beneficial effects of alcohol are small compared with the detrimental effects. Alcohol causes a greater health burden for men than for women. Neuropsychiatric disorders, mainly made up of alcohol use disorders, constitute the category linked to most alcohol-attributable burden of disease, with unintentional injury being the second most important category. Contrary to the assumption by many that cirrhosis is the most important form of alcohol-induced morbidity and mortality, it only contributes to 10% of the burden of disease caused by alcohol. The health burden is considerable both for acute and chronic health consequences.

The highest burden of alcohol-related harm is found in the European Region, followed by the Americas and the Western Pacific Region. In all of these regions there are economically rich sub-regions (Western Europe, North America, Japan, Australia and New Zealand) with relatively higher alcohol consumption. The sub-region with the highest burden of alcohol-related harm is the Eastern part of the European Region, with the Russian Federation as the most populous country. The region with the least alcohol-attributable burden of disease is the Eastern Mediterranean Region, where in many countries alcohol is forbidden by law because of religious reasons. Intentional and unintentional injuries account for a higher proportion of alcohol-caused burden of disease in lower-income countries, whereas alcohol use disorders and cancers account for larger proportions of the burden in higher-income countries. The alcohol burden accounted by cardiovascular disease is highest in Eastern Europe and central Asia and in the lower-drinking poorest parts of the world. The global burden of disease study has limitations, since not all disease conditions where alcohol has a causal impact are included because of lack of data; this is especially relevant for communicable diseases, such as tuberculosis and human immunodeficiency virus (HIV)/acquired immune deficiency syndrome (AIDS).

There is a very close relationship between total alcohol consumption and the prevalence of alcohol dependence, implying that when alcohol consumption increases, so does the proportion of people with alcohol

Table 1.1 Economic development status and alcohol consumption in 2002 (based on population weighted averages of 182 countries)

	Level of mortality/ category of countries	Average GDP PPP in I\$[*]	WHO-regions[†]	Adult total consumption in L/year[‡]	% Drinkers M	% Drinkers F	Consumption per drinker in g/day pure alcohol	Average pattern of drinking[§]
Developing countries	High mortality; lowest consumption	2441	EMR-D, SEAR-D: Islamic Middle East and Indian subcontinent	1.7	19%	2%	33	2.9
	Very high or high mortality; low consumption	2249	AFR-D, AFR-E, AMR-D: poorest countries in Africa and America	7.1	47%	32%	41	3.0
	Low mortality emerging economies	5257	AMR-B, EMR-B, SEAR-B, WPR-B: better-off developing countries in America, Asia, Western Pacific Region	5.7	67%	36%	25	2.5

Table 1.1 (Contd.)

	Level of mortality/ category of countries	Average GDP PPP in I$*	WHO† regions†	Adult total consumption in L/year‡	% Drinkers M	% Drinkers F	Consumption per drinker in g/day pure alcohol	Average pattern of drinking§
Developed countries	Very low mortality	28,405	AMR A, EUR A, WPR A: North America, Western Europe, Japan, Australasia	10.7	81%	65%	32	1.8
	Low child, and low or high adult mortality	6862	EUR B, EUR C: former Socialist countries in Central/Eastern Europe and Central Asia	11.7	77%	59%	37	3.5
World (population weighted from regions)				6.2	55%	34%	30	2.6

Source: World Health Organization 2007.

* GDP: Gross Domestic Product, a measure of the size of a country's economy; PPP: Purchasing Power Parity per capita, the country's per capita purchasing power for an equivalent basket of goods, expressed in International Dollars (I$).

† The regional sub groupings are defined by WHO on the basis of high, medium, or low levels of adult and of infant mortality. A stands for very low child and very low adult mortality, B for low child and low adult mortality, C for low child and high adult mortality, D for high child and high adult mortality, and E for very high child and very high adult mortality.

‡ In litres of pure alcohol per resident aged 15 years and older per year (average of available data for 2001 to 2003); includes recorded and unrecorded consumption

§ Indicator of the hazard per litre of alcohol consumed, composed of several indicators of heavy drinking occasions plus the frequency of drinking with meals (reverse scored) and in public places (1 = least detrimental; 4 = most detrimental).

dependence, and vice versa. Although alcohol policy measures may have a significant impact on alcohol consumption and alcohol-related harms, there are a number of other factors that also affect the level and trends in alcohol consumption, and alcohol-related harms in a population. For example, in recent years there has been an increase in alcohol consumption in a number of low-income countries such as China, India, and South Korea, where abstention rates have been traditionally high, and where an increase in alcohol consumption has implied an increase in the proportion of the population that are drinkers. The consumption increase in these countries probably reflects economic development and increases in consumers' purchasing power, as well as increases in the marketing of branded alcoholic beverages.

Tobacco

Cigarette smoking and other forms of tobacco use are estimated to kill around 5 million people per year around the world. This number is likely to rise.

Smoking is the single greatest reversible risk factor for disease and death in the developed world, and was estimated as the third greatest risk factor (after alcohol and high blood pressure) in low mortality developing countries in 2002. Currently, it kills just less than one in 10 (8.8%) adults worldwide. Among males in developed regions, smoking is believed to cause more than a quarter (26.3%) of deaths.

The prevalence of smoking peaked in many western countries in the 1940s and 50s, when 75% of men and 30% of women smoked cigarettes. It has since declined greatly in response to concerted public health campaigns and legislation. In Australia and some Scandinavian countries the prevalence is now 16–20% of both men and women. Elsewhere in Europe the prevalence of cigarette smoking among males reaches up to 50%.

In contrast to the decline in smoking in the high-income countries, in Southeast and East Asia the prevalence has risen greatly over the past 2–3 decades, more in males, but increasingly also in females. Asia is an unashamed marketing target of the tobacco industry. More than 50% of males in Asia smoke today and one in every three cigarettes smoked in the world today is smoked in China, where there are said to be 1000 cigarette brands. Currently, 82% of the world's smokers live in low and middle income countries, with 38% of the world's smokers based in East Asia and the Pacific.

Lower socio-economic status is also the major risk factor for continuing smoking within developed countries and, similarly, low educational attainment is associated with higher smoking rates. In Australia, where there is a low overall prevalence of smoking, some isolated and disadvantaged Aboriginal communities have smoking rates of up to 80%.

Around the world more men than women smoke. Males in low income countries are more likely to be daily smokers than males in wealthier nations. In contrast, females are more likely to be daily smokers in wealthier nations than in low income nations.

Smoking typically starts before the age of 25, then the prevalence peaks at ages 30–49.

Table 1.2 The impact of alcohol consumption on the worldwide burden of disease, as expressed in the number of healthy life years lost (Disability adjusted life years, DALYs) due to alcohol in 2002

Disease category	Number of DALYs (thousands)	Percentage of the harms due to alcohol (in DALYs) attributed to each disease category
DALYs		
Maternal and perinatal conditions (low birth weight)	94	0.1
Cancer	6054	9.0
Diabetes mellitus	20	0.0
Neuropsychiatric disorders	23,115	34.3
Cardiovascular diseases	6598	9.8
Cirrhosis of the liver	6883	10.2
Unintentional injuries	17,146	25.5
Intentional injuries	7417	11.0
Total 'detrimental effects' attributable to alcohol	67,326	100.0
DALYs prevented		
Diabetes mellitus	−213	13.3
Cardiovascular diseases	−2039	86.7
Total 'beneficial effects' attributable to alcohol	−2351	100.0
Net DALYs		
Net DALYs attributable to alcohol	64,975	100.0
All DALYs	1,490,126	
Net DALYs attributable to alcohol as a percentage of all DALYs	4.4%	

Source: World Health Organization (2007).

Mental health disorders are also a risk factor for smoking. One third of individuals with major depression and a quarter of those with an anxiety disorder are dependent smokers. Persons with alcohol use disorders are more likely to smoke.

Impact of smoking

The World Health Organization estimates that smoking is the cause of 4% of the global burden of disease. One in two long-term regular smokers are likely to die as a result of their smoking. Half these deaths occur in middle age (35–69 years). In developed countries smoking is responsible for much of the mortality gap between rich and poor.

Smoking is a well recognized risk factor for lung cancer, aerodigestive and other cancers, chronic obstructive pulmonary disease, other respiratory diseases and vascular diseases. It is also a risk factor for type 2 diabetes and for renal disease. As well as its chronic health effects, smoking is associated with acute harms from fire injuries.

Tobacco smoking in pregnancy is associated with lower birth weight babies.

Illicit drugs

Worldwide, an estimated 185 million adults use illicit drugs. The burden of disease associated with use of legal drugs outweighs that associated with illegal drugs.

The use of psychoactive drugs has received increasing attention worldwide in recent decades. There is much discussion about the extent of the problem, and drug use is thought to account for a significant share of the global burden of disease given the relatively low prevalence of illicit drug use in many regions of the world.

In this chapter, there is discussion of the major illicit drug types used, the epidemiology of use across the globe, and some discussion of the natural history and burden of disease related to these different drug types. There are differences across drug types in the magnitude and nature of harms.

'Illicit drug use' refers to the non-medical use of a variety of drugs including cannabis, amphetamine type stimulants (including methamphetamine, amphetamine, MDMA (3,4-methylenedioxymethamphetamine, ecstasy), cocaine, and opioids (including heroin) (Table 1.3). There are many other drugs used such as gamma-hydroxybutyrate (GHB), ketamine, and d-lysergic acid (LSD), but these are used by comparatively fewer persons in a more limited number of countries, and both the nature and extent of harm is less well documented, so the present chapter will focus upon the four major drug classes.

Table 1.3 Major illicit drug groups

Cannabis	A generic term for psychoactive preparations (e.g. marijuana, hashish, and hash oil) derived from the cannabis sativa plant
Amphetamines	A class of sympathomimetic amines with powerful stimulant action on the central nervous system
Cocaine	An alkaloid central nervous system stimulant that is derived from the coca plant
Opioids	Derivatives of the opium poppy (such as heroin and morphine), their synthetic analogues, and compounds synthesized in the body, which act upon the opioid receptors in the brain. They have the capacity to relieve pain and produce a sense of euphoria, as well as cause stupor, coma, and respiratory depression

How common is illicit drug use?

The illegality of illicit drug use makes it difficult to quantify the levels of drug use because the drug-users are 'hidden' and thus difficult to identify, and even when they can be located and interviewed, they may attempt to conceal their drug use. The United Nations Office on Drugs and Crime (UNODC) publish estimates of the prevalence of past year illicit drug use, but the quality of the data used varies dramatically from country to country, from high quality national survey data, to key informant and indicator data of uncertain validity. Nonetheless, until there is a concerted attempt to collect high quality data they remain the only source of estimates for some countries.

Cannabis is the most widely used illicit drug and is used in every region of the world. In 2004, around 162 million adults (an estimated 4% of the global adult population) were thought to have used cannabis in the previous year, a 10% increase on estimated rates of global use in the mid-1990s. Patterns of cannabis use have been most extensively studied in developed countries such as the USA, Canada, Australia, and Europe. Europe generally has lower rates of use than Australia, Canada, and the USA. The limited data from low and middle income countries suggest that with exceptions (e.g. South Africa) rates of cannabis use are much lower in Africa, Asia, and South America than in Europe and English-speaking countries. There may be pockets of high level use within a country. For example, in some remote Aboriginal communities in Australia more than 60% of adults are reported to use cannabis regularly.

The term 'amphetamine type stimulants' (ATS) refers to a range of drugs related to amphetamine. Methamphetamine and amphetamine are the major ATS available worldwide, followed by MDMA. The diversion of prescription stimulant drugs such as dexamphetamine has been reported, but this is less of a problem than illicitly produced ATS. Use appears to be increasing in many parts of the world, but many countries have scant or no data on the prevalence, routes and forms of use. Problematic use of amphetamines appears more prevalent in East and Southeast Asia, North America, South Africa, New Zealand, Australia, and a number of European countries.

Cocaine is reportedly the least widely used of the illicit drugs: around 13 million adults were thought to have used cocaine in 2006, with use heavily concentrated in North America, Latin America, and some European countries. The reported prevalence of cocaine use in other high income countries is typically much lower than that in the US.

Illicit opioids are the third most common form of illicit drug use. Globally, illicit opioids were estimated to have been used by around 16 million people in the early 2000s. In high income countries, estimates of dependence are typically below 1% of adults aged 15 or more. Most research on the epidemiology and natural history of opioid use focuses upon dependent users. The distinction between 'use' and 'dependence' is an important one that is briefly discussed below.

Use versus problematic use: an important distinction

Not all drug use causes evident harm to users. Efforts have been made on an international level to classify the behaviours or symptoms associated with use that does cause problems to the user. It is this problematic use towards which most health care interventions are targeted.

The International Classification of Diseases (ICD) distinguishes between 'harmful drug use' and 'drug dependence'. Harmful drug use is defined by clear evidence that the substance use is responsible for physical (e.g. organ damage) and psychological harm (e.g. drug-induced psychosis). In ICD10 drug dependence involves a cluster of behavioural, cognitive, and physiological phenomena that develop after repeated substance use and that typically include a strong desire to take the drug, difficulties in controlling its use, persisting in its use despite harmful consequences, a higher priority given to drug use than to other activities and obligations, increased tolerance, and sometimes a physical withdrawal state.

It is difficult to produce credible estimates of the number of people who make up the 'hidden population' of such dependent or problematic drug users, yet it is this group who probably suffer the bulk of problems related to their drug use and who are in most need of treatment—drug treatment and treatment for general medical health problems. The preferred strategy is to look for convergence in estimates produced by a variety of different methods of estimation. These methods are of two broad types, *direct* and *indirect*. Direct estimation methods attempt to estimate the number of illicit drug users in representative samples of the population. Indirect estimation methods attempt to use information from known populations of illicit drug users (such as those who have died of opioid overdoses or been treated) to estimate the size of the hidden population of illicit drug users.

Examining the harms related to drug use: morbidity and mortality

In the first Global Burden of Disease estimates (1990 and 2001 estimates), there was good evidence suggesting that there had been an increase globally in the extent of mortality related to injecting drug use and dependent use of opioids, cocaine or amphetamines.[1] In the next iteration of these estimates, (see http://www.gbd.unsw.edu.au) attempts will be made to extend estimates to include cannabis given its prevalence of use and the expansion of the evidence on potential harms related to its use.

The best evidence that illicit drug use is a cause of premature death comes from cohort studies of illicit drug users, which have limitations. It is likely that the estimates of disease burden to date have been underestimated because we simply have too little data on the nature and magnitude of harms related to different drugs, and because even where we know drugs cause harm, too few studies have estimated the course of drug use and associated harm over time and across different country contexts. Existing estimates could not estimate morbidity and mortality related to cannabis use; more recently, evidence increasingly suggests that cannabis may increases risks of some cancers (related to smoking of the drug) and motor vehicle accidents.

1 Degenhardt L, Hall W, Lynskey M, Warner-Smith M. Illicit drug use. In: Ezzati M, Lopez AD, Rodgers A, Murray R, eds. *Comparative Quantification of Health Risks: Global and Regional Burden of Disease Attributable to Selected Major Risk Factors*, 2nd edn. Geneva: World Health Organization, 2004; 1109–1176.

Illicit drug use

Cannabis

The best data on the prevalence of cannabis use and its correlates comes from the United States, Canada, and Australia, where the levels of use appear to have been the highest. Rates in Europe have increased over the past decade. Generally, rates of use have been higher among young people in high income countries, but rates of recreational use may be increasing among young people in low and middle income countries.

Studies conducted in the United States suggest that cannabis typically begins in the mid to late teens, and is most prevalent in early adulthood. Most cannabis use is irregular, with very few users engaging in long-term daily use. In the USA and Australia, it is thought that about 10% of those who ever use cannabis become daily users, and another 20–30% use weekly. Transitions in life roles such as entry into full-time employment, getting married, or having children, are associated with reductions in or cessation of use for many people. The largest decreases are seen in cannabis use among males and females after marriage, and especially during pregnancy and after childbirth in women.

Heavy (daily) cannabis use over a period of years increases the risks of experiencing problems. Daily cannabis users are more likely to be male, less well educated, and more likely to regularly use other drugs. Weekly or more frequent use in adolescence appears to carry significant risk for dependence in early adulthood. Population surveys suggest that cannabis use disorders are the most common forms of drug problems after alcohol and tobacco. In Australia, the prevalence of past-year cannabis use disorders has been estimated at around 2%. An estimated lifetime risk of 9% for dependence has been estimated among persons who ever used cannabis.

Risk is not confined to older users. Among a cohort of young people in Australia, the prevalence of cannabis dependence in the past year was 7%, with almost 75% of daily users meeting dependence criteria. In countries such as Australia, New Zealand, and the United States, around one in six young people who ever use cannabis develop symptoms of dependence. Those at highest risk may have a history of poor academic achievement, deviant behaviour in childhood and adolescence, non-conformity and rebelliousness, poor parental relationships, and a parental history of drug and alcohol problems. There is increasing evidence of a substantial genetic contribution to the likelihood of using and developing dependence upon cannabis.

Psychostimulants

The term 'amphetamine type stimulants' refers to a range of drugs related to amphetamine, which share stimulant properties that increase the activity of the central nervous system and produce effects similar to adrenaline. Methamphetamine and amphetamine are now the major ATS available worldwide. ATS have recently become the focus of increasing attention worldwide because of a substantial increase in the production of these drugs over the past decade, and increasing consumption and harm related to their use. After cannabis, ATS are the most widely used illicit drugs, in both high and low income countries.

Because it is derived from a plant, cocaine use has typically been more concentrated in regions where the coca plant is grown or those nearby. The US has had by far the greatest problem with cocaine (and 'crack' cocaine) dependence worldwide, particularly in the 1990s. More recently, there have been increases in the availability and use of cocaine in Western Europe. The use of cocaine is much more uncommon in Asia, Oceania, and African countries.

Psychostimulants are most commonly taken orally, intranasally, the vapours inhaled (smoking), or injected. A dependence syndrome upon amphetamine and cocaine is well described. Dependence has been associated with mental health, physical, occupational, relationship, financial, and legal problems. It is likely that most of the harm related to psychostimulant use occurs among those who have developed dependent use of the drug. Users with a history of other drug and mental health problems may be at greater risk of developing dependence. There has been concern about associations between psychostimulant use and HIV risk, much of which has focused on risky sexual behaviour.

Available data strongly suggest that both route of administration and forms used are important factors affecting the nature and extent of associated harms. The increase in use of the crystalline form of methamphetamine, for example, has been associated with increased problems related to dependent and binge patterns of use. Smoking and injecting have also been associated with a higher risk of dependent or problematic use than swallowing or snorting the drug. There is evidence that 'smoking' crystal methamphetamine and 'crack' cocaine also carries harms related to the inhalation of possibly toxic chemicals and possibly blood borne virus transmission through the sharing of smoking implements.

Few studies have documented the natural history of psychostimulant use, in sharp contrast to the literature on cannabis and even opioids. Our current understanding derives largely from cross-sectional studies, typically involving convenience samples, or treatment or prison settings. US prospective studies have suggested that relapse following treatment for psychostimulant dependence is common. The concentration of work in treatment or prison populations makes it difficult to draw inferences about amphetamine use in the general population, since most users will never come into contact with either treatment or law enforcement agencies. As a result, little is known about the aetiology and consequences of psychostimulant use that does not come to the attention of police or treatment services. This is an area where much more needs to be known given the increases thought to be occurring in the use of these drugs.

Opioids

Cohort studies of dependent opioid users have suggested that users may continue to use opioids for decades, with periods of use interrupted by time spent in treatment, prison, and for some, extended periods of abstinence. Such cohort studies have largely been conducted in high income countries—in Asia, for example, the context of opium (and, more recently, heroin and pharmaceutical opioids) use is quite different from the USA and we know much less about the natural history of opioid use in these countries. Nonetheless, the evidence available to date suggests that opioid dependent persons may struggle to control their use for significant portions of their lives. Data from the US have suggested that one in four persons who use opioids illicitly may develop dependence upon them.

Although opioids are used by far fewer people than cannabis, opioid dependence is associated with substantial mortality and morbidity that appears to far exceed that of cannabis use or dependence. Reviews have suggested that opioid dependent persons may be 13 times more likely to die than peers of the same age and sex. Multiple reasons exist for this: drug overdose, accidents and trauma, suicide, the consequences of blood borne viral infections, such as HIV and hepatitis C virus (HCV), and generally poorer physical health contribute to shorter life expectancy and poorer quality of life for this group. Although heroin has typically been thought to be the primary opioid accounting for problems related to opioid dependence, in many countries (particularly in the United States, South Asia and Eastern Europe) dependence upon pharmaceutical opioids is an increasing problem.

Summary and implications: illicit drugs

The discussion above has attempted to provide a broad overview of the epidemiology of four major drug types. Although we have some data on the scope of the problem, because of the illegal nature of such drug use there is much that we do not understand about the extent, context, and natural history of illicit drugs, particularly in low and middle income countries where drug use seems to be increasing. We still have much to learn about the extent of drug use, and the nature and magnitude of harms that may result.

Although much remains to be understood about illicit drug use, based upon what we do know, several things are certain:
- There is considerable and possibly increasing demand for drugs in the general population
- Demand for and consumption of drugs is dynamic, with current trends suggesting increasing demand for stimulant drugs
- Drug supply may both respond to and drive demand for drugs
- Responses to drug use must reflect these drivers.

From Table 1.4 we see that Australia, New Zealand, USA and Canada rank highest among the prevalence of adult illicit drug users in the world with Singapore, Japan and Sweden the lowest. Cannabis is the most widely used illicit substance in the world.

Although opioid use has plateaued in recent years, the use of amphetamine type substances has increased.

While Tables 1.5 and 1.6 show estimates of prevalence for countries or regions, within any population there are subgroups with far higher prevalence of substance used disorders. Higher rates are particularly common in disadvantaged or marginalized groups. For example, major population surveys in Australia indicate that 2% of the population have, at some time, self injected drugs, compared with 62% of street kids. Among street kids, injecting is epidemic. The most widely injected drugs across Australia were opiates (26%), amphetamines (8-10%), cocaine (2%), and benzodiazepines (2%).

Table 1.4 Percentage of the population aged 15–64 who have used any illicit drug in the past year

	Opiates	Cannabis	Cocaine	Amphetamines	Ecstasy
Australia	0.5	13.3	1.2	3.8	4.0
New Zealand	0.5	13.4	0.5	3.4	2.2
UK	0.9				
England & Wales		10.8	2.4	1.5	2.0
Scotland		7.9	1.4	1.4	1.7
Ireland	0.6	5.1	1.1	0.4	1.1
Italy	0.8	7.1	1.2	0.2	0.4
France	0.4	9.8	0.3	0.2	0.3
Germany	0.3	6.9	1.0	0.9	0.8
Sweden	0.1	2.2	0.2	0.2	0.4
USA	0.6	12.6	2.8	1.5	1.0
Canada	0.4	16.8	2.3	0.8	1.1
Singapore	0.004	0.004	0.0002	0.005	0.004
Japan	0.1	0.1	0.03	0.4	0.1
Russian Federation	2.0	3.9	0.1	0.2	0.1

NB: Data come from different years between 1999 and 2004; the year of the survey may vary between countries and, for different substances, within countries. Data from: United Nations Office on Drugs and Crime. World Drug Report. Vienna, Austria: United Nations 2006. Available at http://www.unodc.org/unodc/en/world_drug_report.html

While illicit drugs attract great public concern, in terms of morbidity, mortality, and social costs, they are far outweighed by the costs from tobacco. For example, in Australia in the late 1990s the annual social cost of tobacco smoking was estimated at AUD 21.3 billion, compared with alcohol AUD 7.6 billion and illicit drugs AUD 6.1 billion.

Table 1.5 Estimated worldwide use of licit and illicit drugs and global burden of disease

	Worldwide use by adults Estimated in 2002	Global burden of disease (DALYs in 2000)	Burden of disease in developed regions (2000)	Deaths worldwide (2000)	Deaths in developed regions (2000)
Licit drugs:					
Tobacco	1.1 billion	4.1%	12.2%	8.8%	18.0%
Alcohol	2 billion	4.0%	9.2%	3.2%	3.9%
Illicit Drugs:	185–200 million	0.8%	1.8%	0.4%	0.5%

Adapted from: Anderson P. Global use of alcohol, drugs and tobacco. *Drug and Alcohol Review* 2006; **25**: 489–502; and Rehm J, Taylor B, Room R. Global burden of disease from alcohol, illicit drugs and tobacco. *Drug and Alcohol Review* 2006; **25**: 503–513.

Table 1.6 Estimated worldwide use of illicit drugs in the early 2000s

Illicit drugs	Any illicit drug: 200 million
Cannabis	146.2–162.4 million
Amphetamines	25–29.6 million
Illicit opioids	15.3–15.9 million
Cocaine	13.3–13.4 million
Ecstasy	8.3–9.7 million

Adapted from: Anderson P. Global use of alcohol, drugs and tobacco. *Drug and Alcohol Review* 2006; **25**: 489–502.

Summary: epidemiology of alcohol, tobacco and illicit drug use
The misuse of licit and illicit drugs increases the burden of disease to the individual, the country, and the world. In addition to criminal activity, injecting use of illegal drugs is a major risk factor for spread of infections, particularly hepatitis C and HIV, secondary to sharing of needles and injecting equipment. However, the health and economic cost of the use of tobacco and alcohol outweighs the cost of illicit substances. It is, in fact, the legal drugs (tobacco and alcohol) that have the greatest cost.

Use of one psychoactive substance often does not occur in isolation. Those with alcohol use disorders are more likely to smoke tobacco; most illicit drug users are polysubstance users and often use non-injectable drugs as well, particularly nicotine, alcohol, benzodiazepines, cannabis, and prescribed and proprietary drugs.

It is difficult to get accurate figures on the prevalence of misuse of many psychoactive substances. For example, it is difficult to differentiate between illicit benzodiazepine use and its prescribed use, and so the true epidemiology of benzodiazepine misuse is unknown. A range of other substances are misused. For example, the misuse of volatile solvents is a problem in many countries particularly among disadvantaged youth, for example petrol sniffing among adolescent Aboriginal and Torres Strait Islander population in remote Australia. A range of proprietary (over the counter) medications are misused, but there are little data on the extent of this.

In the health care setting, substance misuse is commonly encountered, either as overt or covert cause for the consultation, or as an incidental finding. For example, in a primary care setting up to one-third of patients have a disorder related to alcohol and tobacco use, or use of other drugs. In general hospitals, the figure is often greater than this. In mental health services, co-morbid substance use disorders affect half or more of patients.

Further reading

Anderson P. Global use of alcohol, drugs and tobacco. *Drug and Alcohol Review* 2006; **25**: 489–502.

Collins DJ, Lapsley HM. *Counting the cost: estimates of social costs of drug abuse in Australia 1998–1999*, National Drug strategy Monograph series No 49. Canberra: Commonwealth Department of Health and Aging, 2002.

Degenhardt L, Mathers B, Guarinieri M, Panda S, Phillips B, Strathdee S, et al. *The global epidemiology of methamphetamine injection: A review of the evidence on use and associations with HIV and other harm.* Sydney: National Drug and Alcohol Research Centre, University of NSW, 2007.

Ezzati M, Lopez A, Rodgers A, Vander Hoorn S, Murray C. The Comparative Risk Assessment Collaborating Group. Selected major risk factors and global and regional burden of disease. *Lancet* 2002; **360**: 1347–1360.

Rehm J, Taylor B, Room R. Global burden of disease from alcohol, illicit drugs and tobacco. *Drug and Alcohol Review* 2006; **25**: 503–513.

World Health Organization (2007). *WHO Expert Committee on Problems Related to Alcohol Consumption.* Available at: http://www.who.int/substance_abuse/expert_committee_alcohol/en/index.html

Spectrum of substance use and core clinical diagnoses

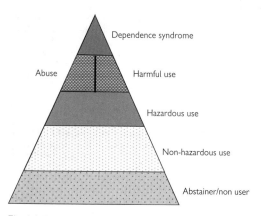

Fig. 1.1 The spectrum of substance use and problems.

Definitions

For any psychoactive substance there is a range of use from that which causes little or no problems through to dependent use. Alcohol and other substance use can be classified conveniently into five categories. These represent the diagnosis made when using international diagnostic systems.

Hazardous drinking or substance use: is repetitive use at levels that places a person at risk of harm of medical or psychological complications.

Harmful drinking or substance use: is a repetitive pattern of use that causes actual physical damage (e.g. liver disease, hypertension, cancers), or psychological harm (depression, anxiety; ICD10).

Substance abuse: repetitive pattern of drinking or use of a substance which results in social complications, e.g. financial, occupational and legal problems (*Diagnostic and Statistical Manual*, 4th edn: DSM-IV).

Dependence: represents an established syndrome of repetitive substance use, which is driven by internal forces. Dependence can be defined as a cluster of psychological, behavioural, and cognitive syndromes that comprise an inner drive to repetitive pattern of drinking or using drugs, pre-occupation with substance use, and sometimes withdrawal symptoms (ICD10 or DSM-IV).

A diagnosis of dependence is made if three or more of the following symptoms have occurred repeatedly within the past year:
- Impaired control over substance use—subjective awareness of an impaired capacity to control use
- A strong desire or sense of compulsion to use—subjective awareness of this compulsion; craving
- Preoccupation with substance use to the neglect of other responsibilities or interests
- Tolerance—increased amounts of the substance are required in order to achieve the desired effects
- Withdrawal symptoms on cessation or reduction of substance use
- Relief or prevention of withdrawal symptoms by further substance use
- Persistence of substance use despite clear evidence of overtly harmful consequences.

(Adapted from ICD10 criteria for dependence)

Dependence exists in various degrees of severity, but craving is a common feature of most forms of dependence and a common reason for relapse. This forms the rationale for use of anti-craving agents in the prevention of relapse. The colloquial term 'addiction' is often used to describe drug dependence just as the term 'alcoholism' is used for alcohol dependence.

Withdrawal syndrome occurs when neurones have adapted to the chronic presence of a psychoactive substance. Cessation of substance use then results in abnormal neuronal function. It only occurs when dependence on that substance is present. However, the extent to which a withdrawal syndrome occurs is dependent on the substance, its level and pattern of use, and on inter-individual differences. Not all dependent users experience withdrawals.

Repetitive use of alcohol or other psychoactive substances may also lead to complications, which may be physical, neuropsychiatric, or social. Furthermore, substance use disorders may co-exist with other underlying illnesses, such as chronic pain, or psychiatric illnesses, such as anxiety disorders, depression, or schizoaffective illnesses ('Dual diagnosis').

Neurobiology of the dependence syndrome

There have been remarkable advances in the neuroscience of drug and alcohol dependence in the past decade. The target sites of action of most misused substances have been identified at the molecular and cellular level, and the brain circuits that underpin drug reward (pleasure) have been identified. Furthermore, the higher level control systems that regulate behaviours, such as planning, wanting, and resisting drug use are becoming understood in humans through the use of techniques such as positron emission tomography (PET) and functional magnetic resonance imaging (fMRI) scanning.

Animal studies—mostly in rodents, although with some key confirmatory ones in primates—have revealed a brain circuit that appears to be common to the rewarding effects of most if not all drugs, as well as other reinforcing behaviours, such as eating, thirst, and sexual drives. This brain circuit comprises a dopamine pathway that runs from the ventral tegmental area into the ventral part of the striatum (the nucleus accumbens) and into the prefrontal cortex. Activation in this pathway is believed to lead to the learning of associations between behaviours and the relevance that they have for the individual. The landmark discovery here was that the self-administration of cocaine to rats is associated with a great release of dopamine in the nucleus accumbens (Fig.1.2a). Subsequently, this group and many others revealed that most other drugs that are misused will also do this (the main exception being the benzodiazepines). From this developed the dopamine theory of addiction—addictive substances release dopamine—this is pleasurable so the behaviour is repeated (reinforced). However, as drugs stimulate greater dopamine release than natural reinforcing activities, such as food, water, and sex, they 'hijack' the system, thus directing motivation and behaviour to drug use, rather than other activities. For instance, rats allowed to electrically stimulate this brain circuit do so relentlessly, not stopping to eat or drink, to the point where they may die unless the electricity is turned off; a phenomenon that has striking parallels with some human binge drug use. In Fig. 1.2b the pathway is shown along with the sites at which drugs act. Some, e.g. cocaine, work at the level of the dopamine terminals to cause dopamine release; others, e.g. the opioids and cannabis, act to switch off an inhibitory gamma aminobutyric acid (GABA) neuron that normally gates the firing of the dopamine neurons, so indirectly lead to dopamine release.

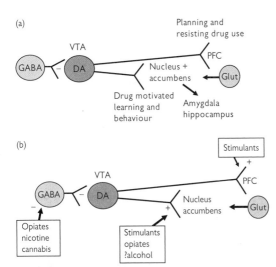

VTA = ventral tegmentalar: PFC = prefrontal cortex DA = dopamine glutamate

Fig. 1.2 (a) The dopamine reinforcement pathway. (b) The dopamine reinforcement pathway: sites of drug action.

More recently, it has been discovered that the state of dopamine neurotransmission may itself influence vulnerability to repeated drug use. A landmark human imaging study by Volkow and colleagues revealed that human volunteers with a lower density of dopamine D2 receptors in the striatum gained more pleasure from IV stimulant administration than those with a higher level. Attempts were made to back-translate this to animal models with remarkable results. It has now been shown both in monkeys and rats that the baseline density of D2 receptors predicts the extent of cocaine use when access is allowed—low levels of receptors before exposure to drug leads to great regular use of cocaine. In mice, low levels of these receptors are associated with alcohol intake and if the level is changed, e.g. by transfecting a virus that adds receptors to the nucleus accumbens, then preference declines. Moreover, repeated use of some drugs, especially stimulants and perhaps alcohol, leads to a reduction in the number dopamine D2 receptors so a vicious cycle of use and repeated use can be predicted (see Fig. 1.3).

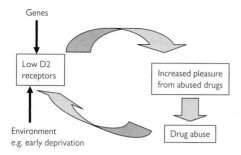

Fig. 1.3 Dopamine can help explain social aspects of addiction also.

One powerful aspect of this dopamine receptor theory is that it can help explain other factors that are known to relate to drug use, e.g. stress and social deprivation, as each of these in animals has been shown to lead to reduced D2 receptor number or function. It also leads to testable predictions about the role of dopamine receptor mutations that may alter neurotransmitter function as vulnerability markers (Fig. 1.3).

It is too simplistic to believe that, in the human, all drug reinforcement can be explained simply in terms of changes in the dopamine system. For instance, not all drugs have been shown to release dopamine in humans, the opioids being the most obvious exception. Also, dopamine blocking drugs, e.g. neuroleptics, have little impact on human drug-taking so it is likely that other neurotransmitter systems play a part in human addiction. There is a good body of evidence to support an involvement of the brain endogenous opioid system—the endorphins—in addiction also. These peptides provide natural reinforcement, as well as regulating pain behaviour and may be released in parallel with, or in place of, dopamine to provide reward, for instance from alcohol and cocaine. There is also good and growing imaging evidence that brain opioid receptors are abnormal in some addictions and that this may be associated with craving and relapse, as well as being a possible vulnerability factor to dependence. The involvement of endogenous opioids in addiction probably explains why opioid antagonists, such as naltrexone and nalmefene have utility in the treatment of alcohol, as well as heroin addiction.

Another critical aspect of drug misuse is the role of high level cortical processing in behaviour. It has been known for a long time that persons who misuse drugs, especially when addicted, have numerous deficits in mental functions, such as attention, memory planning, and impulse regulation. The use of new imaging techniques has revealed that these processes reside in sub-regions of the frontal cortex, particularly the orbitofrontal cortex and its limbic projection regions, especially the amygdala, and clear abnormalities of these brain regions have now been observed in many different addictions. The idea that addiction represents a fundamental remodelling of these pathways leading to long-term consequences for self regulation has been put forward by Volkow and has a lot of support (Fig. 1.4).

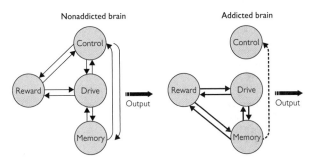

Fig. 1.4 Changed reciprocal brain control relationships in addiction (from Volkow).

The extent to which these reflect predisposing factors or are a consequence of drug induced damage is still under investigation, and both are
likely to be relevant to differing extents in different people. Also there may
well be particular aspects of dysfunction that explain a particular person's
problems, e.g. in one person impulsivity may be the major problem,
whereas in others compulsion to use may predominate. This offers a new
approach to targeting treatments at the major risk factor in a person and
also the prospect of new pharmacological approaches such as cognition
enhancers.

Following repeated drug use, pathways of reward drive and memory
become over-established and detached from higher-level control centres,
so perpetuating drug use.

Underlying conditions and risk factors

When are individuals more likely to become dependent on drugs or alcohol?

Dependence develops on the basis of an interaction between:
- The pharmacological properties of the drug (Table 1.7)
- Individual vulnerability
- The influence of the environment.

Pharmacological properties of drugs that pose a risk for dependence
- Pleasurable effects (rewarding- see previous section)
- Effects are rapid in onset and are, therefore, more positively reinforcing
- Psychoactive substances, including alcohol, which with repeated exposure, induce tolerance as a neuro-adaptive response. More of the drug is required to produce the same effect. This may be due to changes in neurones including receptor properties, ionic flux, and intracellular chemical pathways
- As a consequence of this neuro-adaptation, in many cases withdrawal symptoms occur on cessation or reduction of substance use.
  This provides negative reinforcement of abstinence, is associated with strong craving, and so encourages return to substance use.

Individual vulnerability
Influenced by:

Genetic factors: these are estimated to account for 50–60% of the risk of developing alcohol dependence, particularly in males. In addition, up to half the variance in drinking patterns in non dependent people is genetically determined. Less data is available for illicit drugs, but genetic influences are believed to be involved.

Genetic influences are polygenic, but some influences may be mediated through:
- **Personality traits**: Impulsivity, risk taking and rebelliousness are associated with increased risk of substance use disorders
- **Different metabolism of or response to psychoactive substances**:
  - For example, adolescent boys with a strong family history of alcohol problems show a reduced sensitivity to the effects of alcohol even at the time of their first drinking, so from the very start drink they more than their peers
  - In some Asian populations, an unpleasant flushing reaction to alcohol, based on a deficiency of aldehyde dehydrogenase activity, protects against alcohol dependence.

Psychiatric disorders: e.g. anxiety, depression, schizophrenia, personality disorder, post-traumatic stress disorder (PTSD) are all associated with increased risk of substance use disorders.

Table 1.7 Commonly self administered psychoactive drugs (some common street names in brackets)

CNS depressants	CNS stimulants	Hallucinogens	Other

Alcohol	Amphetamines *(speed; uppers, goey, whiz, velocity)*
	
	 Methamphetamines *(ice, shabu, crystal, yaba, crystal meth)*
		Hallucinogens
		   LSD *(acid)*
		   Mescaline *(magic mushrooms)*
		   Psilocybin *(magic mushrooms)*
			Solvents— e.g. petrol, paint
			
			 Inhalants e.g. amyl nitrite N_2O

Sedatives	Ecstasy—*(MDMA, e, Es, XTC, eckies,)*	Ecstasy— *(empathogenic)*	Anabolic steroids
Benzodiazepines *(benzos, pills)*	Cocaine *(coke; crack; snow, charlie)*		
Z-drugs: zopiclone, zolpidem	Caffeine		
Barbiturates	Nicotine		
Opioids			
Heroin *(chasing the dragon—inhaling heroin vapour)*			
Opioid analgesics			
Codeine Morphine Pethidine Methadone Buprenorphine Oxycodone Pentazocine Dextromoramide Fentanyl			
Cannabis		Cannabis—in high doses *(dope; ganga; yandi; grass; weed; hashish)* May be smoked using a bong (water pipe) or as a joint— cigarette.	
GHB *(fantasy, liquid ecstasy, grievous bodily harm)*			
Ketamine *(special K)*			

Environmental influences
- **Adverse upbringing** including emotional deprivation, physical and sexual abuse, social disadvantage. Also the impact of these major stressors may result in anxiety, depression, or PTSD in later life and then an increased risk of substance use disorders in an attempt to self-medicate
- **Availability of substance**: low cost and ready availability
- **Cultural acceptance**: the degree to which a substance is legally and socially sanctioned, advertisement, traditional practices, and encouragement by peer group can markedly influence substance use
- **Employment**: certain occupational groups, e.g. bar tenders have an increased prevalence of alcohol and other drug misuse. This may be caused by the increased availability of alcohol and constant cues to drinking. Unemployment is an important risk factor for, as well as consequence of substance use
- **Role modelling**: modelling of substance use behaviour by family members, peers and other community members can encourage use.

Natural history of substance use and related disorders

The use of psychoactive substances ranges from single occasion, often experimental, use to the repeated high level use continuing over many years that is characteristic of substance dependence. Natural history of substance use and the core clinical syndromes, such as harmful use, substance abuse, and dependence derives from several sources. These include longitudinal or cohort studies, some being birth cohorts, or those established in childhood or teen years. Another group of natural history studies is based on persons identified as having a substance use disorder in population studies who are followed up over time. A third and relatively numerous type of natural history study comprises clinical populations attending treatment services. Some of these do not receive treatment or have minimal treatment, while others have a range of treatments for their disorder.

Alcohol

In countries with a high prevalence of alcohol consumption, consumption typically starts in the mid–late teens, although this varies according to the legal age for alcohol consumption, which ranges from 16 to 21 years. Young people's alcohol intake tends to be episodic, and consumption of large amounts in a single session has become increasingly common among both young men and young women in many Western countries. Intensity of drinking (number of drinks per session) declines from the mid-20s, but the frequency of consumption per week rises. Approximately 15–20% of the adult population consumes alcohol in a risky or hazardous way and of these, approximately one-third progress to alcohol dependence, with most of the others reducing their consumption to low risk levels by their 30s. Of the 5% of the population who have alcohol dependence, the course is quite variable. About one-third seek treatment within a few years of becoming dependent and this group provides much of our present knowledge of the natural history of this disorder. Untreated alcohol dependence shows a pronounced tendency to progress and following any periods of abstinence, to relapse. Reduction of alcohol consumption in alcohol dependent individuals to low risk levels is highly unusual especially in treatment populations where it is vanishingly small. Overall, untreated alcohol dependence results in the following outcomes over 10 years; 30% achieve recovery from their disorder, based on abstinence, 40% manifest continuing heavy consumption with progressive and continuing features of dependence, and 30% show a progressive downhill course characterized by frequent ever more severe relapse leading to death within this period. The natural history of treated alcohol dependence is influenced by the sociodemographic and cultural background of the person. Typically in people attending comprehensive public sector programmes, 45% have a good or relatively good prognosis, achieving abstinence in the long-term, with intermittent relapses in some cases; 35% show a less favourable course with periods of abstinence interspersed with periods of heavy uncontrolled drinking, while 20% show a progressive downhill course which appears unresponsive to treatment. Among private sector facilities, rates of recovery over 10 years of 50–80% are claimed, although some studies have relied only on telephone interviews without objective measures of recovery status.

The natural history of an alcohol use disorder can be dramatically changed by the presence of physical or neuropsychiatric sequelae, for example, alcohol cirrhosis, one of the most common causes of death inpatients with alcohol use disorders, has an overall mortality rate of 50% at 5 years, comprising 70% of those who continue to drink heavily and 20% of those who abstain. Likewise, alcoholic cardiomyopathy has a bad prognosis with 60% of patients dying within 3 years. Alcohol dependence when complicated by depression, psychosis or suicidal behaviour also has a worse prognosis. The risk of suicide is 50 times greater in alcohol dependent people compared with the general population. Other common causes are motor vehicle accidents (the principal cause in many Western countries), accidental injury, drowning and homicide.

Sedative/hypnotic use

Numerous sedative hypnotic drugs are available on prescription, or in some countries can be purchased in pharmacies or (illegally) over the Internet.

The most commonly used drugs of this type are the benzodiazepines, of which approximately 30 are in common use, with different pharmacokinetic characteristics and clinical effects. Prior to the introduction of these drugs in the 1960s and 1970s, the most commonly available sedative hypnotics were the barbiturates and non-barbiturate drugs, such as methaqualone and chloral hydrate.

Most use of benzodiazepines is short term or confined to use to induce sleep. Approximately 30% of people who start taking benzodiazepines develop dependence on these drugs and this is well described as occurring at therapeutic doses of the equivalent of 15 mg diazepam daily for 3 months. Forty per cent will experience a withdrawal syndrome when the drug is discontinued under double blind conditions; this increases to 70% after 6 months' administration. The risk of dependence increases as the dose extends into supratherapeutic ranges. There is relatively little information on the natural history of benzodiazepine dependence, except that, without intervention, it tends to be long-term and there is a tendency to relapse after a period of non-use. Continuing use is characterized by increasingly levels of dependence, in common with the ever-present risk of the withdrawal syndrome when supply is interrupted. The natural history in treated populations varies widely, with abstinence rates of 70% at 1 year being reported in the people prescribed benzodiazepines legitimately, and also in elderly populations and ranging down to 20% in other studies and lower in street users of these drugs.

The last decade has seen the introduction of the so called 'z drugs', which include zolpidem and zopiclone. Little is known of the natural history of the z drugs other than that they also have dependence potential.

Cannabis

The extent of cannabis use is influenced by the form of cannabis used and several co-morbid factors. Cannabis is the most prevalent illicit drug worldwide. Of those who have ever smoked it, one-third have smoked it in the previous 12 months and approximately 10% have features of cannabis dependence. The natural history of cannabis use varies from the single occasion or experimental use in teenage years to periodic use in parties or other social occasions to regular daily use, which may extend up to 14–16 h of continual smoking per day. Information is scant on the natural history of various levels of cannabis use. Of those who have cannabis dependence, about 50% are still smoking regularly at 5 years and cannabis smoking of 30–40 years is well recognized. Studies conducted in the United States suggest that cannabis typically begins in the mid to late teens, and is most prevalent in early adulthood. Most cannabis use is irregular, with very few users engaging in long-term daily use. In the USA and Australia, it is thought that about 10% of those who ever use cannabis become daily users, and another 20–30% use weekly. Transitions in life roles, such as entry into full-time employment, getting married, or having children, are associated with reductions in or cessation of use for many people. The largest decreases are seen in cannabis use among males and females after marriage, and especially during pregnancy and after childbirth in women.

Opioid dependence

Dependence on opioids can develop from the use of heroin, opium and other illicit opioids, from prescribed or proprietary opioid medications, and from locally or home-produced opioids ('home bake'). Most of our knowledge of opioid dependence is of injecting heroin dependence. Surprisingly little is known of the course of prescribed opioid dependence over the long term.

With heroin use typically starting between the age of 16 and 19 years, heroin dependence typically is evident is at the age of 18–19 years, i.e. after 2 years of use. There is, however, much variation in the rate of development of dependence, which may occur on some people in 6–8 weeks, whereas in others dependence may not develop until many years of intermittent use have occurred.

Among people with heroin dependence, the average duration of dependent heroin use, when untreated, is 10 years, but again there is a wide range and heroin dependence occurring over 20–30 years is well recognized. Heroin dependence thus conforms very clearly to the characteristic chronic and relapsing disorder that is characteristic of untreated established substance dependence syndromes. In the untreated state approximately 30% of heroin dependent individuals will have died at 10 years, most commonly of overdoses, but also of septicaemia and other bacterial complications, HIV/AIDS and hepatitis B- and C-induced liver disease, suicide, trauma, and accidents. Approximately 25% will have recovered, and be abstinent from opiates and other psychoactive substances. Some achieve recovery spontaneously and others through detoxification, other treatment, and involvement with self-help groups. Of the remaining 55%, about half will be using opiates on a regular basis, although in some cases it will have changed to a sporadic pattern of use, based on supply or the finance to purchase it. The other half will be opioid free, but are using other substances in a harmful or dependent manner. Substances mostly used by this group are alcohol, benzodiazepines, and to some extent, psychostimulants.

The natural history of heroin dependence has been modified in recent years by the widespread availability of opioid substitutes, such as methadone and buprenorphine, and also by ready access in many (but not all) countries to sterile injecting equipment provided as part of a harm reduction approach. Opioid substitution reduces the death rate by 75%, so the mortality rate among IV heroin users is now under 10%. Sterile injecting equipment also reduces mortality and also morbidity from infections including blood borne viruses. By contrast, some forms of treatment are associated with no change or increased mortality and so the practitioner working with heroin-dependent people needs to select treatment very carefully. For example, naltrexone treatment with or without prior or rapid detoxification reduces opioid use, but mortality is the same as in an untreated population because of the risk of relapse into an opioid naïve state after treatment ceases. Periodic detoxification is associated with an increase in mortality rate of with the untreated state with 1-year death rate of up to 7% compared with 3% among untreated populations.

Psychostimulant use

Psychostimulant dependence in Western societies is a more recent phenomenon than opioid or cannabis dependence, and consequently less information is available on its natural history, especially in the long term.

Few studies have documented the natural history of psychostimulant use, in sharp contrast to the literature on cannabis and even opioids. Our current understanding derives largely from cross-sectional studies, typically involving convenience samples, or treatment or prison settings. US prospective studies have suggested that relapse following treatment for psychostimulant dependence is common. The concentration of work in treatment or prison populations makes it difficult to draw inferences about amphetamine use in the general population, since most users will never come into contact with either treatment or law enforcement agencies. As a result, little is known about the aetiology and consequences of psychostimulant use that does not come to the attention of police or treatment services. This is an area where much more needs to be known given the increases thought to be occurring in the use of these drugs.

Amphetamine dependence occurs in 30–40% of people who start using amphetamine repeatedly. Uptake of amphetamine use occurs typically from the ages of 17–25 years and dependence develops after an average period of use of 3–4 years, again with much variation. The natural history of amphetamine use differs according to the route of administration. The most common methods are smoking, per nasal use ('snorting') and intravenous use. In Australia, most amphetamine is injected, but the opposite applies in most European countries.

When people have developed amphetamine dependence, the course is again typically a chronic one with periods of non-use and episodes of relapse. Approximately 60% will still be amphetamine-dependent after 3 years, but the long-term natural history (over 10–20 years) has still to be determined. At 3 years, mortality is 5% with most of the deaths occurring from accidents, suicide, and homicide, and a smaller proportion as a result of blood borne infections.

Cocaine dependence develops in approximately 55% of people in Western societies who use cocaine repeatedly. As described earlier, cocaine is used in various forms, as in coca leaf in which the leaves are mixed with an alkali, chewed, and left to rest in the mouth. This is characteristic of its use in indigenous populations in South America. In Western societies, cocaine is used in two main forms, as purified cocaine hydrochloride that may be produced illicitly or obtained from medical supplies, and cocaine freebase, various forms of which are available including 'crack' cocaine. Purified cocaine tends to be used by more socio-economically advantaged people, while crack is used by lower socio-economic and often homeless people.

What can we do about alcohol and other substance use problems?

A range of prevention and intervention measures are available. As with any health problem, intervention may aim to prevent a problem, provide early intervention and treatment; or provide treatment or harm reduction in a well established disorder. The main body of the book is concerned with practical ways in which doctors and health care professionals can diagnose the various forms of alcohol and substance use disorders and provide practical assistance and treatment to people with a view to helping them recover or at least reduce the risk of harmful consequences. However, we should note that at a societal level, the most effective strategy to reduce alcohol and substance-related harm derives from population level approaches, such as legal controls on availability, random breath testing to reduce drink driving and public policies such as no smoking zones, supported by public and school-based education.

Other population-based strategies have specifically targeted blood borne viral infections, e.g. HIV/AIDS and, in more recent years, hepatitis C and B infections. Many countries have in recent years established campaigns and programmes to reduce the harm caused by alcohol and other substance use at a population level. These include the Australian National Campaign Against Drug Abuse and the UK 10-year drug strategy. An important role of doctors and health care practitioners is to support these broad community based measures within their own spheres of influence, while recognizing that the bulk of their work will be concerned with the practical issues of assessment, diagnosis, and treatment of their patients.

Where do we see the role of doctors and health care professionals in prevention? The main body of this text book will deal with the assessment, diagnosis and treatment of people with known or suspected substance dependence, and its related problems. In many cases, treatment is orientated to the goal of abstinence from substance use. In others the goal is maintenance on a substitute medication. Doctors and other health professionals also have an important role to play in early intervention for non-dependent substance use disorders. The following sections summarize the four main components of health care:

Prevention (primary intervention)

Aims to prevent hazardous alcohol and other substance use in the general population, e.g. by controls on availability (supply reduction), media, or school education campaigns (demand reduction), work place policies and addressing underlying risk factors, such as social disadvantage or psychiatric disorders, or by enhancing protective factors such as establishing links with family or community. In terms of practical health care, primary intervention can also be taken as intervention by a general practitioner or health care worker at the point of first contact with a patient who is drinking or using substances hazardously.

Early intervention (secondary intervention)

Actively identifies persons with hazardous alcohol or other substance use before dependence, or physical or psychosocial complications have arisen, and enables them to cease or reduce substance use. Advice or brief counselling at point of first contact is typically used. All health care professionals, including General Practitioners, hospital doctors, and nurses play a major role in early intervention. Early intervention has the potential of being the most effective approach to reduce substance-related harm in the population as a whole.

Treatment (tertiary intervention)

Aims to provide treatment for patients with established dependence or who have already experienced harm caused by substance use to help them cease substance use or be placed on maintenance medication in a therapeutic setting.

Harm reduction and palliation (quaternary intervention)

Involves providing health education and other measures (e.g. supply of clean injecting equipment, ignition interlocks to stop drink driving), to reduce the risk of physical, psychiatric, or medical complications among those who are still using alcohol or other substances in a risky manner. Harm reduction approaches may be used when an individual is trying to change their substance use, but still experiencing slips or relapses. It is also very important in the individual who is not yet able or willing to engage with treatment or to change their substance use. Harm reduction can not only reduce risk to the individual, but also to broader society (e.g. through reduced prevalence of blood borne viruses by means of needle and syringe exchange programmes, hepatitis B vaccination, and treatment of chronic hepatitis C infection).

In some individuals (e.g. those with well established alcohol-related brain damage who continue to drink) there may be little realistic prospect of cure. Palliation and harm reduction measures form an important part of treatment. With respect to alcohol dependence, thiamine is used to reduce the impact of alcohol on the central nervous system in an effort to reduce brain damage. Such an approach aims to relieve symptoms and maintain function and independence to the greatest extent possible. Provision of supervised accommodation is another example of harm reduction.

Chapter 2

Assessment and diagnosis: general principles

Assessment is the first step in the diagnosis and management of patients with alcohol and other drug problems. The assessment allows development of a therapeutic relationship and enables the clinician to demonstrate concern for the patient and the problems they face and so is itself part of the therapeutic process.

A thorough history of the patient's alcohol and substance use is required, together with a medical, psychiatric, social and family history. The patient's readiness to change is gauged and screening or assessment instruments may be used. Clinical examination is performed and investigations of blood measures may be ordered.

Who should be assessed?

Hazardous or harmful drug and alcohol use is so common that all patients seen in any setting (medical, surgical, psychiatric, general practice, specialist rooms) should have a routine and quick screen for alcohol and other substance use. When there are clues to substance use disorders, a more detailed history will be required.

History taking

Good interview and history-taking skills

The alert physician: A high level of awareness of the possibility of an alcohol or other substance use disorder is required. Insomnia, anxiety, depression or other psychiatric symptoms are common clues to substance misuse; similarly physical or social problems can be reminders of the need for a more detailed history.

Examples of clues that might alert the clinician to the possibility of substance misuse

In history
- Insomnia
- Anxiety
- Depression
- Other psychiatric conditions, e.g. aggression, violence, suicidal tendency
- Repeated injuries (especially with alcohol use disorders)
- Clusters of chronic physical conditions that could be related to alcohol
- Repeated social problems, e.g. relationship problems, job loss, frequent changes of job.

In general appearance
- Smell of alcohol
- Restlessness, anxiety (e.g. withdrawal from alcohol or benzodiazepines, stimulant use)
- Drowsiness, slow speech (benzodiazepine, opioid, or cannabis use)
- Attempts to obscure the antecubital fossae (e.g. long sleeves in hot weather, carefully placed tattoos)
- Unprofessional tattoos (may reflect time in prison)
- Unkempt or thin/malnourished (in more severe dependence).

In behaviour
- Drug seeking
- Repeated requests for medical certificates.

On physical examination
- Hypertension or atrial fibrillation (alcohol)
- Needle track marks (injecting drug use) (see Fig. 2.1 p. 43)
- Pin-point (opioid overdose) or dilated pupils (opioid withdrawal).

On blood tests
- Isolated elevation of alanine aminotransferase (ALT, hepatitis C)
- Other unexplained liver function tests (LFT) elevation (alcohol or viral hepatitis).

Establish good rapport with the patient. Some patients are reluctant to discuss alcohol and other substance use problems for fear of prejudice, so an empathic and non judgemental approach and sensitivity to the patient's current life situation and cultural background will increase accuracy of the history.

The assessment process should:
- Effectively engage the patient and develop a therapeutic relationship
- Deal with the presenting issue appropriately and professionally, in a flexible and non-judgemental manner
- Use an appropriate questioning style and content
- Be non-confrontational, show empathy and sensitivity to the patient's cultural background
- Place onus of denial on the patient where there is suspected or alcohol or substance misuse, e.g. to encourage a more open answer ask 'how often do you drink/use recreational drugs' (rather than do you ever?)
- Persevere and be alert to diversionary tactics, and do not abandon taking an appropriate substance use history. If the patient is becoming uncomfortable, the line of questioning can temporarily move to another related topic, then gently come back to the issue of substance use. The clinician can explain that these questions are routine and important to get the full background to any current health concerns.

What are the presenting problems/symptoms and history of presenting illness?

What is the reason for presentation? Whether the patient is presenting for help with drug and alcohol problems, or an incidental issue, it is important to be clear on the reasons for presentation, e.g.
- Medical complications or an unrelated medical issue
- Psychiatric complications or psychiatric co-morbidity, e.g. anxiety, depression
- Family pressure, relationship difficulties, work, financial, or other social complications
- Legal or forensic complications, e.g. drink driving offence or a pre-court assessment
- Pregnancy
- Drug seeking.

Why is the patient presenting now? Having clarified the reason for presentation, you then need to understand why the patient is presenting *now* (e.g. has there been a recent crisis?) and what type of assistance, if any, is being sought:
- Treatment and/or withdrawal management
- Entry to an opioid maintenance programme, e.g. methadone, buprenorphine
- Entry to rehabilitation programme/ therapeutic community
- Psychotherapy (e.g. cognitive behavioural therapy), supportive counselling
- Advice or information
- A hospital bed for some time out or accommodation
- Other help with accommodation or financial issues
- A legal report

- Medical certificate
- Prescription for drugs, e.g. benzodiazepines, opioids.

The clinician needs to determine if the presenting symptoms reflect

- Alcohol and/or other substance intoxication
- Alcohol or other substance dependence and/or withdrawals (related to one or more drugs)
- Hazardous or harmful alcohol and/or other substance use
- Any medical, psychiatric or social complications arising from the patient's alcohol and/or other substance misuse.

Drug and alcohol history

Take a systematic history in order to establish the nature, extent and pattern of use:

- Make it easy for patients to admit to substance use problems:
  - Introduce alcohol consumption as an everyday occurrence or as any other health risk factor
  - Suggest a relatively high level of consumption where you suspect an alcohol use disorder: 'How often do you drink a case of beer?' 'How many bottles of wine do you get through?'
  - For a known illicit drug user, ask about recency and frequency of use, rather than a more general question '*When did you last* use heroin?' or 'How often have you used heroin in the last month?', rather than '*Have you used* any heroin?'
- A substantial proportion of patients use more than one drug. Thus, history taking should include use of benzodiazepines, cannabis, heroin, prescription opioid analgesics, psychostimulants (amphetamines, cocaine, ecstasy), and other illicit drugs.

Record for each psychoactive substance:

- The quantity and frequency of use:
  - Alcohol use must be quantified. Terms such as 'social drinker' have widely variable meanings.
- Pattern of use (episodic versus daily)
- Duration of use
- Time or date of last use
- Route of use:
  - Many illicit drugs can be taken by different routes. Heroin may be inhaled (chasing the dragon) or injected; others such as amphetamines can be taken orally, injected, or snorted. In addition to being ingested, tablets such as benzodiazepines or opioids are sometimes crushed and injected.

Establish whether a diagnosis of substance use disorder can be made: Where there is a suspected alcohol or drug use disorder, core diagnosis in relation to each substance needs to be established. Establish whether the patient is drinking, or using substances, hazardously or harmfully, or whether the patient is dependent (p. 18).

A diagnosis of dependence is made when the answer is 'yes' to three or more of the following questions pertaining to the past 12 months:

- Is there impaired control? Is the patient drinking or using substances in larger amounts than intended?
- Is there a compulsion or craving to drink or use substances?

- Is the patient preoccupied with drinking or using substances, and has it 'taken over' his/her life? Have important family, social, or work responsibilities or interests been neglected?
- Is the patient drinking more and more, or taking more and more of the substance, in order to get the same effect? (tolerance)
- When stopping, or reducing intake:
  - Have there been withdrawal symptoms? This includes early morning withdrawal symptoms experienced by daily heavy drinkers and the withdrawals a heroin dependent individual feels when overdue for a hit. OR
  - Does the patient drink or use substances to prevent withdrawal symptoms?
- Does the patient continue to drink or use substances despite clear evidence of harm?

The diagnosis of dependence is strengthened when there is a past history of attempts to stop drinking or using substances by means of detoxification, pharmacotherapies, involvement with self-help groups, such as Alcoholics Anonymous (AA), Narcotics Anonymous (NA) and other rehabilitation services.

Periods of abstinence: e.g. for a long-term drug user ask 'Since you started using, how many years have you been clean?'. Similarly, for long-term dependent drinkers 'Since you started drinking daily/having problems with your drinking, how many years have you been dry?' 'What treatment helped?'

Precipitating factors for relapse: Ask 'In your view what caused you to relapse this time?'

Past medical and psychiatric history

- Medical illnesses and operations:
  - Consider whether any health problems experienced could be complications of alcohol and other substance misuse—in particular, cardiovascular disease, hypertension in heavy drinkers, liver disease, chronic airway limitation (common in cigarette smokers), seizures (may be related to alcohol and benzodiazepine withdrawals), head injury, obstructive sleep apnoea.
  - Specifically ask about the more common or earlier complications of alcohol or drug misuse, e.g.
    — hypertension or liver damage in drinkers
    — blood-borne viruses in injecting drug users: HIV, Hepatitis B and C status; if present, has hepatitis C been investigated or treated? Has hepatitis B vaccination course (3 injections) been completed? When were LFT's last checked? What were the results?
  - Consider whether or how any coexisting medical problems are likely to be impacted on by substance use.
- Primary underlying psychiatric disorders or psychiatric complications of alcohol and other substance use:
  - Anxiety, depression, psychosis, post traumatic stress disorder
  - Past history of suicide attempts, including deliberate overdoses
  - Childhood issues, e.g. 'Can your childhood be described as positive, negative, or mixed?'; 'Did you have any distressing experiences

during childhood?' Consider the possibility of a past history of childhood sexual or physical abuse.

Family history
- Alcohol and other substance misuse
- Major medical or psychiatric illnesses.

Social history
The depth of social history will depend on the time available, but some sense of the patient's context is vital in forming a realistic treatment plan. Further details on how the individual's alcohol and/or substance use has impacted on self, family, or friends is important, but often may be acquired at follow up appointment, e.g. who do they drink/use drugs with?

Information obtained as early as feasible
- Living arrangements:
    - Alone, with partner, friends, relatives
    - Children under care
    - Family violence
- Do other adults in the house or key friends misuse alcohol or other substances? If so, this does not augur well for short-term prognosis.
- Available support.

Information that may be obtained in successive consultations
- Domestic and allied problems—marital conflict, separation, divorce, relationship status
- Highest schooling or training
- Work experience:
    - Employment skills and recent employment history
    - Absenteeism, poor work performance, unemployment
- Financial—debts, gambling
- Legal status:
    - Drink driving offences, loss of licence, motor vehicle accidents
    - Robbery, violence, assault, criminal activity,
    - Incarceration
- Sex work, risks of sexually transmitted infections
- Further detail on social situation.

Medications
- Prescribed medications: in addition to other prescribed medication, specifically inquire about use of:
    - Benzodiazepines and other sedative/hypnotics (Ask 'Do you sleep well?' If not, 'Do you need sleeping pills to sleep?')
    - Opioid analgesics (particularly patients with a history of chronic pain or previous heroin use)
    - Antidepressants
    - Antipsychotics
    - Non-steroidal anti-inflammatory drugs (risk of gastric erosions in alcohol use disorders)
- Over-the-counter preparations (codeine, paracetamol, antihistamines, etc.), which may be misused deliberately or unconsciously (see p. 278 on pharmacy drugs).

Clinical examination

General appearance

In many patients with hazardous or harmful drinking or drug use, physical examination may be normal.

With dependent alcohol or substance use, the appearance may provide more clues to the diagnosis:

- Is the patient unkempt, malnourished?
- Is there alcohol on the breath and other signs of intoxication? Or of withdrawals?
- Face: flushing, telangiectasia, periorbital oedema, parotid swelling (alcohol misuse)
- Are there nicotine stains on the fingers? (cigarette smoking)
- Are there needle track marks? If so are they fresh or old? (injecting drug use; see Fig. 2.1)
- Signs of skin infections—thrombophlebitis, skin abscesses (Fig. 2.2)
- Pallor, fever, flushing
- Tremors (alcohol or benzodiazepine withdrawals)
- Sweating (benzodiazepine or alcohol withdrawal, also in-patients on methadone maintenance treatment)
- Conjunctival injection, i.e. red eyes (alcohol, cannabis)
- Jaundice (alcoholic liver disease, hepatitis C)
- Bruises of different ages (alcohol in particular)
- Excoriations (stimulants, liver disease)
- Dental: bleeding gums, caries (opioids), tooth grinding (stimulants)
- Signs of injury or other trauma.

Systematic examination of body systems

In particular look for:

Respiratory system

- Chronic airways limitation in smokers
- Pneumonia or other respiratory infections
- Tuberculosis (poor self care, poor living conditions, or suppressed immunity)
- Other infections, HIV
- Pulmonary oedema.

Cardiovascular

- Hypotension (opioid overdose) or hypertension (stimulant use, chronic alcohol excess, withdrawal states)
- Tachycardia (stimulant use, withdrawal states)
- Tachyarrhythmias (alcoholic cardiomyopathy, alcohol-induced atrial fibrillation, stimulant use)
- Cardiac failure
- Heart murmurs (bacterial endocarditis, cardiomyopathy).

Gastroenterological

- Hepatomegaly (signs of hepatitis, fatty liver, or chronic liver disease)
- Splenomegaly, portal hypertension, signs of hepatic decompensation.

(a)

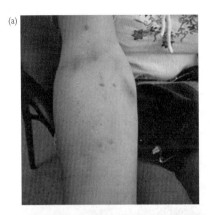

(b)

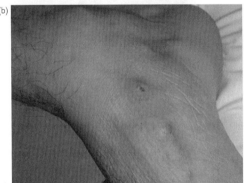

(c)

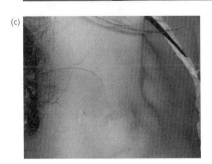

Fig. 2.1 (See colour plate 1–3) Needle track marks. (a) Arm, (b) Ankle, (c) Neck.

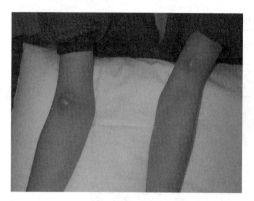

Fig. 2.2 (See colour plate 4) Abscesses at injecting site.

Musculoskeletal system
- Scars, fractures (recent and/or old)
- Muscle weakness or wasting (alcoholic myopathy, chronic liver disease).

Neurological
- Is the patient intoxicated, drowsy, confused, or agitated?
- Pupil size and equality: (dilated in opioid withdrawal) or constricted (in opioid use)
- Peripheral neuropathy (pain, diminished sensation, absent reflexes; with alcohol dependence)
- Cerebellar signs in alcohol dependence
- Diplopia/lateral gaze palsies/nystagmus (one or more may occur in Wernicke's encephalopathy)
- Speech (slurred with alcohol or benzodiazepines; may be slow with opioid or cannabis intoxication, or rapid or pressured with stimulant intoxication)
- Gait (ataxia with alcohol or benzodiazepine intoxication or alcoholic cerebellar damage).

Mental state examination

The Mental State Examination (MSE) is a systematic assessment of the features of the patient's presentation, behaviour and psychological experiences at the time of the interview. There are several key areas to explore.

Appearance and behaviour: General description of the patient, general reaction to the interview (e.g. friendly, co-operative, withdrawn, uncommunicative, hostile, guarded), physical appearance (level of self-care, unkempt, well dressed), abnormal motor activity (sweating, tics, tremor, restlessness, physical agitation, psychomotor retardation).

Speech: May help point towards neurological or psychiatric problems. Assess the rate (e.g. slow, hesitant, rapid), the volume (e.g. loud, soft, inaudible), the quantity (e.g. poverty of speech). Note any abnormal articulation, e.g. stuttering or slurred speech.

Mood and affect

Mood—the patient's subjective experience of their emotional state (depressed, angry, anxious, sad, fearful, elated).

Affect—objective and what you observe of the person's emotional state by noting their appearance, level of movement, posture, and general behaviour (normal, restricted, flat, anxious etc).

Form of thought: The patient's amount and rate of thoughts (vague, poverty of ideas, slow, hesitant), order of thoughts (logical, distractible, loosening of associations, tangential); disturbance of language (incoherent)—helps assessment of co-morbid problems.

Thought content: Look for delusional beliefs; false beliefs, delusions of control, anxiety states, phobias, obsessional thoughts, preoccupations, depressive thought content if mood is depressed, including excessive guilt and self-blame; hopelessness, helplessness worthlessness. Suicidal thoughts (ascertain whether the patient has any current thoughts, plans or intention to self harm or commit suicide. (Refer also to section on the suicidal patient (refer to pp. 46–47) and thoughts of harm to others (ascertain whether the patient has any current thoughts, plans or intention to harm others (refer to the section on the violent patient).

Perception: Abnormal perceptual experiences such as illusions (distortions of real external stimuli) and misinterpretations (true perceptions, the meaning of which is misinterpreted), and hallucinations (the person hears, sees or smells something, but there is nothing there).

Hallucinations—may be auditory, visual, tactile (formication is a form of tactile hallucination commonly experienced with excessive use of methamphetamine or cocaine), gustatory, olfactory, or somatic. Consider drug-induced psychosis (psychostimulant intoxication/psychosis; heavy cannabis use), co-morbid schizophrenia; alcohol withdrawals (delirium tremens), benzodiazepine withdrawals.

Cognitive state: Cognitive testing can be brief in a patient whose cognitive state appears to be intact and there are no factors in the history to suggest that cognitive impairment is likely. Patients with alcohol-related brain damage should have more detailed assessment by the Mini Mental State Examination (p. 443). Key areas to examine are:

- **Level of conscious awareness:** is the patient alert, drowsy, showing a fluctuating level of consciousness? Confused or delirious? (Think of alcohol or benzodiazepine withdrawals; Wernicke's encephalopathy; hepatic encephalopathy, hypoxia, infections, head injury)
- **Orientation:** does the patient know who they are, where they are, what day it is, and what the date is (i.e. are they orientated in time, place, and person)?

- **Attention and concentration:** this is assessed based on their general behaviour during the interview and can be examined more formally using specific tests including:
  - Simple arithmetic
  - Serial sevens (take 7 away from 100 and keep taking it away):
    — if serial sevens are too difficult, give the months of the year backwards
    — if this is too difficult, give the days of the week backwards
- **Memory:** three areas should be tested:
  - Immediate and short-term memory
  - Recent memory
  - Long-term memory.
- **Intelligence:** this can be assessed by the patient's performance in the interview, their educational and occupational level, their general knowledge. Tests for general information and knowledge can also be given including the name of the current prime minister, the capital of their country, the president of the USA, etc.

Insight and Judgement: Insight refers to the patient's awareness of their psychological state; the impact of their behaviour on others; their under-standing of their illness, its likely causes, consequences and treatment.

Assessing the patient's judgement provides information about their ability for rational problem-solving and decision-making. The level of the patient's judgement is often apparent as the history is taken.

Rapport: This describes the level of relatedness or connection between the patient and the health professional during the interview. Difficulties in establishing rapport may provide clues about the difficulties the patient is having in establishing relationships with others, e.g. through mistrust, hostility, irritability, lack of warmth. The interviewer's reaction often pro-vides a sense of what disorder the patient may be suffering from. For example, if the interviewer is laughing with the patient, they may be manic or hypomanic. If the interview feels sad, the patient may be depressed or grieving. If the interviewer feels frightened, they may be with a dangerous, hostile patient, and they should end the interview and leave the room. If the interviewer feels totally confused by what the patient is saying, the patient may be psychotic with loosening of associations.

Should the patient be scheduled/compulsorily detained: Refer to the Mental Health Act section, Chapter 15, p. 414.

Suicide risk assessment

The overall assessment of suicide risk should take into account **Risk,** as well as **Protective Factors**.

Common examples of Protective Factors include:
- Strong perceived social supports including good relationships with family and friends
- Good coping and problem-solving skills
- Ability to seek and access help
- Positive values and beliefs.

Suicide risk assessment is particularly important in patients who are in the crash phase of psychostimulant use or withdrawing from alcohol or benzodiazepines.

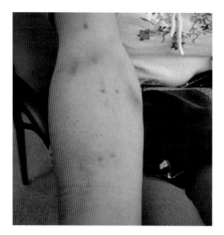

Plate 1 (Also see Fig. 2.1) Needle track marks, (a) Arm.

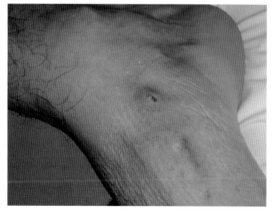

Plate 2 (Also see Fig. 2.1) Needle track marks, (b) Ankle.

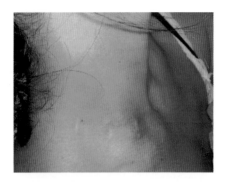

Plate 3 (Also see Fig. 2.1) Needle track marks, (c) Neck.

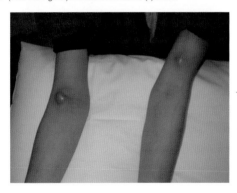

Plate 4 (Also see Fig. 2.2) Abscess at injecting site.

The purpose of the assessment is to:

- Determine the nature and severity of the patient's problems. This includes looking at past and current psychiatric history, as well as mental state assessment
- Determine the potential risk of harm to self or others
- Determine whether or not the patient should be referred for a more detailed risk assessment and for more intensive management because of the level of risk.

Findings from the patient's current mental state examination should be combined with findings in the patient's history to determine the patient's current level of risk (high, medium, or low) and to allow for effective treatment planning to manage this risk.

Questions to ask about suicidal thoughts should include

- Have things been so bad for you lately that you've felt that life is not worth living?
- Do you have any current thoughts about harming yourself or taking your life?
  - If yes—have you made any plans to try to harm yourself or end your life? Can you tell me about those plans? (Ask in detail, e.g. if the patient has had thoughts of shooting themselves with a gun, ask if they have access to a gun. If they have had thoughts of hanging, have they attempted to make a noose?)
- Do you feel it is likely you will try to carry those plans out?
  - If yes—can you tell me when you plan to do this?
    If no—what are some of the things that are stopping you from harming yourself or taking your life?

A modified form of the acronym 'SAD PERSONS' (Preskorn 1999) can be used to identify some of the key risk factors for suicide in any individual (see p. 397).

Laboratory investigations

- Breath or blood alcohol concentrations
- Urine drug screens may provide useful information even though results may not be available for more than 24 h. (Results may help confirm suspected substance use, and/or use of more than one drug—which is common.)

Routine investigations (see pp. 100–105**)**

- Full blood count
- Liver function tests (LFTs)—(especially GGT, AST, ALT)
- Coagulation tests (INR/APTT)
- Urea and electrolytes—focusing on sodium, potassium levels
- Magnesium (for alcohol dependence)
- Glucose—increased or decreased with heavy drinking; DD of delirium or coma.
- Viral serology: in injecting drug users screening for hepatitis C, B and HIV is important (p. 220, 371).

Other laboratory tests depending on clinical presentation

- ESR /CRP
- Serum B12 and folate, if MCV elevated, or malnutrition is suspected
- Thyroid function tests (TFTs)
- Creatine phosphokinase (CPK, rhabdomyolysis from psychostimulant use or in patients who may have had a long period of coma)
- Cardiac enzymes (cocaine induced myocardial infarction)
- Blood cultures (septicaemia, bacterial endocarditis following IV drug use)
- Sexually transmitted infections screen, e.g. including syphilis serology, chlamydia PCR, VDRL.

Other investigations

- Brain CT/MRI (head injury, subdural haematoma, first seizure)
- ECG (atrial fibrillation from acute heavy alcohol use or alcoholic cardiomyopathy, psychostimulant-induced arrhythmias)
- Chest X-ray (aspiration and other pneumonias)
- Oximeter readings or blood gases (asthma/CAL/hypoxia).

Table 2.1 Some common presentations of alcohol and other substance use disorders

Clinical problem	Presumptive diagnosis	Alcohol and other substance use-related diagnosis
Gastrointestinal system		
Dyspepsia, heartburn	Peptic ulcer; hiatus hernia	Alcohol-induced gastritis, oesophagitis
Vomiting, diarrhoea	Gastroenteritis	Alcohol withdrawals Opioid withdrawals
Upper gastrointestinal bleeding	Oesophagitis Gastritis Peptic ulcer NSAIDs ± alcohol Carcinoma	Alcohol-induced: – Gastritis/oesophagitis – Mallory Weiss syndrome – Oesophageal varices
Lower gastrointestinal bleeding	Diverticular disease, polyps Carcinoma Inflammatory bowel disease	Cocaine intoxication (bowel ischaemia from vasoconstriction)
Abdominal pain ± jaundice	Viral hepatitis Cholecystitis Pancreatitis	Alcoholic hepatitis/cirrhosis Viral hepatitis (hepatitis C, B secondary to IDU) Alcoholic pancreatitis
Cardiovascular system		
Palpitations, SOB, ankle swelling	Ischaemic heart disease, Tachyarrhythmias Congestive cardiac failure (CCF)	Alcoholic cardiomyopathy Stimulant intoxication
High blood pressure	Essential hypertension	Alcohol-induced hypertension Stimulant-induced hypertension
Chest pain	Myocardial infarction, ischaemic heart disease	Cocaine induced ischaemia/myocardial infarction
Neuropsychiatric		
Anxiety, tremor, sweating, insomnia	Anxiety disorder	Alcohol (and/or sedative) withdrawal Stimulant intoxication
Depression	Major depressive illness	Stimulant 'crash' or withdrawal
Blackouts	Vasovagal or cardiac syncope Concussion—head injury	Alcohol intoxication
Seizures	Hypoglycaemia Epilepsy Cerebral neoplasms Head trauma Cerebral infections Hypoglycaemia Hypomagnesaemia, Hypocalcaemia Hyponatraemia	Alcohol withdrawal seizures Benzodiazepine withdrawal seizures Stimulant-induced seizures

Table 2.1 (Contd.)

Clinical problem	Presumptive diagnosis	Alcohol and other substance use-related diagnosis
Confusion	Hypo- or hyperglycaemia Infections, etc. (As below for delirium)	Alcohol intoxication Alcohol withdrawal (mild to moderate) Benzodiazepine withdrawal Wernicke's encephalopathy
Delirium	Infections Hypoxia Trauma—head injury, subdural haematoma Post-ictal Hypo- or hyper glycaemia Hypo- or hyper thyroidism Electrolyte disturbances Cardiac failure Cerebrovascular accidents Hepatic encephalopathy Uraemia Cerebral neoplasm HIV/AIDS	Severe alcohol withdrawals/delirium tremens Severe benzodiazepine withdrawals Wernicke's encephalopathy
Cognitive impairment	Dementia Alzheimer's disease Chronic subdural haematoma Syphilis HIV/AIDs Cerebral neoplasm Cerebrovascular disease Thiamine or B_{12} deficiency	Alcohol related brain damage Wernicke–Korsakoff syndrome
Coma	Trauma—subdural haematoma, head injury Hypo- or hyperglycaemia Cerebrbrovascular accident Cerebral and other infections Epilepsy Cerebral neoplasm	Alcohol intoxication. Opioid overdose Benzodiazepine overdose
Paranoid delusions and hallucinations	Schizophrenia	Alcoholic hallucinosis Delirium tremens Stimulant-induced psychosis Cannabis-induced psychosis

Screening and brief assessment instruments

A number of screening and brief assessment instruments and questionnaires can often help the practitioner extract the salient points in the history (e.g. AUDIT and CAGE variants for alcohol problems; ASSIST is a combined screen for drug and alcohol misuse developed by WHO). These typically include 10 items or fewer and are suitable for self completion while in the waiting room or hospital clinic. The Hospital Anxiety and Depression Scale (HADS) is also a useful brief screening tool for patients with underlying anxiety or depression.

More detailed assessment instruments such as SADQ (Severity of Alcohol Dependence Questionnaire), ASI (Addiction Severity Index), SDS (Severity of Dependence Scale), SODQ (Severity of Opiate Dependence Questionnaire), and quality of life questionnaires (SF14, SF36, SF96) are also sometimes used in specialist practices.

Diagnostic schedules

Complex interview based schedules, such as CIDI (Composite International Diagnostic Interview), SAM (Substance Abuse Module), HoNOS (Health of the Nation Outcome Scales), SCAN (WHO Schedules for Clinical Assessment in Neuropsychiatry, DIS (Diagnostic Interview Schedule, National Institutes of Mental Health) cover a range of alcohol and substance use disorders from which validated diagnosis can be made. These are used by trained researchers for research purposes and are rarely used in clinical practice.

Collateral and corroborative information

Some patients with alcohol and other substance use disorders are reluctant to divulge information about their substance misuse for fear of prejudice or develop defence mechanisms to explain, understate or rationalize their use to themselves and others. In many cases, the clinician will be faced with inconsistencies in the patient's history or the patient's report is at odds with the clinical signs or laboratory test results. In such cases, obtaining collateral or other corroborative information is important. These days one would seek the patient's consent to approach relatives or their GPs within the ethical framework for obtaining information. Other corroborative information comes from previous medical records/case notes, letters, and information from social service agencies, ambulance officers and police.

In some emergency situations (e.g. acute overdose, acute psychosis, delirium), seeking the patient's consent is not possible. It is important that the ethics and implications of potentially revealing previously undisclosed information about the patient's substance use be carefully kept in mind.

Formulating a working diagnosis and differential diagnosis

- Having performed the assessment, information needs to be synthesized for a clear provisional diagnosis for each substance or group of substances, and for medical, psychiatric and social complications and co-morbid conditions
- In general, the clinician seeks the most parsimonious diagnosis. Alcohol and other substance use can explain a range of seemingly unrelated problems or conditions
- Diagnosis in alcohol and substance use disorders is not typically a spot diagnosis. In some cases, in the initial consultation a definitive diagnosis cannot be made, and the diagnosis is reviewed at follow-up interviews
- Always be open to new information. Repeated and incremental assessment is necessary to receive, process, and appraise new information, particularly if there is concern that the patient is understating or minimizing use, and the impact it is having on him or her.

Establishing a final diagnosis

A definitive diagnosis is made after putting together all incrementally obtained relevant information.

Diagnosis is based on the following core clinical syndromes:

- Alcohol and/or other substance dependence or non-dependent hazardous/harmful use/abuse or use?
- Alcohol and/or other substance withdrawal syndromes?
- Alcohol and/or other substance intoxication
- Medical complications of alcohol or other substance use
- Psychiatric complications of alcohol or other substance use
- Social complications of alcohol or other substance use
- Co-morbidity—medical or psychiatric.

Polysubstance use is common among patients who misuse alcohol or other substances, so consider whether a substance use disorder is present for each major group of substances.

In addition the following information can be noted:

- Are there major psychosocial stressors which are likely to impact on the treatment plan?
- Antecedent factors for alcohol and other substance misuse:
  - Genetic factors:
    — Personality traits—impulsivity, risk taking, rebelliousness
    — Family history of alcohol and other substance use disorders.
    — Family history of psychiatric problems
    — Differences in metabolism of psycho-active substances (e.g. rapid opioid metabolizer)
  - Primary or underlying mental health disorders, e.g. anxiety, depression, psychosis
  - History of childhood sexual or physical abuse
  - Environmental factors: peers/partners who drink excessively or use substances
- Perpetuating factors for alcohol and substance misuse:
  - Missed or incorrect diagnosis of alcohol or substance use disorders, and inappropriate management
  - Missed or incorrect diagnosis of medical, psychiatric, and social complications of alcohol and other substance misuse, or co-morbidity, and inappropriate management
  - Lack of appropriate medical, psychiatric or psychological treatment services
  - Psychological factors—boredom, low self-esteem, stress
  - Environmental factors: lack of family or social support, peers/partners who drink excessively or misuse substances.

Approaches to management

Alcohol and substance use disorders cover a wide spectrum from simple mild to moderate problems, associated with non-dependent hazardous or harmful drinking, or substance use, that are readily dealt with in primary care, to severe, entrenched dependence and complicating problems that require referral to specialist drug and alcohol services.

Underlying principles of treatment

Provide education and information about the nature of substance use disorders, and allow the patient to develop an understanding of this.

The treatment goal depends on the diagnosis. In general, if the diagnosis is hazardous or harmful drinking, the goal of treatment is controlled drinking. If the diagnosis is alcohol dependence, or dependence on other drugs, the recommended goal of treatment is abstinence. However, this is not always feasible or acceptable to the patient initially.

The treatment of alcohol and substance use disorders is based on an understanding of the individual's freedom to exercise personal responsibility and choice in relation to his/her alcohol or substance use.

In negotiating a management plan, it is important to understand what the patient is seeking and what his/her motivation is. Sometimes the patient is not yet ready to consider change and the short term treatment goal may involve enhancing his/her motivation to change and attempting to move the patient towards an acceptable negotiated goal. (See Motivational Interviewing, p. 62–64)

Management of non-dependent hazardous or harmful drinking, or other drug misuse

Following the establishment of the diagnosis, early and brief intervention techniques are employed. In the case of alcohol use disorders, early intervention has been demonstrated to be effective (see p. 91–95 for more detail on brief intervention for alcohol problems). Similar evidence is not yet available for most illicit substances. The general principles of alcohol brief interventions can be applied to providing opportunistic interventions for other substances (e.g. when the illicit drug user presents for treatment of an injecting site infection).

The steps of brief intervention—FLAGS acronym

F—Feedback problems experienced. This feedback attempts to link the patient's alcohol and substance misuse with any medical and/or psychosocial complications experienced.
L—Listen: to readiness to change.
A—Provide unequivocal advice to change.
G—Negotiate goals to reduce drinking or substance use.
S—Set out strategies and discuss practical methods for achieving goals.

Treatment of alcohol dependence or other drug dependence

To guide our practice we have adopted a 10-step approach to management of dependence. The key components of management are:

Information/education: Provide education, information, and advice regarding the nature of dependence, and provide feedback and education (where needed) on the medical, psychiatric, and social complications of substance use that the individual has already experienced or risks experiencing.

Explain that dependence is a chronic relapsing disorder and that if they resume drinking or taking substances they are likely to rapidly return to their previous levels of use.

Recognition and acceptance: Let the patient digest the information provided and consider what point they are at. The dependent patient must then reach a point of acceptance of the need to stop and develop a commitment to stop drinking or using substances.

Detoxification: A necessary first step. This allows the patient to cease alcohol or substance use in a comfortable and non-distressing manner. It may involve symptomatic management of withdrawal symptoms. Detoxification may be medicated or non-medicated depending on the severity of withdrawal. It can be conducted on an ambulatory or in-patient basis. Ambulatory detoxification requires the patient's commitment and close liaison between the medical officer, general practitioner, and psychologist/counsellor. Ambulatory detoxification may not be feasible if there is an unsuitable home environment (e.g. unstable or with high level of substance use). Also, individuals who are dependent on more than one drug (e.g. benzodiazepine plus alcohol), or who have significant medical or psychiatric co-morbidity often require in-patient detoxification.

Pharmacotherapy: To suppress the internal driving force of dependence.

Pharmacotherapies used to treat substance dependence

Smoking
- Substitution therapy:
  - Nicotine replacement (patches, gum)
  - Nicotinic partial agonists—Varenicline
- Anti-craving agents
  - Bupropion
  - Varenicline.

Alcohol dependence
- Anti craving agents
  - Acamprosate
  - Naltrexone
  - Nalmefene
- Alcohol sensitizing drugs:
  - Disulfiram.

Opioid dependence
- Substitution therapy:
  - Methadone
  - Buprenorphine
    — Suboxone®
- Opioid antagonists:
  - Naltrexone.

Psychological treatments: This very important component of treatment includes:

Brief advice (as described above): Simple medical advice may be used to help engage the patient with ongoing treatment. However, in general for substance use dependence, ongoing counselling or support is desirable.

Counselling: this may provide general support, but increasingly also employs specific psychotherapies, as set out below.

Motivational enhancement therapy (p. 62–64)

Cognitive behavioural therapy (CBT): Aims to reshape thinking and develop skills to prevent relapse. It may include:
- Development of skills in:
  - Coping, and problem solving
  - Communication and assertiveness
  - Relaxation and stress management
  - Anger management
  - Alcohol and drug refusal, finding alternative ways to cope with triggers to substance use
- Behavioural self-management and modification programmes
- Cognitive restructuring
- Behavioural treatments to deal with impaired cognition.

Treatment of co-morbidity and complications of alcohol and other substance dependence

Parallel treatment of:

Medical complications or co-morbidity (e.g. see pp. 80 and 367): on treatment of complications of injecting and on complications of alcohol dependence). Individuals with ongoing alcohol or other drug dependence will often find it difficult to engage with the full range of specialist services, so the general practitioner or addiction medicine specialist has an important role in monitoring medical complications and facilitating, or in some cases providing, treatment.

Psychiatric co-morbidity or complications (pp. 87 and 295): treatment for any underlying or complicating psychiatric conditions is necessary to improve the prognosis for the substance use disorder. A psychiatrist therefore plays a vital role in the management of patients.

Support of, and from, family and friends: The patient is treated within the family and social context. Families and friends of users require support, assistance and advice on how to support and help the user and on how to deal with a very difficult situation. Mutual help groups such as AlAnon, Nar-Anon and Al Ateen have been established to support families.

Self-help programmes/12-step fellowship: In many countries mutual help groups such as AA and NA exist to support the dependent user. Regular attendance at meetings with abstinence as a goal has been found to be useful in achieving and maintaining abstinence. These are based on the 12-step programme on the principle that alcohol and substance dependence is a physical, mental, and spiritual disease, which requires lifelong abstinence and participation in a recovery programme.

Continuing follow-up/after care (and residential rehabilitation in some cases): Treatment of dependence is not just a brief one-off event. Regular follow-up, ongoing review, re-evaluation, and re-negotiation of treatment goals and management plans play a very important role. In the process support is provided, motivation boosted, and brief cognitive behavioural or other psychotherapy may be provided. Close collaboration between the patient's own GP and the specialist Addiction Medicine team can greatly increase integration of treatment and maximize the chance of success.

Residential in-patient treatment and rehabilitation programmes: Patients with severe alcohol or/and other substance dependence who fail to respond to multiple in-patient detoxifications and outpatient treatment programmes, and who repeatedly relapse are referred to a more intensive residential treatment or rehabilitation programme which may last weeks to months. Patients are most often referred to such services by specialist drug and alcohol treatment units. Other criteria for referral to residential in-patient treatment programmes include:

- Lack of ability to adhere to treatment
- Homelessness and lack of social support
- Severe life crises
- Concurrent medical or psychiatric illnesses.

Patients with severe cognitive impairment or major psychiatric or medical co-morbidity who are unable to participate in intensive in-patient rehabilitation programmes may require longer-term supervision or care, for example in a residential facilities or a nursing home (also see p. 414 on guardianship).

Life style and environmental change: Changes at work, home and environment to deal with antecedent or perpetuating factors may be necessary, e.g. if the patient lives with family or friends who are heavy drinkers or substance users, moving house may be a key to success. Many individuals who use illicit drugs find that the only way they can avoid drug use is to limit or eliminate contact with using friends. Adopting a healthy life style with regular healthy meals and exercise are important in restoring health.

A reality check is required at this point. Some patients with severe and complicated alcohol and substance use disorders are unwilling or unable to cease use. Most patients will not be able to totally avoid slip ups or relapses when they engage with treatment, even though they may be striving to cease their substance use.

Harm reduction and palliation

Measures to reduce the harms of any slip ups are important (e.g. discussing how to avoid drinking and driving should a relapse occur in alcohol dependence; treatment of chronic hepatitis C and hepatitis B vaccination for injecting drug users).

It is still possible to engage and work with individuals who are unwilling or unable to cease substance use (at least at the current point of time) using the principles of harm reduction, assisting them to reduce the physical or psychiatric complications of their substance use. This approach can also reduce harms to the family and community around the user, e.g. by reducing spread of sexually transmitted infections and spread of hepatitis C by encouraging treatment, and reducing risk of violence and suicide by appropriate psychiatric intervention. In some cases where the prognosis is very poor (e.g. alcohol dependence in a person with advanced alcohol-related brain damage) the principles of palliation are employed, to maximize the individual's quality of life, and also efforts are made to diminish the impact of their use on family and community.

Motivational interviewing: enhancing the process of change

Most patients with alcohol or other drug problems have difficulty changing their behaviour. Building an effective therapeutic relationship is an important component in motivating the patient to reduce or give up alcohol or drug use. Basic counselling skills, such as empathic listening, reflecting, summarizing, re-framing, and exploring options form the basis for an effective therapeutic alliance. In therapy, behaviour change is due to:

- The patient's own strengths and resources (40%)
- The patient's perception of the relationship with the clinician (30%)
- Hopefulness and expectation (15%)
- The particular therapeutic technique employed (15%).

To enhance the patient's own strengths and resources for change

- Assess and summarize for patients their strengths (e.g. persistence, intelligence, resilience, ability to survive) and resources (e.g. family, friends, work colleagues)
- Ask patients about their beliefs regarding the problem
- Select interventions that are compatible with the patient's beliefs.

To enhance therapeutic alliance: Once goals have been negotiated, accept the patient's goals, rather than challenging them or altering them to fit a particular theoretical model:

- Tailor the therapy to the individual patient
- Negotiate and collaborate with patients, rather than dictating to them
- Explore issues that are relevant to the patient
- Regularly follow-up, review and renegotiate goals and strategies.

To enhance hope and expectation

- Convey an attitude of hope and possibility without minimizing the problem or the pain that accompanies it
- Encourage patients to focus on present and future possibilities, instead of focusing exclusively on past problems.

To enhance the effectiveness of a therapeutic technique, choose one that

- Capitalizes on the individual patient's strengths and resources
- Is considered empathic, respectful, and genuine by the patient
- Fits with the patient's goals and beliefs
- Increases hopefulness, expectancy and sense of personal control.

When individuals attempt to change a problem behaviour, a lapse is highly probable. As well as dealing with biologically-based cravings, patients in treatment for problematic substance use are attempting to change what has become an automatic response to a particular situation. For them, using a substance has been a solution to another problem (depression, anxiety, anger, stress, boredom, discomfort, grief, loss, etc.). Until patients find alternative solutions for these problems, they will be at risk of relapsing.

The change cycle

Prochaska & DiClemente (1986) developed a model for assessing the patient's 'stage of change' in relation to their substance use. This involves progression through five stages.

Table 3.1 Stages of change

1. Pre-contemplation: The patient is not aware that there is a problem and is not yet considering change.

2. Contemplation: The patient is more aware of problems associated with substance use and contemplates change, but is ambivalent about changing. Motivational interviewing may help the patient to explore this ambivalence and move towards making a decision to change.

3. Preparation: The patient understands that the negative consequences of substance use outweighs the benefits and prepares to do something about it. Negotiate a goal.

4. Action: The patient actively attempts to reduce or cease substance use. Support the patient. Find ways to overcome obstacles or set less ambitious goals.

5. Maintenance: The patient has changed and continues to focus on maintaining the change. Relapse prevention strategies are important during this phase.

6. Relapse: Both the clinician and the patient need to understand that relapse is part of the change cycle. Even after patients have found an alternative solution to drugs or alcohol they may have trouble remembering to use it. Altering an automatic behaviour is difficult. Help your patients to see that failure is only the point at which we stop trying. If we are still trying, we haven't failed. We can learn from our set-backs and ultimately succeed.

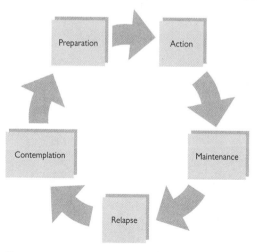

Fig. 3.1 The cycle of stages of change.

Individuals typically recycle through these stages several times before termination of the addiction.

Facilitating change

Motivation can arise from interaction between people. Confrontation tends to strengthen addictive behaviours because the ambivalent patient takes the contrary view to the confronting clinician. It is much more effective to explore the patient's ambivalence, looking for discrepancies between deeply held values and current behaviours. For example, if a father becomes aware that he is behaving as if alcohol were more important to him than his children, this may trigger the start of his cutting back or abstaining from alcohol.

Empathize with the patient about the losses that come with abstaining from alcohol or drugs. For them it will be like losing a friend that was always there for them, even though it was a damaging relationship.

Further reading

Asay TP, Lambert MJ. The empirical case for the common factors in therapy: quantitative findings. In Hubble MA, Duncan BL & Miller SD (Eds). *The Heart and Soul of Change: What Works in Therapy.* Washington, DC: American Psychological Association, 1999.

Geldard D. *Basic Personal Counselling: A Training Manual For Counsellors* 5th edn. Sydney: Pearson Education, 2005.

Marlatt GA, Witkiewitz K. Relapse prevention of alcohol and drug problems. In Marlatt, GA & Donovan, DM (Eds) *Relapse Prevention: Maintenance Strategies in the Treatment of Addictive Behaviors.* New York: Guilford Press 2005.

Miller WR, Rollnick S. *Motivational Interviewing: Preparing People For Change.* New York: Guilford Press, 2002.

Morawetz D. What works in therapy: what Australian patients say. *Psychotherapy* 2002; **9**: 66–70.

Prochaska JO, DiClemente CC, Norcross JC. In search of how people change. Applications to addictive behaviours. *American Psychologist,* 1992; **47**: 1102–14.

Alcohol

Introduction

Alcohol dependence is a serious and lingering disorder with a remitting and relapsing course, in which there is strong psycho-physiological drive to consume alcohol and to do so even in the face of serious alcohol-related harm. In a few countries the treatment of alcohol dependence is the province of the Addiction Specialist or specialist treatment agency. However, in most, primary care practitioners will need to offer a range of treatments. In this section we indicate what these are, and also describe the treatment that can be provided in more specialist settings.

Alcohol dependence is a clinical syndrome in which there is a prominent physiological drive to consume alcohol. It develops over many months or years and if untreated usually shows a progressive or chronic relapsing course. Because of the neurobiological midbrain changes, people with alcohol dependence are intensely reactive to various triggers or cues. These may be environmental ones such as the sight of a bar, internal ones such as distressing or negative emotions, or interpersonal ones such as a difficult interaction with someone.

There is a wide range of treatments and supports for people with alcohol use disorders. Treatment has developed considerably over the past decade; there are well-established detoxification (withdrawal management) procedures and several prescribed medications have become available. Psychological therapies are well developed and support therapies and involvement with self-help (mutual help) groups have much to offer.

There was a time when alcohol use disorders were considered to be poorly responsive to treatment and many practitioners developed a sense of pessimism about patients affected by them. Treatment is recognized as being increasingly effective. Importantly, it is also cost effective, as has been demonstrated in numerous outcome studies.

Most patients with alcohol dependence can abstain from alcohol for short periods and may do so spontaneously without treatment or support. However, 70–80% of patients with established alcohol dependence will relapse within the first year. The prognosis with treatment is better overall; approximately 30–40% are abstinent at 10 years and, in some treatment programmes, rates of 70% are achieved.

Epidemiology

Alcohol is the fifth most important risk factor for the burden of disease and disability in the world, as ranked by World Health Organization's years of life lost from disability. It is the source of great suffering, both to the individual with an alcohol use disorder and those close to them.

Approximately 15% of hospital in-patients have a disorder that is directly related to excess alcohol consumption. A further 15% may drink above recommended limits or have other alcohol related problems. In the family practice setting, up to one in six patients may have evidence of an alcohol use disorder.

Excessive alcohol consumption may cause harm either by its chronic effects on health, including its effects on the liver, or by the acute effects of intoxication, which may be apparent even in the young, infrequent or episodic drinker. Alcohol is associated with up to 80% of suicides and deaths from fire, half of murders, and 30% of fatal road traffic accidents. Alcohol is a common factor in injuries of every type: at home, at work, or on the roads. Because of its disinhibiting effect, it is often involved in crime. In young people there is a linear association between excess alcohol consumption and risk of death, especially from violent causes.

While there is some evidence of specific health benefits from low to moderate drinking in middle aged or older adults, with reports of reduction of ischaemic heart disease, chronic alcohol use above recommended limits is a risk factor for a wide range of conditions. Despite public awareness on the role of alcohol in liver damage, there is less awareness that excessive drinking contributes up to 30% of cases of hypertension. Alcohol is also a risk factor for cancers in various sites and accentuates the risk of liver damage from causes such as obesity and hepatitis C.

Alcohol use disorders can occur across a wide range of cultures, and in any social class and age group. However, those with psychiatric illnesses or who are disadvantaged may be at greater risk. Alcohol use disorders peak in adults in their 20s and 30s, so when complications, chronic disability or death occur, they do so in relatively young people. There are also clear genetic influences on the risk of developing alcohol dependence.

Because of the high prevalence and impact of alcohol use disorders, accurate diagnosis and management of alcohol use disorders, including early stage problems, are an important part of every clinician's work. Failure to diagnose alcohol problems at an early stage leads to delayed diagnosis, unnecessary investigations, inappropriate and ineffective treatment and needless costs.

Pharmacology

Ethyl alcohol or ethanol is water soluble and readily absorbed from the upper small intestine (80%) and to a lesser extent (20%) from the stomach. Peak blood concentrations are reached after 30–60 min. Absorption is delayed by food or drugs which delay gastric emptying.

Alcohol is widely distributed throughout the body. Volume of distribution is roughly equivalent to total body water. As women have a lower proportion of body water and a higher proportion of fat, blood alcohol concentrations are higher in women than in men after ingestion of equivalent amounts of alcohol.

Metabolism is mainly in the liver, but a smaller amount of ethanol is also metabolized in the stomach wall (gastric first pass metabolism). Ethanol is primarily broken down by the enzyme alcohol dehydrogenase to acetaldehyde. This step is rate limiting. Women have 20% lower gastric alcohol dehydrogenase activity than men. A healthy 70 kg person metabolizes approximately one standard drink [10 g ethanol) per hour (approximately 0.015 g% (or 15 mg %) blood alcohol concentration (BAC) per hour).

Acetaldehyde is, in turn, metabolized by aldehyde dehydrogenase to acetate which enters the Krebs cycle, and is ultimately oxidized to carbon dioxide and water (Fig. 4.1). Some individuals, especially those of Japanese and Chinese origin, have a sub-functioning form of the aldehyde dehydrogenase enzyme so experience higher levels of acetaldehyde for any given alcohol intake. This leads to adverse effects (as seen with the disulfiram reaction), including flushing, headaches and nausea after small amounts of alcohol. These individuals have a much lower risk of alcohol dependence.

A CYP2E1 cytochrome P-450 dependent liver microsomal ethanol oxidizing system (MEOS) also metabolizes a smaller amount of ethanol (3–5%) in healthy subjects. This system may be induced in chronic daily drinkers and alcohol-dependent individuals.

As a result of oxidation of alcohol, hydrogen equivalents are produced, which fuel several subsidiary reactions leading to the production of lactic acid, ketone bodies, and neutral fats. Metabolism of alcohol also leads to depletion of glutathione, induction of oxidative stress, and the generation of free radicals, which can damage cell membranes.

A small percentage (2–3%) of alcohol is excreted unchanged in the urine, expired air and sweat. This can be detected in breath, urine or by transdermal alcohol assays.

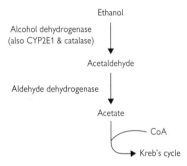

Fig. 4.1 Ethanol conversion.

Pathophysiology

Neurobiology of alcohol intoxication and dependence

Alcohol has strong reinforcing properties and rewarding effects including mild euphoria and anxiolysis. The mesolimbic dopamine 'reward' system in the brain (ventral tegmental area, nucleus accumbens, amygdala, and prefrontal cortex) is involved in this process. Pharmacologically, alcohol is a central nervous system depressant/sedative. These effects are due to potentiation of GABA-A receptor-mediated inhibitory function in the brain and, at higher concentrations, inhibition of glutamatergic N-methyl-D-aspartate (NMDA) excitatory function in the brain. The effects on other neurotransmitters are probably indirectly mediated by changes in these two as they are so widely distributed in the brain.

Other neurotransmitters that have been implicated: The rewarding or positive reinforcing effects of alcohol are also thought to reflect a mixture of mesolimbic dopaminergic function and endogenous opioid release. A relative deficiency of serotonin (5HT) has been reported in young males with early onset alcohol dependence. During withdrawal there is considerable over activity of central and peripheral noradrenaline systems.

Alcohol dependence can develop as a result of chronic excessive ingestion of alcohol. This is associated with several adaptive neurochemical and physiological changes, a process known as 'neuro-adaptation'. With ongoing exposure, the brain attempts to compensate and restore glutamate function by decreasing the number of GABA-A receptors and increasing the number of NMDA receptors, leading to tolerance. Once drinking stops, the relative deficit of GABA-A and excess of NMDA function explains the hyperexcitability of the alcohol withdrawal syndrome. Only patients who are alcohol dependent will experience the withdrawal syndrome.

Alcohol dependent individuals are often magnesium depleted. As magnesium is the brain's natural glutamate antagonist, magnesium depletion in conjunction with the relative over activity of the NMDA system during alcohol withdrawal can increase brain excitability and so predispose to withdrawal seizures. Magnesium deficiency may also impair thiamine utilization.

Pathophysiology of acute complications

Alcohol intoxication causes impaired co-ordination, impaired judgement, slowed reaction time and accordingly is associated with increased risk of injury. The disinhibition associated with intoxication means individuals may take risks they otherwise would not take, for example unprotected sex or drug taking. Some are more likely to become violent. Intoxication may also leave a person vulnerable and less able to protect him or herself, for example from sexual or physical assault.

Pathophysiology of organ damage

Chronic alcohol excess causes damage to multiple organs. These harms are thought to result from a wide variety of mechanisms, as follows:

- Acetaldehyde, (a breakdown product of metabolism of alcohol):
  - Is a highly reactive molecule with potential to cause oxidative harm
  - Can form adducts with proteins, which can then be the subject of an immune attack
  - Can combine with small molecules, including amine neurotransmitters, to produce compounds with brain activity, e.g. salsalinol—that may contribute to dependence and withdrawal.
- Alcohol's effects on membrane permeability. This includes increased absorption of endotoxins from the gastrointestinal tract.
- Alcohol impairs thiamine absorption and utilization; thiamine deficiency may result in a range of neurological and other organ disorders.

The pathophysiology of chronic complications is also discussed briefly where each complication is described.

Further reading

Lingford-Hughes A, Nutt D. Neuropharmacology of ethanol and alcohol dependence. In: Heather N, Peters T, Stockwell T (Eds) *International Handbook of Alcohol Dependence*. Chichester: John Wiley & Sons Ltd., 2001.

Nutt D. Alcohol and the brain: pharmacological insights for psychiatrists. *British Journal of Psychiatry* 1999; **175**(8): 114–119.

The spectrum of use and misuse

What are safe levels of drinking?

Guidelines for drinking limits are typically based on epidemiological data on the levels at which risk of harm begins to increase above the risk levels for non-drinkers or light drinkers.

Excessive drinking on a one-off or regular basis has well documented risks for health However, low to moderate alcohol consumption (for example, up to 1 or 2 drinks per day for a man, and one per day for a woman) has been reported to have some benefits to health in middle aged and older people, in particular in relation to ischaemic heart disease. Clinicians do not generally recommend that abstainers commence drinking because of the concern that a propensity to dependence may be unmasked. It is considered that there are safer ways to reduce the risk of ischaemic heart disease than by alcohol use.

Recommended limits for drinking vary around the world, but there is a general consensus on a low level. Below are some examples, typically expressed in standard drinks or units.

What is a standard drink?

A standard drink or unit is defined differently in different countries. For example, a unit contains 8 g ethanol in the UK; a standard drink is 10 g in Australia and 14 g in the USA. It is therefore important to convert ethanol content to grams when interpreting results from the international literature.

Alcoholic beverages are often served in sizes larger than the 'standard' drink. For example, the standard 'small' glass of wine in the UK is now 175 mL instead of 125 mL, while a unit of 12.5% wine is 80 mL. In addition, home-poured drinks may be 50% (or more) larger than the standard drink size. Heavy drinkers may drink spirits in 200 mL serves (shots), rather than the standard 30-mL nip. Most commonly consumed alcoholic beverages in Australia contain the equivalent of 1.5 Australian standard drinks: e.g. 1 can or 'stubby' of standard beer (375 mL), or a schooner (425 mL), or a restaurant-poured glass of wine (180 mL). In the UK it is possible to buy 500 mL cans of strong (8–9%) lager (beer), each can delivering 4 units of alcohol.

Beverages such as wine have tended to become higher in ethanol content in recent years, so standard drink sizes in some cases have reduced accordingly. For example, in Australia in the 1980s a standard drink of wine was 120 mL, when wine contained 10–11% ethanol (i.e. 10 g ethanol/100 mL beverage). The typical ethanol content has since increased to 12–14%, so a standard drink of wine has reduced to 100 mL, so that it still approximates 10 g ethanol.

Table 4.1 Examples of standard drink sizes from around the world

	Australia	NZ	UK/Ireland	France	Netherlands	USA	Canada
Standard drink (SD) size (in g ethanol)	10 g	10 g	8 g	12 g (for beer), 8 g (for wine)	9.9 g	13 g	13.6 g
Beverage serving size in mL (oz)							
Beer (5%)	285 mL (10 oz)	330 mL can	285 mL (½ pint) 330ml bottle 440ml can	250 mL	300–330 mL (varies)	341 mL (12 oz)	341 mL (12 oz)
Wine (12%)	100 mL (4 oz)	100 mL	175 mL standard glass (7 oz)	125 mL	125 mL	142 mL (5 oz)	142 mL (5 oz)
Fortified wine (25–26%)	60 mL (2 oz)	Not described	One standard measure: 50 mL	70 mL	Not described	Not described	Not described
Spirits (38–40%)	30 mL (1 oz)	30 mL	One small standard measure: 25 mL Large measure: 35 mL	25 mL	Not described	43 mL (1.5 oz)	43 mL (1.5 oz)

Super strength lager available in UK (9+%)

Table 4.2 Examples of recommended drinking limits from around the world (g/ethanol)

Recommended limits for	Australia	NZ	UK/Ireland	France	Netherlands	USA	Canada
Adult male							
Per day (regular)	40 g	30 g	24–32 g; not regularly more than 3–4 units per day	20–60 g	40 g	14–28 g	27.2 g
Per week (p.w.)	2 alcohol-free days, i.e. max 200 g p.w.; Max 60 g per occasion	Some alcohol-free days, max 210 g p.w. Max 60 g per occasion	Max 168 g/week (UK) Max 210 g/week (Ireland)	No weekly limits given	2 alcohol-free days p.w. No weekly maximum given	Max 196 g p.w. (14 units)	Max 190 g p.w. (14 units)
Adult female							
Per day (regular)	20 g	20 g	16–24 g; not regularly more than 2–3 units per day	20–30 g	20 g Women with low body weight should drink less	14 g (~1 unit)	17.5 g (1.25 units)
Per week	2 alcohol free days, i.e. 100 g p.w. Max 40 g per occasion	Some alcohol-free days; max 140 g p.w. Max 40 g per occasion	Max 112 g (UK) 140 g (Ireland)	No weekly limits given	2 alcohol-free days p.w. No weekly max given	98 g (7 units)	Max 116 g (9 units)

Table 4.2 (Contd.)

Recommended limits for	Australia*	NZ	UK/Ireland	France	Netherlands	USA/Canada
Pregnant women	Abstinence is safest; max 10 g per day	No alcohol at all	Avoid alcohol altogether. Never more than 1 or 2 units per week if pregnant or trying to conceive	No alcohol at all	No alcohol at all	No alcohol if pregnant, planning to be, or breast feeding
Risky situations (e.g. driving, operating machinery))	Avoid alcohol	Restrict or avoid alcohol when operating machinery or on the water	Not stated	No alcohol at all	No alcohol at all	Avoid alcohol when driving, using machinery, taking medications, etc.
Source of recommendation	National Health and Medical Research Council, 2001	Alcohol Liquor Advisory Council (ALAC)	Department of Health www.dh.gov.uk/ publication 277506/ How much is too much: adults	1. Ministry of Health, Youth & Sports 2. National Academy of Medicine	Sundhedsstyrelsen [National Board of Health (NBH)]	Centre for Addiction & Mental Health Dept of Agriculture & Dept of Health & Human Services

Note: the recommendations above have been expressed in g ethanol, to facilitate international comparison.
* At the time of writing, Australian consumption guidelines are under review.

Core clinical syndromes

Intoxication

The effects of alcohol depend on the level of tolerance in the drinker. At low BACs alcohol causes euphoria and has a disinhibiting effect. At higher levels it impairs co-ordination and at BACs above 0.2 g% it can depress the level of consciousness. In the non-tolerant drinker, BACs above 0.3 g% are associated with risk of death from respiratory depression (Table 4.3).

Table 4.3 Levels of impairment in non-tolerant drinkers by blood ethanol concentration

Signs and symptoms of intoxication	BAC in novice drinkers		
	mmol/L*	mg/100 mL	g%*
Euphoria, disinhibition, garrulousness, impaired attention, impaired judgement	6.5	30	0.03
Increased risk of accidents, injuries, violence	10.9	50	0.05
Dysarthria, ataxia, confusion, disorientation 0.15	32.6	150	0.15
Increased risk of falls, fractures			
Altered state of consciousness, stupor, blackouts	43.5	200	0.20
Inhalation of vomitus, asphyxiation, coma, death	65.2– 108.7	300– 500	0.30– 0.50

* 1 g% = 1 g/100 mL. 1 mmol/L = (1 mg/100 mL)/4.6 = (1 g% * 1000)/4.6.

Non-dependent alcohol use disorders

Hazardous alcohol use

An individual who regularly drinks above recommended limits, but has not yet experienced any harms from drinking, is described as a hazardous drinker.

Harmful alcohol use

A person who is already experiencing physical or psychological harms because of their drinking, but is not dependent on alcohol (or 'addicted') is described as a harmful drinker.

Alcohol abuse

Alcohol abuse occurs when a person's drinking is causing repeated social harms to that individual and/or to others, e.g. drink-driving, relationship problems, failing to fulfil important obligations, or when they are repeatedly drinking in situations that place them at risk physically

NB: A person with alcohol abuse may also experience physical harms from drinking and so be a harmful drinker. Abuse is a DSM term, while harmful drinking is an ICD term (see Fig. 4.2).

> The diagnostic terms of abuse and dependence are mutually exclusive when referring to the same time period.

Alcohol dependence

Alcohol dependence is the clinical term used to describe a person who has become 'addicted' to alcohol. The colloquial term 'alcoholism' is typically used by the public to refer to someone with severe alcohol dependence, and is still used in the name of the self-help group Alcoholics Anonymous.

Alcohol dependence represents a cluster of psychological, behavioural and cognitive syndromes fuelled by an inner drive to a repetitive pattern of drinking of alcohol. It develops over many months or years, and if untreated usually shows a progressive or chronic relapsing course.

Establishing whether a person is dependent or not on alcohol is clinically very important, as it determines the goal and methods of treatment.

Dependent drinkers have typically lost control of their drinking, may experience withdrawal symptoms on cessation of intake and should aim for a goal of abstinence. They will usually need support and treatment to achieve this goal. Individuals with alcohol abuse or hazardous/harmful drinking, on the other hand, will often able to cut down on their drinking with less support or treatment, some even requiring only a 'brief intervention'.

A diagnosis of current alcohol dependence is made if three or more of the following symptoms have occurred repeatedly within the past year (Table 4.4).

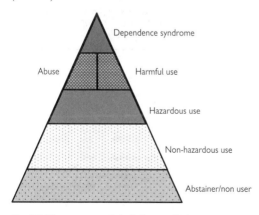

Fig. 4.2 The spectrum of alcohol use and misuse.

Table 4.4 Criteria for a diagnosis of alcohol dependence

Features common to both sets of criteria	ICD-10	DSM-IV
Impaired control	Subjective awareness of an impaired capacity to control drinking	Drinking larger amounts or longer than intended
Craving/compulsion	Awareness of a strong desire or sense of compulsion to drink/craving	Persistent desire or unsuccessful attempts to cut down
Drinking 'taking over' life	Preoccupation with drinking to the neglect of other responsibilities or interests	Much time spent seeking alcohol, drinking, or getting over alcohol's effects
		Important social or work activities reduced or given up
Tolerance	Tolerance—increased amounts of alcohol are required in order to achieve the desired effects	Increased drinking to achieve the same effect
Withdrawal or withdrawal relief	Withdrawal symptoms on cessation or reduction of alcohol intake; or using alcohol to relieve or prevent these	Withdrawal signs or symptoms, or drinking to relieve or prevent these
Persistent use despite harm	Persistence of alcohol use despite clear evidence of overtly harmful consequences	Use despite physical or psychological consequences

'Alcohol use disorders' is used as a summary term to include hazardous/harmful drinking, abuse or dependence on alcohol.

All of the above diagnoses can be current, i.e. the last 12 months, or past.

Further reading

American Psychiatric Association. Diagnostic and Statistical Manual of Mental Disorders, 4th edn. (DSM-IV-TR). Washington, DC: American Psychiatric Association, 2000.

World Health Organization. The ICD-10 classification of mental and behavioural disorders. Clinical descriptions and diagnostic guidelines. Geneva: World Health Organization, 1992. Available online at: http://www.who.int/substance_abuse/terminology/ICD10ClinicalDiagnosis.pdf

See Chapter V, the subsection entitled 'Mental and behavioural disorders due to psychoactive substance use'.

The alcohol withdrawal syndrome

The alcohol withdrawal syndrome is a cluster of symptoms involving central nervous system hyperactivity, which occurs when an alcohol-dependent person ceases to drink or markedly reduces their level of consumption. Not all dependent drinkers experience physical withdrawal symptoms and, when present, withdrawals may range in severity from mild to severe, mirroring the severity of alcohol dependence.

Simple alcohol withdrawal is typically self-limited, involving overnight insomnia and morning 'edginess', which lasts until the first drink of the day. In more severe cases, symptoms may increase in severity over the next 48–72 h, and include anxiety, tremor, sweating, tachycardia, increased temperature, and pulse. In the most severe cases, withdrawal symptoms progress to delirium (delirium tremens), a life-threatening illness if not identified and treated early (see diagnosis and management of withdrawal syndrome, p. 110–118).

Complications of alcohol use

The complications of drinking may result from acute intoxication or chronic excessive drinking. Alcohol affects almost every system of the body and risk of chronic alcohol-related organ damage increases with increasing levels of alcohol intake and with duration of drinking, particularly when drinking has continued for 5 years or more.

Acute complications

Complications of acute intoxication may be medical, neuropsychiatric, or social.

Medical

- **Coma and respiratory depression**: alcohol intoxication is a potentially lethal condition because of the risk of respiratory depression in non-tolerant drinkers. Many young people in particular present to the Emergency department with an acute 'overdose' of alcohol or 'alcohol poisoning'
- **Drug overdose**: the risk of respiratory depression is increased if alcohol and other CNS depressants such as benzodiazepines or opioids are taken at the same time, either accidentally or intentionally in a suicide attempt
- **Aspiration pneumonia** may complicate severe intoxication
- **Trauma**: Intoxication predisposes to accidents particularly in episodic heavy drinkers, e.g. motor vehicle accidents, acts of violence, falls and fractures (ribs/long bones). Subdural haematoma may occur after head injury
- **Burns**
- **Drowning**
- **Sexual risk-taking**, and consequent risk of HIV and other sexually transmitted infections and unwanted pregnancy
- **Upper gastro-intestinal bleeding** from gastritis, oesophagitis, Mallory Weiss tear or when alcohol is taken in conjunction with NSAIDs
- **Acute pancreatitis**—(p. 82)
- **Atrial fibrillation** (p. 83) may be induced by an acute excessive consumption of alcohol during an acute alcoholic binge in an otherwise healthy heart—the 'holiday heart' syndrome. Alcohol is a common cause of atrial fibrillation in persons under the age of 65 who are otherwise healthy.

Neuropsychiatric

- **Confusion and disorientation** occur at a BAC of around 0.15 g% in healthy, non-tolerant drinkers, but can occur at relatively low BACs in vulnerable individuals, such as the elderly.
- **Amnesic episodes** (alcohol induced blackouts; memory blackouts):
  - A period of anterograde amnesia during heavy drinking. These occur when a high blood alcohol interferes with the acquisition and storage of new memories (i.e. the person cannot remember what they did after the onset of severe intoxication)

- The person may appear intoxicated, but there are no observable cognitive abnormalities; they may find him/herself in unknown surroundings on recovery
- Realization of amnesic episode occurs on recovery
- **Acute nerve pressure palsies**, especially of the brachial plexus ('Saturday night palsy')
- **Suicide attempts**: because of its disinhibiting effect, and its effect on mood (depression), alcohol is commonly associated with suicide attempts.
- *Wernicke's encephalopathy* (p. 84).

Social

Acute intoxication can cause a range of social problems often arising from disinhibited behaviour or from short-term neglect of alternative responsibilities. Alcohol intoxication may trigger gambling or impair judgement as to when to stop. Gambling losses in turn may trigger drinking (see problems described under chronic social problems, p. 88).

Chronic complications

Medical complications

Alcohol has the capacity to cause widespread damage, affecting almost every system of the body.

Alcoholic liver disease

Alcohol remains a prominent cause of liver disease in many developed countries and it is one of the commonest causes of morbidity and mortality from liver disease in the world. Alcoholic hepatitis and alcoholic cirrhosis occur in a significant minority of heavy drinkers. Alcohol is also an important aggravating factor in other liver disorders including hepatitis C, B, haemochromatosis. It is important to remember that regular users of illicit injectable drugs may also be consuming excess alcohol. Alcohol also exacerbates the course of obesity-related liver damage.

The clinical presentations of alcohol related liver disease include:

- **Alcohol-related fatty liver**: most people consuming alcohol at hazardous levels develop a degree of hepatic steatosis, a metabolic consequence of regular alcohol ingestion. This is usually a reversible and relatively benign condition, but may progress to fibrosis without passing through the phase of classical alcoholic hepatitis. Abstinence or marked reduction in alcohol intake will result in a reversal of fatty liver. However, if an inflammatory response has been invoked (evidenced by an elevation of AST and ALT), fatty liver may not always subside with abstinence.
- **Alcoholic hepatitis**: alcoholic hepatitis is a serious form of alcohol-related liver disease, formerly associated with a mortality of 30–50%. Nowadays, with hospital admission and active treatment, mortality rates are low. These individuals typically present with jaundice, fever and pain in the right hypochondrium. Occasionally, patients will present with signs of marked liver impairment, bruising and signs of liver failure. Severely ill patients may develop liver failure with the attendant risks of bleeding varices and the hepatorenal syndrome. Only 20–25% of heavy drinkers develop alcoholic hepatitis and consequent cirrhosis.

- **Alcohol-related cirrhosis**: this form of cirrhosis remains one of the most common in the developed world. It evolves from alcoholic hepatitis in most cases, but occasionally from alcohol-related fatty liver. Because many patients have bouts of heavy drinking and flares of acute inflammatory alcohol-related disease, this condition is characterized histologically by micro and macro nodules, fatty change and as it evolves, peri-cellular and peri-central fibrosis is a classical feature. Once established, alcohol-related cirrhosis is largely irreversible and is a predisposing factor for the development of liver cell carcinoma.

Pathogenesis of alcohol related liver injury: Only a minority of heavy drinkers progress to alcoholic hepatitis and cirrhosis. Genetic factors may determine a predisposition to alcohol-related liver disease of the more severe types. Alcohol-related liver disease is due to a number of factors including alcohol toxicity, nutritional deficiencies and immune mechanisms. Alcohol metabolism generates a degree of oxidative stress with its attendant potential for injury, but it also initiates cytokine release which contributes to injury. Immunological factors play a role in the evolution of liver injury in alcohol consumers, as do increased release of endotoxins from the gut.

Alcohol's effect on other liver diseases: Alcohol-induced liver disease can co-exist with other forms of liver disease and the presence of one exacerbates the course of the other.

Injecting drug users are at increased risk of contracting hepatitis C, B, and D, and they also are at risk of direct drug-related hepatotoxicity. Alcohol consumed at hazardous levels will increase the rate of progression of liver disease in patients with hepatitis C and hepatitis B. Alcohol appears to encourage hepatitis C viral replication, as well as causing additive harm.

Similarly, alcohol use disorders, which in their own right contribute to increased iron absorption and deposition, also appear to increase the rate of fibrosis development in patients with genetically determined iron storage disease (haemochromatosis). Conversely, excessive iron appears to increase the level of fibrosis in patients with alcoholic liver disease.

Other gastrointestinal disease

- Glossitis, angular stomatitis
- Gastro-oesophageal reflux disease
- Oesophagitis/gastritis with mucosal erosions and bleeding secondary to binge drinking. Alcohol causes back diffusion of hydrochloric acid through the gastric mucosa.
- Mallory Weiss tear—upper gastrointestinal bleeding in a setting of repeated vomiting
- Oesophageal varices, with risk of bleeding, in the presence of cirrhosis
- Alcohol is a risk factor for *H. pylori* infection and for peptic ulcer disease. It also increases the risk of perforation or haemorrhage from peptic ulcer.
- Small bowel dysfunction resulting in diarrhoea and malabsorption
- Gastrointestinal cancer—chronic excess alcohol consumption is a risk factor for carcinoma of the oropharynx, oesophagus, and colorectum.

Acute pancreatitis: Alcohol is a risk factor in 20% of cases. Alcoholic pancreatitis typically presents with severe alcohol epigastric or upper abdominal pain within 12–24 h after heavy drinking. The pain radiates to the back and is relieved by sitting forward. Nausea and vomiting may progress to fluid loss, hypotension, shock, renal failure or respiratory failure. There is a 10–15% mortality rate if not diagnosed and appropriately treated.

Chronic pancreatitis: Mainly occurs after persistent consumption of excess alcohol for more than 10 years. It is characterized by chronic epigastric or upper abdominal pain following intake of alcohol. The pain radiates to the back and is relieved by leaning forward. May be associated with weight loss, malabsorption, steatorrhoea, diarrhoea and diabetes mellitus.

Cardiovascular disease

- **Hypertension**: up to 30% cases of 'essential' hypertension may be related to alcohol excess. Alcohol is also an important cause of morbidity and mortality by predisposing to cerebrovascular accidents. Hypertension does not respond to antihypertensive agents if the patient continues to drink excessively, but generally improves on abstinence or when alcohol consumption is substantially reduced. Hypertension also occurs during acute alcohol withdrawal.
- **Tachyarrhythmias**: supraventricular and ventricular arrhythmias; atrial fibrillation in 'holiday heart syndrome'
- **Cardiomyopathy**: dilated cardiomyopathy is typically seen in middle-aged men who have been drinking alcohol in excess of 80 g/day for a decade or more. Patients present with gradual onset of heart failure with breathlessness on exertion, nocturnal dyspnoea, pulmonary, and peripheral oedema. Atrial fibrillation is common. There is a high incidence of thrombus formation in the chambers and up to 40% of patients will experience systemic embolism within 3 years. Patients may also be jaundiced with hepatomegaly and ascites. With continued heavy drinking 80% are dead within 3 years, so abstinence from alcohol is crucial
- **Beri Beri**: high output cardiac failure with oedema (wet beri beri) or neuropathy (dry beri beri) due to thiamine deficiency
- **Reported *cardioprotective effects*:** while heavy drinking has deleterious effects on the cardiovascular system, drinking at low levels has been reported to protect against ischaemic heart disease in middle-aged men and post-menopausal women. The protective effect of alcohol is thought to be due to increased HDL cholesterol, inhibition of thromboxane and platelet aggregation, and enhancement of clot lysis.

Haematological disorders

- **Anaemia**: associated with gastro-intestinal blood loss
- **Macrocytosis**: due to a direct toxic effect of alcohol on bone marrow, seen in up to 50% of alcohol-dependent individuals. Up to one-third have co-existing folic acid deficiency due to impaired absorption of folate from the small intestine
- **Thrombocytopaenia**: due to a direct toxic effect of alcohol on the bone marrow, decreased platelet survival time, and aggravated by cirrhosis (including reduced thrombopoetin production) and hypersplenism. May be an early warning of advancing liver disease.

Musculoskeletal disorders

- **Acute myopathy**: pain, swelling and tenderness of skeletal muscles
- **Acute rhabdomyolysis**: after a prolonged period of immobility is associated with myoglobinuria and may lead to acute renal failure if not diagnosed. Increased CPK levels may be noted

- **Chronic myopathy**: associated with weakness and wasting of skeletal muscles, especially proximal muscles. It improves with abstinence, but in some cases recovery is slow and incomplete
- **Osteoporosis**: affecting the spine, may result in wedge fractures and back pain and risk of dependence on opioid drugs
- **Avascular necrosis** of the hip
- **Gout** caused by accumulation of uric acid.

Respiratory disease

- **Aspiration pneumonia**
- **Pulmonary infections**: lobar pneumonia, lung abscess, tuberculosis. Alcohol depresses T-cell function; associated smoking is common, there may also be poor nutrition
- **Obstructive sleep apnoea**.

CNS and neuropsychiatric complications

- **Wernicke's encephalopathy**: Is an acute reversible neuropsychiatric condition, which presents in alcohol-dependent individuals due to acute deficiency of thiamine. It is most common in single, elderly and malnourished individuals and those with malabsorption or repeated vomiting and diarrhoea. Thiamine deficiency is due to low thiamine intake, impaired thiamine absorption and impaired thiamine utilization. Thiamine is an essential co-factor for many enzymes in the glycolytic and pentose phosphate pathways. Thiamine deficiency may be precipitated by a carbohydrate load, prolonged vomiting or upper gastrointestinal disease. Wernicke's encephalopathy represents a medical emergency with an estimated mortality of 10–20%.

  Acute Wernicke's encephalopathy is characterized by the classical triad of cerebellar ataxia, ocular abnormalities (nystagmus, ophthalmoplegia—commonly external recti, manifested as diplopia) and a global confusional state (disorientation, inattention, poor responsiveness). However, more often the full triad of symptoms is not present. Patients may present with nausea, vomiting and confusion, and rarely, hypothermia, hypotension and coma may be present. The diagnosis is frequently missed. Neuropathological studies show that Wernicke's pathology is present in 12.5% of those who misuse alcohol, and often has not been diagnosed *in vivo*. The pathology is 20 times more common than the classical triad.

  Wernicke's encephalopathy is less common than it used to be, because of thiamine supplementation of bread, but still occurs in malnourished alcohol-dependent patients given a carbohydrate load without pretreatment with thiamine.

  Most patients who do not recover promptly within the first 48–72 h will develop Korsakoff's syndrome. Prompt treatment with adequate doses of parenteral thiamine is vital (p. 119).

- **Korsakoff's syndrome**: The sequel to untreated or inadequately treated Wernicke's encephalopathy with resulting structural changes in the brain (in the area of the hippocampus, mamillary bodies, mamillo-thalamic tract and thalamus). Korsakoff's syndrome is a largely irreversible condition characterized by short-term memory loss, decreased learning ability, and compensatory confabulation. Cued recall is better than spontaneous recall. Long-term memory is typically preserved. In some individuals there will be overlapping features of Korsakoff's and cortical pathology (with cortical atrophy and ventricular dilation, especially involving the frontal lobes).

- **Alcohol withdrawal seizures**: alcohol withdrawal also reduces the seizure threshold in epilepsy (see alcohol withdrawal seizures, p. 117).
- **Strokes**: excess alcohol, especially episodic heavy drinking or binge drinking, is a risk factor for haemorrhagic strokes
- **Subdural haematoma**: secondary to head injury, particularly if there is co-existing thrombocytopenia. May be overlooked if the patient is intoxicated
- **Cerebellar degeneration**: typically affects the vermis leading to truncal ataxia, dysarthria, uncoordinated movements, frequent falls
- **'Reversible alcoholic cognitive deterioration'**: This term has been used to refer to those cognitive impairments which are mild to moderate and tend to resolve with abstinence
- **Cerebrocortical degeneration/cortical atrophy**: can be seen on CT of the brain. Abstinence will arrest the progression of alcoholic dementia and may lead to gradual improvement in some neuropsychiatric functions and brain scan results.
- **Frontal lobe syndrome**: commonly caused by heavy episodic drinking and characterized by disinhibition, defective conceptualization and abstract thinking, impaired organization and strategic planning, concreteness in thought, personality change and, in advanced cases, perseveration and long tract signs. Diminution of critical insight leads to further reduction in control over drinking and perpetuation of the drinking problem. Intelligence and verbal skills may remain intact until very late. Late features include serious intellectual impairment, memory impairment and marked loss of judgement. There is no evidence of benefit from specific therapies, but abstinence from alcohol, thiamine supplements, an adequate diet, and a structured environment may be helpful
- **Alcoholic dementia**: 50–70% of severe chronic heavy drinkers show evidence of ventricular dilatation, cortical shrinkage, or both on neuroimaging. Alcoholic dementia typically presents as a presenile dementia in a patient with a history of heavy drinking, personality change, and memory deterioration. Examination reveals global impairment of all mental functions. Involvement of the frontal lobes is particularly common with or without dementia, and may result in affective changes (apathy, euphoria or emotional lability), impaired judgement, and poor appreciation of social cues
- **Central pontine myelinolysis**: a rare demyelinating disease of the pons seen in alcohol-dependent patients following rapid correction of hyponatraemia. Patients present with quadriplegia and pseudobulbar palsy
- **Peripheral neuropathy**: with glove and stocking tingling and numbness, sensory impairment and absent ankle jerks. Hypersensitivity of soles of feet may be an early sign. Some recovery may occur with lengthy abstinence (over 1 year).

Nutritional disturbances
- **Protein-calorie malnutrition**
- **Vitamin deficiencies**: a range of vitamin deficiencies may occur due to dietary deficiency, impaired absorption and/or utilization:

- Thiamine deficiency: an important cause of Wernicke's encephalopathy and Beri beri (see above)
- Other vitamin deficiencies:
  — Folate
  — Niacin deficiency (Pellagra)
  — Vitamin C deficiency
  — Impaired fat absorption, with associated impairment of absorption of fat soluble vitamins: for example, Vitamin A (night blindness) and D (osteoporosis)
  — Deficiencies of Vitamins A, C, D, E, K, and the B vitamins, may result in reduced wound healing
- **Mineral deficiencies**: deficiencies may occur due to a range of factors, lower consumption, impaired absorption, increased excretion, or deficiency of other nutrients:
  — Magnesium. Reduced magnesium levels may lower seizure threshold. Some clinical features of magnesium deficiency such as tremor, confusion, agitation, hallucinations and seizures may resemble acute alcohol withdrawal. Magnesium deficiency may also impair thiamine utilization
  — Zinc (night-blindness, skin lesions).

Metabolic disorders
- **Hyperlipidaemia:** although moderate consumption increases HDL-cholesterol, heavy drinking leads to low density lipoprotein (LDL) hypercholesterolaemia and hyperlipidaemia
- **Hyperuricaemia:** gout
- **Hypoglycaemia**: may be induced by a single large dose of alcohol on an empty stomach. Elevated NADH to NAD ratio by metabolism of alcohol impairs gluconeogenesis and may deplete liver glycogen
- **Hyperglycaemia:** repeated heavy drinking can also lead to increased insulin resistance, which is reversible (in contrast low level drinking may improve insulin sensitivity); diabetes may be a consequence of pancreatic damage
- **Alcoholic ketoacidosis**: this follows a heavy drinking bout typically with reduced food intake and dehydration. There is elevated beta hydroxybutyric acid and lactic acid, and a large anion gap.
- **Lactic acidosis**: particularly in diabetic patients on biguanides
- **Porphyria**: alcohol may precipitate acute intermittent porphyria.

Endocrine disorders
- **Gonadal atrophy**: affects both sexes resulting in subfertility and reduced spermatogenesis in men
- **Pseudo-Cushings syndrome**: caused by excessive glucocorticoid production. Distinguished from true Cushings by being transient, resolving with abstinence, and by more ready suppression of cortisol levels by dexamethasone.

Cutaneous disorders
- **Porphyria cutanea tarda**: photosensitivity—alcohol causes abnormal porphyrin metabolism in genetically predisposed individuals
- **Psoriasis**: alcohol exacerbates psoriasis

- **Discoid eczema** (especially on the palms of the hands and the soles of the feet)
- **Cutaneous infections**: particularly fungal infections, due to reduced T cell function and sometimes reduced self-care.

Malignancies

An increased rate of malignancies in a variety of organs, including oro-pharynx, larynx, oesophagus, colon, rectum, breast, and liver.

Infections

- Alcohol may increase risk of infections due to concomitant nutritional deficiency and reduced T cell function
- Due to its disinhibiting effect, alcohol increases high risk behaviour, and is a risk factor for HIV and other sexually transmitted infections.

Foetal alcohol spectrum disorders

Now recognized as one of the two commonest causes of mental retardation in the developed world. The mean IQ of affected children is 70. Children with the full foetal alcohol syndrome have characteristic face with depressed bridge of the nose, thinning of the upper lip and absent philtrum, and low-set ears. Cardiac abnormalities and behavioural disturbances are common. Lesser grades of presentation also occur (see 'Drugs in pregnancy section', p. 316).

The risk is greatest in the first trimester of pregnancy, often before the woman knows she is pregnant; hence, women of childbearing age should greatly restrict their drinking if they are likely to become pregnant. It follows that young women who drink heavily, even episodically, should be on reliable contraception that does not rely on a regular daily routine, e.g. implant or intrauterine device.

There are no internationally agreed safe limits for drinking in pregnancy. Many countries recommend total abstinence.

Psychiatric complications/co-morbidity

Anxiety: Symptoms of uncomplicated alcohol withdrawal can mimic anxiety and panic disorder. Within hours of the blood alcohol level dropping, the individual may feel anxious and agitated, with a range of symptoms due to over-activity of the autonomic nervous system, which can mimic an anxiety attack. These symptoms include tachycardia, high blood pressure, sweating, tremor, insomnia, anorexia, nausea, and vomiting. Symptoms usually begin within hours of the last drink, peak on day 2 or 3, and subside within 5 days.

Once detoxification from alcohol is completed, many individuals will experience a protracted post-withdrawal phase. This may last for some months, and symptoms may resemble an anxiety disorder with irritability, restlessness, dysphoria, insomnia, hyperventilation and distractibility. Almost any form of anxiety can occur for 3–12 months following cessation of drinking, including generalized anxiety, panic attacks and social anxiety. These symptoms typically abate or reduce over time without treatment. However, a small number of patients will have a history of an anxiety disorder preceding heavy drinking, and this may need specific treatment.

Anxiety disorders are a common reason for excessive and inappropriate alcohol intake. It has been estimated that up to a quarter of young men with alcohol dependence have untreated social anxiety disorder. Likewise many individuals with PTSD turn to alcohol to help them sleep, dull flashbacks, and obliterate memory of the traumatic event. In these individuals alcohol withdrawal often worsens symptoms so a cyclical pattern of worsening of both disorders ensues.

Depression: With prolonged heavy drinking, around to 80% of individuals will develop depressive symptoms, and around 30–40% of individuals will have symptoms resembling a major depressive episode. In most cases depressive symptoms improve significantly during the first few weeks of abstinence, even without antidepressant medication.

Alcohol withdrawal hallucinosis: Withdrawal hallucinosis, usually visual or tactile, occurs in around 25% of people with alcohol dependence. It is more common in the first 48 h after cessation of alcohol, but can occur up to days 4 or 5. It may occur without other preceding withdrawal symptoms and is often intermittent and self-limiting. Distinct from delirium tremens, it occurs in a state of clear consciousness and the sufferer may have insight about the perceptual disturbance.

Alcoholic hallucinosis and alcoholic paranoia: Both of these are variants of alcohol-induced psychotic disorder (DSM-IV). Chronic ingestion of alcohol can cause suspiciousness which can develop into paranoid delusions ('alcoholic paranoia'). Alcohol can also cause persistent hallucinations ('alcoholic hallucinosis'). These are usually auditory, and may consist of unformed noises or snatches of music, but typically take the form of voices (single or multiple). At times the hallucinations can be visual or tactile. They may be accompanied by misidentification, delusions, ideas of reference and an abnormal affect, and resemble acute paranoid schizophrenia.

Both disorders can develop during a drinking bout, during alcohol withdrawal, or can occur within several weeks of the cessation of drinking. They occur in a state of clear consciousness.

Other addictive behaviours: Patients with alcohol use disorders may also exhibit other substance use disorders and/or pathological gambling. These behaviours may be triggered by intoxication or may compromise co-morbid disorders.

Social complications

Alcohol can cause or exacerbate a wide range of social problems. These can affect:

Family: reduced sexual functioning, relationship problems, family and marital problems, domestic violence, separation, divorce, loss of friends. The alcohol-dependent patient often becomes moody, unpredictable, withdrawn, and isolated from family and friends. The family and children around the dependent drinker may be exposed to severe stress, and in some cases neglect, violence, or abuse.

Occupation: absenteeism, poor work performance, lack of career advancement, industrial accidents, frequent changes of employment, early retirement, unemployment.

Financial status: unemployment and expenditure on alcohol lead to failure to pay bills, borrowing money, and going into debt. Impulsive gambling while intoxicated may precipitate or exacerbate financial problems.

Legal problems: drink-driving offences, motor vehicle accidents, loss of driver's licence; physical or sexual assault (the drinker can be victim or perpetrator), including assault on children, and homicide.

Natural history of alcohol use disorders

In countries where drinking is prevalent, alcohol consumption typically starts in the teenage years. Episodic consumption is a common pattern and this has become increasingly heavy in the late teenage years in many countries. In the mid-20s the quantity consumed per occasion typically starts to diminish and the frequency of drinking may increase. Approximately 15–20% of adults consume alcohol in a risky way. Of these, around one-third progress to alcohol dependence, with most of the others reducing their consumption to low risk levels by their 30s.

Approximately 5% of the population have alcohol dependence. Without treatment, alcohol dependence shows a strong tendency to progress. During relapse, following periods of abstinence, there is rapid reinstatement to the previous levels of drinking and dependence ('back where they started').

Alcohol dependent individuals rarely manage to reduce their alcohol consumption to low levels (about 5% in the community and extremely rare in treatment populations).

When individuals with untreated alcohol dependence were followed over 10 years, 30% achieved stable abstinence, 40% continued to drink heavily, and 30% had a progressive downhill course and died within this period. Among persons with alcohol dependence attending comprehensive public sector treatment programmes, the prognosis is improved, with 45% achieving long-term abstinence, some with intermittent relapses; 35% showing a less favourable course with periods of abstinence interspersed with periods of heavy drinking, while 20% showing a progressive downhill course which appears unresponsive to treatment. It should be noted that no long-term follow-up figures are yet available for modern treatments that include pharmacotherapies for alcohol dependence, but early outcome figures suggest these are likely to be improved. Among private sector facilities, higher rates of recovery over 10 years (50–80%) are claimed, although in some cases evaluation has not been rigorous.

In those unable to achieve long-term abstinence, alcohol dependence typically follows a chronic relapsing course. Maintaining long-term abstinence is very challenging. A variety of forms of treatment has demonstrated short- to medium-term success, and many drinkers report great assistance from mutual aid programmes, such as AA. Treatment is associated with a reduction in alcohol-related problems in 60% of dependent drinkers.

The highest risk of relapse occurs in the first 3 months after cessation of drinking, with the risk reducing thereafter for up to a year. Without pharmacotherapy, the majority (70–80%) relapse within the first year. The use of pharmacotherapy is associated with a reduced risk of relapse, but this may, nevertheless, still be as high as 60% despite strong motivation. It should be noted that any remission provides the individual with physical and psychological relief from drinking, and provides relief to family, friends and supporters.

The presence of complications of alcohol use, for example, alcohol-related liver disease can impact significantly on ongoing drinking, and can greatly shorten the life span (see specific complications). For example, alcohol cirrhosis has a mortality rate of 50% at 5 years (comprising 70% of those who continue to drink heavily and 20% of those who abstain). Likewise, of those with alcohol cardiomyopathy, 60% die within 3 years. Alcohol dependence complicated by depression, psychosis or suicidal behaviour also has a worse prognosis. The risk of suicide is 50 times greater in alcohol-dependent people compared with the general population. Other common causes of death are motor vehicle accidents, accidental injury, drowning and homicide.

Identification and brief intervention for (non-dependent) hazardous or harmful drinking

Brief intervention is a pro-active approach to detecting and intervening in hazardous or harmful drinkers. It is typically delivered when the drinking problem has been detected opportunistically, for instance in the primary care setting. A brief intervention involves the offering of structured advice to cut-down on alcohol intake, and is typically given over 5–20 min.

Why a brief intervention?

Although 15–30% of patients seen in general practice or the general hospital setting have an underlying alcohol use disorder, less than one-third of these are diagnosed. The earlier the diagnosis is made and intervention offered, the better the prognosis. Identification of hazardous or harmful drinking (at risk drinking) should be an active process, as drinkers are not likely to divulge this information spontaneously. Problem drinkers do not tend to seek help until they have advanced dependence and often associated complications. At a minimum each patient should be asked one question about drinking and this should give an idea of the quantity consumed.

'How often do you drink more than six standard drinks on one occasion?' (or four standard drinks for a woman), will allow identification of both regular and episodic excess drinkers (sometimes known as 'binge drinkers').

Where possible, three simple questions should be asked:
• 'How many (standard) drinks do you have on a day when you are drinking?'
• 'How often do you have a drink containing alcohol?'
• 'How often do you have 6 (4) or more standard drinks on one occasion?'
In many societies, heavy drinking is largely confined to Friday or Saturday nights, and drinking may be lighter on other days. Questions can be adapted to the clinician's own style and to the circumstances. An alternative to the third question is 'How much do you drink if you are going out, or on special occasions?'

Terms such as 'social drinker' or 'occasional drinker' should be avoided in the recorded history, as they do not provide useful information. Different people use these terms differently, e.g. for some patients 'social drinker' means they don't consider themselves a 'closet alcoholic'.

Similarly patients (and health professionals) use the term 'binge' differently. Some drinkers use it to describe a period of relapse in alcohol dependence, whereas others use it to describe a short period of drinking heavily (e.g. 1–3 days, which may occur in a non-dependent drinker).

Screening tools

A wide variety of brief screening questionnaires is available, that can be used to screen for alcohol use disorders (dependent or non-dependent), and some also assess the severity of a particular disorder. These can be as short as 1–3 questions, and may be used as part of the routine admission paperwork for hospital in-patients, to screen all new family practice patients before seeing the doctor, or can be incorporated into the routine clinical interview.

Laboratory tests help in screening for alcohol problems, but in most populations are far less sensitive than self-report of alcohol use. For example, GGT, the most sensitive of the traditional blood tests for alcohol use detects only around 30% of those drinking 60 g ethanol or more daily in a community setting, while the 10-item AUDIT questionnaire detects around 75%. Shorter versions of the AUDIT such as the 3-item AUDIT-C have been found to detect only slightly fewer cases than the full questionnaire. A range of other brief screening questionnaires have been developed e.g. the TWEAK which is a variant of the original CAGE questionnaire. Some validated examples are included in Appendix, p. 416.

Effectiveness of brief interventions

Brief structured advice or counselling for excessive drinking is effective in reducing drinking in non-dependent (hazardous or harmful) drinkers. Randomized controlled trials have shown that such advice results in a significant reduction in alcohol consumption and related problems in treatment groups compared with untreated control groups. Reductions in alcohol consumption of the order of 30% are typically achieved, although not all patients will reduce their drinking to within recommended limits. Interventions as short as five min have been found to be effective. Benefits of brief intervention include reduced drinking and decreased days of admission to hospital.

While doctors worry that patients will resent them asking about alcohol consumption, patient surveys have shown that patients expect to receive advice from their doctor on drinking and other lifestyle issues from their doctor.

Treatment of the non-dependent problem drinker is far easier than treatment for the dependent drinker, as the former patient generally has a relatively intact social support system, does not experience withdrawal symptoms when they reduce their drinking, and most importantly, retains some control over their drinking. Whilst some excessive drinkers may not be prepared to change their lifestyle, many are unaware they are placing their health at risk and are willing to learn how to optimize their health. It is the responsibility of health practitioners to arm patients with the information they need in order to make informed decisions about health, and to support and encourage them when they wish to change their drinking. On the other hand, it is important to acknowledge the individual has the right to choose their own lifestyle.

Brief interventions are indicated for individuals who are found to be drinking above recommended limits, or are for some other reason experiencing alcohol-related problems or are at risk because of their drinking. For non-dependent drinkers, a brief session of structured advice can result in reduced alcohol consumption. Providing follow-up where appropriate or providing a booster session of advice at a later date may increase the chance of success of the intervention.

Components of brief intervention

The components of an early and brief intervention for non-dependent drinkers can be summarized by the acronym **FLAGS.**

Feedback: on problems experienced
Listen: to readiness to change
Advice: unequivocal advice to change drinking
Goals: negotiate goals
Strategies: discuss practical methods for achieving goals

- **Feedback**: provide brief feedback on any alcohol-related harms the individual may have experienced. The patient may be unaware of the possible role of alcohol in causing or exacerbating physical problems (such as insomnia, injuries, hypertension, raised GGT level). Also, the role of alcohol in social and psychological problems can be reviewed in an empathic manner. This discussion is conducted in a non-judgemental manner, helping the patient to understand their situation. For those who have not experienced any harms, the feedback will be on the risks of harm if drinking continues at this level
- **Listen**: to the patient's response and readiness to change. This may include any past attempts to address drinking
- **Advice**: provide clear and unequivocal advice to change. This can include describing the benefits that are likely to follow this, such as improved fitness and sleep, and reduced expenditure on alcohol
- **Goals**: typically, the clinician will suggest the patient reduces drinking to within recommended limits. The patient may accept this goal, or another compromise goal
- **Strategies**: discuss practical strategies to reduce drinking, such as switching to low-alcohol beer, alternating alcoholic with non-alcoholic drinks, reducing drink size. A self-help pamphlet and/or drink-diary may be used. Planning an alternative focus for socializing or unwinding; or identifying high-risk situations and practical ways to deal with these may be useful. The patient may be offered follow-up or further help, or information if appropriate.

This basic model can be adapted to different patients. For example, in those not yet motivated to change their drinking, the principles of motivational interviewing can be incorporated into the feedback of harms. The clinician can assist the patient to weigh up the good and bad aspects of their drinking. (See 'Motivational interviewing', p. 62.)

Brief intervention to engage dependent drinkers in further treatment

A brief intervention alone is not a sufficient treatment for the dependent drinker, but can be an effective method to engage them into further discussion about their drinking, and hopefully further treatment. This approach is particularly useful in a busy family practice, emergency department, or when alcohol is being discussed as part of an incidental finding in a ward round.

Heavier drinkers (e.g. 60g alcohol or more per day, or AUDIT score ≥13) identified through screening or routine clinical interview, should be assessed for dependence (p. 95), and will require physical examination, blood tests and fuller intervention (see p. 124 on management of alcohol dependence).

Summary: brief intervention

For (non-dependent) hazardous or harmful drinkers, an early and brief intervention provided by the patient's treating doctor serves as simple and immediate treatment, which can help prevent or lessen harms from excessive alcohol consumption. It is often the only treatment that is required.

Comprehensive assessment of alcohol use disorders

Here we cover the more detailed assessment of a patient with an alcohol use disorder. This is particularly relevant where there are clues to alcohol misuse. It also indicates the type of assessment that would be undertaken by a specialist practitioner or treatment agency. It includes the assessment of intoxication, of dependence on alcohol, risk of withdrawal, or complications of alcohol use.

General principles of taking an effective alcohol and drug use history have previously been described (see pp. 36–41), including effective interviewing styles.

The history
The alcohol history
Establish the quantity, frequency and pattern of drinking

> Home poured drinks are often larger than a standard drink and it is necessary to ask the glass size and the level of drink in the glass.

- If the patient mentions one type of alcohol, e.g. beer, ask about other forms of alcohol (e.g. wine and spirits)
- Making the patient feel comfortable admitting to heavy drinking helps elicit a more accurate response: e.g. 'How often do you get through a carton of beer?' Or, if you suspect heavy drinking, and the patient appears reluctant to put a figure to the amount consumed: 'Would you get through 20 drinks per day?'
- If the patient is having difficulty recalling their alcohol use a 'retrospective diary' style approach can be useful. Work backwards from the current time. 'What have you had to drink before you came here today? What were you doing yesterday, what did you drink then? What were you doing the day before... what did you drink then? ...' etc., for up to a week. Pinning drinking to events assists recall.

Is the patient dependent on alcohol?
Where the patient has experienced clear alcohol withdrawal, you can be confident that they will fulfil at least three criteria for a diagnosis of alcohol dependence.

Where clear evidence for dependence has not emerged, the criteria for alcohol dependence can be operationalized into questions to help clarify the diagnosis (see Table 4.2).

Does the patient experience alcohol withdrawals?
Check for overnight alcohol withdrawal: e.g. insomnia or morning tension that resolves with the first drink. (see p. 110 for assessment of alcohol withdrawal.

Time of last drink: To assist in predicting or assessing the timing and severity of any withdrawal.

Table 4.5 Eliciting evidence of dependence on alcohol

ICD/DSM criterion	Question
Impaired control	How easy is it for you to avoid or stop drinking, if you have something important on?
Craving/compulsion	If you don't have alcohol around, do you think about it a lot?
Drinking 'taking over' life	What does your typical day involve?
Tolerance	How much do you need to drink before you feel unsteady on your feet?
Withdrawal or withdrawal relief	How do you feel in the morning when you wake up, before your first drink?
Persistent use despite awareness of harm	[If necessary, clarify if the patient was aware that any reported harms were linked to their drinking]

Overview of lifetime drinking history
Some simple questions can elicit an overview in the dependent drinker:
- 'Of the last 10 years, how many years overall have you been drinking daily?'
- 'What is the longest time that you've had dry?'
- 'How did you achieve this?'

In most cases in the initial history an overview is required, rather than great detail.

Complications of drinking
- Dependent or heavy drinkers should be asked about any liver disease (alcohol-related or other)
- The general medical history (below) acts as a screen for history of complications in any system.

Desire to change drinking:
If this does not emerge spontaneously in the interview, it should be explored:
- Elements of motivational interviewing can be used to assess the desire to change and at the same time, may help develop motivation in the ambivalent patient: e.g. 'What do you like about your drinking? What problems does it cause you?'
- 'Have you thought about changing your drinking?'
- 'Have you ever tried to change your drinking?'

Current treatment for alcohol use disorders and past interventions
(for the dependent drinker)
For example, 'Have you had help for your drinking before?'
Past medications, counselling (and type of counselling), engagement with AA or other support.

History of other substance use (prescribed, alternative, licit and illicit). As described in the assessment chapter (p. 35). Assessing benzodiazepine use is important, because of cross-tolerance with alcohol and benzodiazepines, and because benzodiazepine dependence or withdrawal can complicate alcohol dependence or withdrawal.

Medical history including all body systems, to elicit systems affected by alcohol, thus providing an overview of health including co-existing conditions that can be affected by alcohol (see complications of alcohol, p. 80).

Psychiatric history: including depression, anxiety, any admissions to psychiatric hospitals.

Screen for depression and anxiety in particular. Where present, assess their nature and severity, including how much they interfere with function.

Check for presence of suicidal ideation: does it ever get so bad you think of harming yourself?

Relationship to drinking: was depression/anxiety a problem before you started drinking regularly? If there has been a past remission from drinking: What was your depression/anxiety like when you had been dry for 6 months/12 months?

Other current medications: These give an indication of health, and also of potential alcohol drug interactions.

Family history of alcohol or drug problems.

Social

Current living arrangements/social setting
- Do other people at home drink heavily? Do key friends and family drink?
- Employment status

Forensic history: History of drink driving, assaults
(See p. 108 for assessment of the intoxicated or confused patient.)

Physical examination

> In many persons with alcohol use disorders, signs may be minor or non-existent.

General appearance
- Obesity
- Poor nutrition
- Poor self-care
- Facial stigmata of alcohol dependence (telangiectasia, rhinophyma, coated tongue, glossitis, parotid enlargement, facial erythema, facial or peri-orbital puffiness resembling Cushing's syndrome, acne rosacea):
  - The distribution of alcohol-induced facial telangiectasia includes the cheeks and the angle of the jaw. In contrast telangiectasia from sun exposure tends to be greatest on areas with greatest sun exposure, e.g. forehead, nose and cheek bones, and less in the shadow of the jaw
- Conjunctival injection
- Signs of injury (old and new)

- Evidence of intoxication (smell of alcohol, slurred speech, ataxia)
- Alcohol withdrawal signs (anxiety, restlessness, tremor, sweating, increased pulse, temperature and blood pressure; p. 110).

Focused examination of all body systems with an emphasis on acute or chronic alcohol-related harm.

Cardiovascular

- Blood pressure (increased with chronic alcohol use or in withdrawal; may be reduced with intoxication)
- Pulse increased with withdrawal, blood loss
- Heart failure in cardiomyopathy
- Arrhythmias.

Respiratory

- Chronic airways disease—due to concomitant smoking (particularly important when sedation is to be considered)
- Infections (impaired immune system)
- Aspiration pneumonia.

Gastro-intestinal

- Tender epigastrium—gastritis
- Signs of alcohol-induced liver disease:
  - Cutaneous signs of liver disease—spider naevi on face, upper trunk and arms, liver nails
  - Dupuytren's contracture
  - Palmar erythema
  - Parotid enlargement
  - Gynaecomastia, loss of body hair
  - Hepatomegaly—of variable degree may occur in-patients with fatty infiltration, alcoholic hepatitis, fibrosis and cirrhosis
  - Splenomegaly, ascites, distended abdominal wall veins
  - Check for asterixis if hepatic encephalopathy is suspected
  - Testicular atrophy, hirsutism in females
  - Excessive bruising related to thrombocytopenia.

Musculoskeletal

- Gout
- Muscle wasting with proximal myopathy.

Neurological

- Pupil size (e.g. if possible head injury)
- Ophthalmoplegia (diplopia), nystagmus, ataxia, confusion (Wernicke's encephalopathy)
- Cerebellar signs, truncal ataxia (cerebellar involvement)
- Gait disturbances
- Evidence of alcohol related brain damage; frontal lobe impairment, memory loss, and impairment of cerebellar function
- Mental state examination (p. 44)/mini mental state examination (pp. 443–445)
- Peripheral neuropathy.

Laboratory tests (see Tables 4.6 and 4.7)

When to do blood tests in assessing alcohol use and its complications

In many hazardous drinkers seen in the community setting (e.g. drinking just over the recommended limits, with no evidence of harms from alcohol, dependence or co-existing medical conditions no blood tests are indicated. Brief intervention is an appropriate response.

For men drinking 60 g ethanol or more a day, or women drinking 40 g ethanol or more a day, or those where complications of drinking are suspected, blood tests should be ordered to assess the physical harms of alcohol, particularly the presence of alcohol related liver injury.

Because of the relatively low prevalence of significant liver damage even in heavy drinkers (20–25%), liver enzymes may be normal in a majority of cases seen in family practice. Alcohol can cause significant health and social problems without any detectable liver damage, particularly in persons under 30 years of age.

In pre-test counselling the patient should be advised that in most cases the blood tests will be normal, even where there are major problems from alcohol. The tests are only being done to check for evidence of significant liver damage. This warning is important, to prevent the patient from taking 'consolation' from normal results, and feeling that the results negate the clinician's advice about alcohol.

In cases presenting to a family practice or clinic blood tests usually include:

- **Biochemical screen**: Electrolytes, urea, creatinine, liver function tests (enzymes, albumin)
- Full Blood Count
- INR/APTT in heavier drinkers.

In those presenting with confusion, with significant alcohol withdrawal, or with complications, a wider range of laboratory tests may be indicated (see p. 113 for investigations of alcohol withdrawal, and below for investigations of complications p. 104).

When elevated at baseline, GGT results are useful in monitoring progress and in providing feedback and encouragement to the patient who is doing well. In those without underlying liver disease, GGT and transaminases typically return to normal in the 4–6 weeks following abstinence. MCV takes up to 4 months to return to normal.

Other laboratory markers for recent alcohol consumption e.g. CDT are used in research settings, but are not broadly available. These include for example the ratio of 5-hydroxytryptophol: 5-hydroxyindoleacetic acid; and ethyl glucuronide.

Further reading

Conigrave KM, Davies P, Haber P, Whitfield J. Traditional markers of excessive alcohol use. *Addiction* 2003; **98**(Suppl. 2): 31–43.

Table 4.6 Laboratory tests used to assess alcohol use

Investigations	Results	Interpretation and comments
Blood alcohol	Raised with recent intoxication	Recent intoxication. Urine alcohol levels stay positive longer than blood levels. Passive breathalysers provide a breath alcohol reading on those not capable or willing to blow into a breathalyser. High correlation between breath and blood alcohol.
FBC	Macrocytosis More sensitive among women, and drinkers aged >30 years Long half life of 60 days after reduction/cessation of drinking (red cell survives 120 days)	Increased red cell volume (MCV) in 20–30% of heavy drinkers in the community and 50–75% of heavy drinking in-patients. Due to direct toxic effect of alcohol on the bone marrow and in a minority, folate deficiency. Other causes of macrocytosis include: 　Folate or B12 deficiency, including through malabsorption 　New red blood cells (reticulocytosis): e.g. bleeding, haemolysis 　Bone marrow disorders 　Hypothyroidism 　A range of medications, in particular anticonvulsants (phenytoin) 　Smoking.
Liver function tests		
GGT	Elevated. More sensitive among men, and >30 years of age. Half life of 2 weeks with abstinence if no underlying liver disease	Elevated in only 30–50% of heavy drinkers in the community and 50–80% of medical in patients GGT is the most sensitive of the traditional markers. Other causes of elevation: 　Liver and biliary diseases

		Diabetes Pancreatitis Hypertriglyceridaemia Wide range of medications e.g. Anti-convulsants (phenytoin) NSAIDs Smoking.
AST & ALT	Elevated half life of 2 weeks with abstinence if no underlying disease	Transaminases are relatively insensitive: only 20% of those drinking 60 g+ of ethanol in the community have elevated results. Raised levels tend to reflect histological change/impairment of hepatocyte cell membrane integrity AST and ALT levels are high, and typically greater than GGT. AST/ALT ratio > 2 is indicative of alcoholic hepatitis.
Uric acid	Increased serum uric acid	Gout may be precipitated by alcohol consumption.
Cholesterol	Increased HDL cholesterol	An incidental finding rather than one of major diagnostic value.
Carbohydrate deficient transferrin (CDT)	Raised half life 17 days with abstinence	Isoforms of serum transferrin, which are lower in carbohydrate content increase with regular heavy drinking. CDT reflects recent alcohol use (past 2–4 weeks); higher specificity than liver enzymes, and higher sensitivity in dependent drinkers. GGT and CDT tend to be elevated in different drinkers, so can be used together. False positives in advanced cirrhosis of other causes, and in primary biliary cirrhosis. In pregnancy absolute levels need to be interpreted in relation to total transferrin. Available in some centres only and can be more expensive than liver enzymes.

Table 4.7 Laboratory tests used in assessing suspected complications of alcohol use disorders and common differential diagnoses

Investigations	Results	Interpretation and comments
FBC	Low Hb	Anaemia, e.g. nutritional, due to gastrointestinal blood loss, haemolysis in cirrhosis, or bone marrow suppression.
	Microcytosis	Iron deficiency secondary to overt or silent GI blood loss.
	Red cell abnormalities	Spur cells or other red cell abnormalities in advancing liver disease.
	Raised WCC Reduced WCC	Infections secondary to poor self-care or reduced T cell function, lung infections secondary to smoking. Pancytopaenia in advanced liver disease.
	Reduced platelets	Falling platelets may be a warning sign of advancing cirrhosis with or without hypersplenism; liver is a source of thrombopoetin; in advanced liver disease there may be pancytopaenia.
Electrolyte, urea creatinine	Electrolyte abnormalities	Hyponatraemia, hypokalaemia.
Minerals	Reduced magnesium	Alcohol impairs absorption and increases urinary excretion. Low Mg may lower seizure threshold or resemble alcohol withdrawal.
	Zinc deficiency	
Blood sugar	Raised	Differential diagnosis of confusion. Reversible insulin resistance with repeated heavy drinking. Diabetes as a consequence of pancreatic damage.
	Low	Differential diagnosis of confusion.
LFTs	AST and ALT	AST/ALT ratio of >2 is indicative of alcoholic hepatitis.(or other drug related liver disease), rather than immune or viral hepatitis. In a heavy drinker where ALT elevation predominates, consider hepatitis B or C as a possible co-existing diagnosis. In uncomplicated alcoholic hepatitis ALT and AST levels seldom exceed 250 IU/L.

Table 4.7 (Contd.)

Investigations	Results	Interpretation and comments
		Where ALT or AST exceeds 300 IU/L consider other causes of liver disease including viral hepatitis and drug induced liver injury, e.g. paracetamol.
	ALP Elevated	May be an early indicator of alcohol induced liver disease. A minimal elevation of ALP is commonly the only abnormal LFT in alcoholic cirrhosis,
	Albumin reduced	Reduced synthetic function, or dilution in fluid overload/ascites
INR APTT	Raised Raised	Reduced production of clotting factors in advancing cirrhosis.
Serology for viral hepatitis		In assessing differential diagnosis and/or additive factors in cirrhosis, particularly if there is a past history of injecting drug use (hepatitis C), or patient born in a country with high prevalence of hepatitis B (see pp. 370–371; 220–221).
α Foetoprotein	Raised	Elevated in some cases of hepatocellular carcinoma as a complication of cirrhosis.
Serum B12/folate	Low serum folate Low serum B_{12}	Reduced absorption of folate, nutritional deficiency. Nutritional deficiency, reduced absorption.
Serum amylase/lipase	Elevated	Acute pancreatitis.
CPK	Raised	Traumatic muscle necrosis, acute myopathy or acute rhabdomyolysis—especially if comatose. Increased risk of acute renal failure.
TFTs	Raised Low	Hyperthyroidism in differential diagnosis of an excitatory state. Hypothyroidism in differential diagnosis of macrocytosis.
Urine drug screens		May help detect other drug use, especially in a person with altered consciousness. Results may not be available for several days.
Beta hydroxybutyric acid; lactic acid	Raised	In alcoholic ketoacidosis there is elevated beta hydroxybutyric acid and lactic acid, and a large anion gap. Blood sugar is often low or low normal, but may be slightly elevated.

Investigations in alcohol related motor vehicle accidents

In some countries there may be a medicolegal requirement to measure a blood alcohol level in persons involved in a motor vehicle accident who are presenting for treatment. For example, in Australia all drivers in motor vehicle accidents who present to hospital must have a specially collected blood alcohol level sent for forensic testing (see drink driving, p. 400).

Laboratory tests used in assessing suspected complications of chronic alcohol excess

See p. 102 and 106 ; see also Tables 4.7 and 4.8.

Laboratory test results in alcohol related liver disease
Alcohol-related fatty liver
- When uncomplicated, liver tests are typically normal or isolated GGT elevation
- May be minimal elevation of ALP
- Abstinence over a period of 4–6 weeks should lead to normalization of liver function tests.

Alcoholic hepatitis
- Usually raised GGT, often with a slightly raised ALP
- Elevations of AST and ALT, with AST/ALT ratio of >2, and ALT and AST levels usually no more than 250 IU/L.
- Albumin may be low and bilirubin raised by the time of presentation.

Alcoholic cirrhosis
- May have normal liver function tests or minimal elevation of alkaline phosphatase (ALP) may be the only abnormality
- As hepatic synthetic function falls, albumin may fall and bilirubin rise, while the prothrombin time becomes prolonged.
- Falling platelets may be a warning sign of worsening liver damage
- In advanced liver disease there may be pancytopaenia.

Liver cell cancer
Liver cell cancer complicates 15% of cases of cirrhosis. Elevations in ALP, GGT are expected and α-foetoprotein will become elevated in a proportion of cases. In patients with cirrhosis, α-foetoprotein should be monitored twice yearly and abdominal ultrasound done at the same time.

Other investigations for complications of alcohol use disorders
- Endoscopy: for upper abdominal pain, gastritis, peptic ulcer, oesophageal varices
- Abdominal ultrasound and/or CT scan (with or without contrast); TC sulphur colloid scan (uncommon now).

Indications for liver biopsy
Where there is no suspicion of a cause of liver disease other than alcohol, liver biopsy is rarely required.

Biopsy can assist with differential diagnosis or establishing the relative impact of co-existing causes of liver disease. For example, it is useful when there is lack of improvement of LFTs, despite documented abstinence from alcohol, or the pattern of LFT abnormalities is atypical for alcoholic liver disease. In some countries, liver biopsy is performed to confirm the presence of cirrhosis or to stage its progression.

Suspected acute pancreatitis

Acute pancreatitis, when severe, is a medical emergency. Investigations for suspected acute pancreatitis should include serum amylase and lipase levels, electrolytes, plain X-ray of the abdomen, chest X-ray and abdominal ultrasound. CT abdomen and blood gases are usually undertaken subsequently.

Chronic pancreatitis

Liver function tests (raised serum alkaline phosphatase), Glucose tolerance test (diabetes mellitus), stool tests for faecal fats (steatorrhoea). Plain X-ray abdomen (pancreatic calcification), abdominal ultrasound, CT abdomen. Refer to gastroenterologist; may require endoscopic retrograde cholangiopancreatography (ERCP) or surgery.

Establishing a diagnosis

Having taken a history, performed physical examination and ordered any necessary investigations, it is important a formal diagnosis is reached in relation to the alcohol use disorders, and any complications.

Diagnosing whether or not the person is dependent on alcohol is particularly important. Presence of dependence determines the treatment plan, e.g. whether the goal needs to be abstinence and the potential need for withdrawal management and for relapse prevention strategies.

The diagnosis should include:
- Diagnosis of the alcohol use disorder
- Diagnoses of any complications of this:
  - Medical
  - Neuropsychiatric
  - Social
- Diagnosis of antecedent or co-existing conditions (physical, neuropsychiatric, and relevant major social stressors)
  - Including diagnoses of other substance use disorders
  - Major antecedent factors or factors perpetuating ongoing drinking may be listed.

Diagnosis in the ICD general medical system

In the ICD (general medical) system, the principal diagnosis is listed first.

Table 4.8 Other investigations for assessing complications and differential diagnoses of alcohol use disorders

Investigation	Finding	Interpretation/comment
Abdominal (liver spleen) ultrasound	Altered texture or organ size	Can give an indication of the presence of cirrhosis (irregular texture, altered size) and secondary splenomegaly.
		Fatty liver and cirrhosis give rise to increased echotexture but ultrasound cannot definitively diagnose cirrhosis.
		A screen for hepatocellular carcinoma.
Abdominal CT	As above	Evidence of abnormal or changing liver size and texture or secondary splenomegaly.
		Evidence of hepatocellular carcinoma.
Liver biopsy	Nature of liver disease	If diagnosis is uncertain or to stage the severity of liver disease. Not routinely indicated.
Endoscopy	Varices, reflux, gastritis, oesophagitis	All newly diagnosed cirrhotic patients should have an endoscopy to determine if varices are present, to allow prophylactic therapy to reduce risk of bleeding.
Abdominal X-ray	Calcification in the pancreas	Chronic pancreatitis.
Chest X-ray	Pneumonia, TB	Aspiration pneumonia following heavy intoxication; lobar pneumonia secondary to smoking; increased risk of TB in alcohol dependence (decreased T cell function, poor living conditions)
		If a chronic heavy smoker (e.g. lung hyperinflation on chest X-ray) be cautious in use of benzodiazepines in alcohol withdrawal.
	Cardiomegaly, pulmonary oedema	Cardiomyopathy.

Oximeter readings, Blood gases	Chronic airways limitation, hypoxia, respiratory acidosis	If a chronic heavy smoker with co-existing chronic airways obstruction/pneumonia. Look for hypoxia, particularly in the confused or sedated patient, or where benzodiazepines are to be administered.
ECG	Atrial fibrillation	Alcohol induced atrial fibrillation secondary to acute intoxication or to cardiomyopathy.
Cardiac ECHO	Four-chamber dilatation and hypokinesis with low ejection fraction—mural thrombus, mitral or tricuspid regurgitation	Cardiomyopathy.
Brain CT	Space occupying lesion; atrophy	Important to detect possible subdural in a person with decreased level of consciousness; differential diagnosis of first withdrawal seizure or atypical seizure; assessment of reducing level of cognitive function.
EEG		To help differentiate epilepsy from alcohol withdrawal seizure.

Example of a diagnosis in ICD general medical system

Diagnoses
- Harmful alcohol use
- Complicated by hypertension and depression
- Family history of early onset alcohol dependence
- Nicotine dependence
- Complicated by chronic airways limitation
- Hyperthyroidism: stable and treated
- Difficult social environment: living with alcohol-dependent sister, drink driving case pending.

Table 4.9 Example of a diagnosis in psychiatry (DSM) diagnostic system

Axes	Description of axis	Sample diagnosis
Axis I	Primary mental illness	Alcohol dependence
Axis II	Personality disorder	Borderline personality disorder
Axis III	Co-existing physical disorders	Fractured femur secondary to intoxication
Axis IV	Psychosocial stressors	Recent divorce
Axis V	Global assessment of functioning (GAF) (90-point scale)	80

Diagnosis in the psychiatry (DSM) diagnostic system
In the DSM IV system, there is a multi-axial diagnostic formulation. Alcohol use disorders fall within Axis I, the mental health disorder. Axis II is used for any personality disorder which may be present. Axis III includes physical disorders, which may be either complications of drinking or coincident.

Management of alcohol intoxication

Alcohol intoxication or alcohol poisoning can be a life-threatening condition, particularly in a non-tolerant individual. In many developed countries young people frequently present with alcohol overdose, for example, around New Year's Eve.

Alcohol intoxication is a differential diagnosis in-patients presenting with abnormal mental states, confusion, ataxia, or coma. It may be complicated by overdose with other drugs, e.g. benzodiazepines, opioids, tricyclic antidepressants, paracetamol, stimulants, ecstasy. The person presenting in an intoxicated state may also have other medical or surgical illnesses, which are often missed.

Assess and monitor:
- Vital signs—temperature, BP, PR, breathing
- Neurological observations: Glasgow coma scale should be monitored hourly, and mental state should be monitored for features not consistent with intoxication alone, e.g. confusion, disorientation, anxiety, panic, psychosis, suicidality
- Breath or blood alcohol levels
- Urine or plasma drug screen.

If the patient is drowsy, confused or has reduced level of consciousness:
- General supportive measures, to ensure that vital signs are stable and monitor airways, breathing, and circulation
- Protect from falls/aspiration.

If the patient is unconscious, in addition:
- Place in coma position to avoid aspiration
- Assisted respiration may be necessary
- Avoid prolonged immobility to prevent rhabdomyolysis
- Maintain fluid balance and urine output; give intravenous fluids and replace electrolytes/magnesium/glucose as necessary.

> Always give thiamine parenterally before the administration of glucose solutions where there is a suspicion of chronic heavy alcohol use to avoid precipitating Wernicke's encephalopathy.

When the patient improves:
- If intoxication was acute (e.g. in a young person), provide brief intervention
- If intoxication was part of a chronic alcohol problem:
  - Place on alcohol withdrawal scale
  - Review need for treatment for alcohol dependence (see later)
  - Discuss/arrange follow up at the alcohol and drug services.

Examination of the confused patient

While confusion and disorientation occur in non-tolerant individuals at blood alcohol levels over 0.15% (i.e. 150 mg/dL), these symptoms may occur at lower doses for those with other vulnerabilities (e.g. the elderly, those with pre-existing brain disorders, those taking sedative medication). In these vulnerable individuals confusion may take days or weeks to clear. Medical conditions need to be excluded (differential diagnosis or coincident diagnoses; see p. 112, Table 4.10).

Look for other causes of impaired level of consciousness, for example, trauma including fractures or head injury or evidence of any medical illness that may be masked by intoxication. In a person with probable alcohol dependence, consider a diagnosis of Wernicke's encephalopathy (see below) until proven otherwise.

> It is important to exclude other causes of confusion, including head injury, metabolic abnormalities, medical illnesses, and Wernicke's encephalopathy (see Table 4.10).

Diagnosis and management of alcohol withdrawal

The alcohol withdrawal syndrome is a central nervous system hyperactivity syndrome which occurs when a dependent drinker either chooses to stop or cut down on drinking, or is prevented from drinking by an illness or lack of availability of alcohol.

When a person goes into alcohol withdrawal at home, an early symptom is overnight insomnia and morning 'edginess', which lasts until the first drink of the day. Some patients may present to hospital with withdrawal symptoms which may be mild and inconsequential. In others, the symptoms may increase in severity, and progress to severe and life-threatening delirium tremens if not identified early and treated appropriately.

The severity of alcohol withdrawal is increased by old age, higher amount of alcohol consumption and duration of drinking, co-existing medical disorders, concurrent sedative (benzodiazepine) dependence, recent anaesthesia and in malnourished patients or those with severe vomiting or diarrhoea.

Where withdrawal is anticipated and treated early, complications should be rare. However, some patients present to the emergency department already in advanced withdrawal, or with complications.

Features of the alcohol withdrawal syndrome

Onset: 6–24 h after the last drink.
Peak: 24–48 h after the last drink.
Duration: 5–7 days.

Clinical features
Autonomic hyperactivity
- Sweating
- Tremor
- Tachycardia
- Raised blood pressure
- Raised temperature
- Apprehension, anxiety, irritability, agitation, insomnia.

Gastrointestinal
- Nausea
- Vomiting.

Alcohol withdrawal seizures may occur in 2–5% cases of withdrawal
Seizures may herald the onset of delirium tremens.

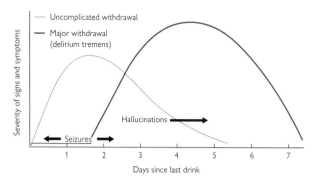

Fig. 4.3 Time course of the alcohol withdrawal syndrome.

Rating and monitoring the alcohol withdrawal syndrome

Regular monitoring of the severity of alcohol withdrawal is important. Two scales are commonly used to rate the severity of key signs of alcohol withdrawal, these are the Alcohol Withdrawal Scale (AWS) and the Clinical Institute Withdrawal Assessment for Alcohol, Revised Version (CIWA-AR). These are designed to assist in early detection and monitoring of alcohol withdrawal (see Appendix pp. 430–435).

However, both are rating scales, rather than diagnostic instruments, and a variety of other medical conditions can cause elevated scores.

Delirium tremens

Delirium tremens ('the DTs') represents very severe alcohol withdrawal with an alcohol withdrawal score about 15 or more on AWS and about 20 or more on CIWA-AR. It occurs in about 5% patients in alcohol withdrawal, often in medically compromised patients with a long history of dependence who cease heavy alcohol use. If good screening and treatment policies are implemented, DTs should never occur when alcohol withdrawal supervenes in the hospital setting. DTs are still seen when patients present to hospital in a state of advanced withdrawal.

Delirium tremens is a potentially life threatening condition. All alcohol-dependent patients require regular monitoring for alcohol withdrawal and to be appropriately treated at an early stage in order to avoid DTs.

Delirium tremens

Onset: 48–72 h after the last drink (may occur up to 5 days after)
Duration: 3–10 days
Generally preceded by other signs of alcohol withdrawal
Seizures may herald the onset of delirium tremens

Clinical features
- As per severe alcohol withdrawal:
    - Autonomic hyperactivity: tachycardia, sweating, tremor, hypertension, fever
    - Severe anxiety, marked agitation
    - Dehydration, electrolyte imbalances may be present
- Plus:
    - Clouding of consciousness/delirium (disorientation and confusion, fluctuating mental state)
    - Hallucinations: typically visual or tactile
    - Paranoid delusions.

Cardiovascular collapse may occur.
Untreated delirium tremens has a mortality of up to 15%.

Differential diagnosis of the alcohol withdrawal syndrome

A range of medical disorders may mimic or co-exist with alcohol withdrawal. Co-existing medical conditions need to be identified and treated concurrently. In particular, infection, hypoxia, gastro-intestinal bleeding, hepatic encephalopathy, head injury, subdural haematoma, and metabolic disturbances should be considered.

A differential diagnosis of benzodiazepine withdrawal or concurrent benzodiazepine withdrawal should also be considered.

Table 4.10 The differential diagnosis of confusion/acute organic brain syndrome

• Severe alcohol withdrawal delirium tremens	• Drug intoxication
• Wernicke's encephalopathy	• Metabolic disturbances:
• Benzodiazepine withdrawals (may occur concurrently with alcohol withdrawals)	• Hypo- or hyperglycaemia
	• Hypo- or hyperthyroidism
• Hypoxia	• Fluid and electrolyte imbalances
• Infections (e.g. urinary tract, pneumonia, sepsis)	• Hypokalaemia
	• Hyponatraemia
• HIV/AIDS	• Hypo or hypercalcaemia
• Hepatic encephalopathy, GI bleeding	• Hypomagnaesaemia
• Head injury, subdural haematoma,	• Renal failure, uraemia
• Cerebrovascular accidents	• Acute psychotic illness (schizophrenia, drug induced psychosis)
• Cerebral neoplasms	
• Post-ictal state	

Investigations for the management of the alcohol withdrawal syndrome

Investigations are directed to excluding metabolic imbalances and assessing or excluding co-morbid or complicating medical conditions (See Table 4.10 on p. 112).

Routine tests

- Full blood count: e.g.
  - Low Hb (anaemia, bleeding)
  - Leucocytosis (infection)
  - Macrocytosis (excess alcohol, B12, folate deficiency)
  - Thrombocytopaenia
  - Liver function tests (LFTs)
  - Low albumin (chronic liver disease)
  - Raised GGT (excess alcohol)
  - AST/ALT ratio >2 (acute alcoholic hepatitis)
- Urea and electrolytes—dehydration,
  - Hypokalaemia
  - Hyponatraemia
- Serum magnesium levels (hypomagnesaemia)
- Blood glucose—hypoglycaemia or hyperglycaemia.
- BAC—if withdrawal signs and symptoms are present with relatively high BAC, withdrawal is likely to worsen significantly
- Urine drug screens—if suspicion of other drug use, e.g. benzodiazepine or opioid dependence.
- **If clinically indicated**, tests to exclude other pathology, e.g.:
  - CPK levels (if rhabdomyolysis is suspected)
  - Serum calcium levels
  - Serum B$_{12}$/folate
  - Thyroid function tests
  - CXR—pneumonia
  - Arterial blood gases—hypoxia, hypercapnia
  - Brain CT or MRI—head injury, subdural haematoma
  - ECG, cardiac ECHO
  - EEG—epilepsy.

At what blood levels do withdrawal start and when to administer benzodiazepines?

For most patients significant withdrawal symptoms only occur after blood alcohol levels have fallen below 0.05 g/dL. However, if the patient is tolerant to particularly high BAC, e.g. 0.3 g/dL withdrawal signs and symptoms can occur with relatively high blood alcohol concentrations (e.g. 0.15 g%).

Thus, diazepam is generally administered when the blood alcohol levels have fallen below 0.05 g%. However, if a person has a history of complicated withdrawal (e.g. seizures, DTs) prophylactic diazepam can be considered once BAC has fallen to 0.15 g%, at which stage they are typically in a mild withdrawal.

Management of the alcohol withdrawal syndrome

The alcohol withdrawal syndrome may range from simple and mild withdrawal to severe or very severe withdrawal (delirium tremens). An accurate history of alcohol use at the time of admission, including presence of dependence and of past withdrawal or seizures, and the time of last drink, can allow earlier treatment and prevention of complications of withdrawal.

Skilled nursing is the key to management of the alcohol withdrawal syndrome. Nurse the patient in a quiet, dimly lit room, provide constant reassurance and regular reorientation.

Regular monitoring of the withdrawal state: All patients in withdrawal, or at risk of withdrawal, or known or suspected of drinking more than 60 g ethanol per day should be monitored with the Alcohol Withdrawal Scale or CIWA–AR every 2–4 h (see pp. 430–435), and implement sedation early if withdrawal symptoms are experienced (see below). For severe withdrawal/delirium tremens monitor 2 hourly.

Close monitoring by 2–4-hourly alcohol withdrawal (AWS) or the Clinical Institute Withdrawal Assessment for Alcohol, revised version (CIWA-AR) is recommended for patients:
- Drinking more than 60 g ethanol per day for several years
- With a previous history of alcohol withdrawal
- Presenting with a high BAC without signs of intoxication
- With a history of seizures and suspected heavy drinking.

The alcohol withdrawal scale is NOT a diagnostic instrument.

Other medical conditions and withdrawal from benzodiazepines may cause similar clinical signs.

Thiamine: Vitamin deficiency, particularly thiamine deficiency, is common in alcohol-dependent patients especially those who are malnourished or have been sick with vomiting or diarrhoea.

Always consider Wernicke's encephalopathy in a patient with alcohol dependence and administer parenteral thiamine (at least 100 mg intramuscularly or intravenously).

The dose of thiamine is increased to at least 100 mg tds intramuscularly or intravenously if the patient is malnourished and there is suspicion of Wernicke's syndrome (pp. 119–120).

In the UK, Pabrinex® ampoules should be administered once daily for 3–5 days (see pp. 119–120) as prophylaxis.

Do not administer intravenous dextrose solutions until the patient has first received parenteral thiamine.

Administer thiamine 100 mg daily intramuscularly or intravenously daily for 3–5 days then orally thereafter. Oral multivitamin supplementation is also recommended.

In the United Kingdom thiamine is available as a preparation called Pabrinex®. It is recommended that one pair of high-potency Pabrinex® ampoules be administered once daily for 3–5 days as prophylaxis (pp. 119–120).

Sedation with benzodiazepines: For simple, uncomplicated alcohol withdrawal (e.g. AWS 1–4), rest and reassurance may be all that is required. However, if the alcohol withdrawal scale rating reaches or exceeds the threshold (AWS ≥5 or CIWA-AR ≥10) administer regular benzodiazepines, titrated against the withdrawal scale. Benzodiazepines have been shown to reduce withdrawal symptoms, and prevent complications such as seizures and delirium tremens.

Depending on the severity of withdrawal symptoms, the following is an example of benzodiazepine dose regimes that may be administered, titrating the dose according to the individual patient's response.

An equivalent regime using chlordiazepoxide is often preferred in the UK, because it is thought to have less of a predisposition to dependence than diazepam.

Diazepam loading may be required for patients whose withdrawal score is rising, despite the diazepam doses above, or who present, or are detected in moderate to severe withdrawal that does not respond to the regime above.

Maximum dose of diazepam should not exceed 120 mg in 24 h. If more diazepam is required, seek specialist advice. However, provided that there are no concurrent problems (see Precautions) and a specialist has first been consulted, up to 240 mg diazepam may be administered in the first 24 h.

Delirium tremens is a medical emergency.
Intravenous diazepam may be required in patients in severe withdrawals or DTs.

NB: If intravenous benzodiazepines are considered necessary, the patient should be nursed in a high dependency unit or intensive care unit.

Once the patient is stabilized and able to take oral medications, they can resume the oral dose regimes described above.

Table 4.11 Benzodiazepine dose regimes

Severity of alcohol withdrawal	Diazepam regime (Australia)	Chlordiazepoxide regime (UK)
Mild withdrawal (e.g. AWS 1–4; CIWA <10)	Rest and reassurance	Rest and reassurance
Mild to moderate withdrawal (e.g. AWS 5–9; CIWA 10–14)	5–20 mg orally 3–4 times a day reducing by 5–10 mg a day to zero over 5–7 days	10–20 mg four times daily, reducing gradually over 5–7 days
Moderate to severe withdrawal (e.g. AWS 10–14; CIWA 15–20)	20 mg four times daily orally with supplementary doses of 10–20 mg if required until patient is calm and mildly sedated. Then reduce by 5–10 mg a day to zero or Diazepam loading: 20 mg orally every 2 h until patient calm & mildly sedated	30–40 mg four times a day reducing gradually over 7–10 days
Severe withdrawals/ **delirium tremens** (DTs) (e.g. AWS ≥15; CIWA >20)	Diazepam loading: 20 mg orally every 2 h until patient calm and mildly sedated or IV Diazepam 10 mg slowly, repeat after 30 min if necessary Once patient is stable, continue oral dose regimens as described for moderate to severe withdrawal	Day 1: 40 mg four times a day + 40 mg prn Day 2: 40 mg four times a day Day 3: 30 mg four times a day Day 4: 25 mg four times a day Day 5: 20 mg four times a day Day 6: 15 mg four times a day Day 7: 10 mg four times a day Day 8: 10 mg three times daily Day 9: 10 mg twice daily Day 10: 10 mg nocte

Precautions in use of benzodiazepines

In patients with chronic air flow limitation without respiratory failure, the dose of diazepam should be either be reduced or a shorter acting benzodiazepine, e.g. oxazepam be considered. Monitor oximeter readings before and after each dose of benzodiazepine.

If there is respiratory failure, DO NOT sedate in a general ward. Urgent referral to a high dependency or intensive care unit is recommended.

In patients with cirrhosis and hepatic decompensation (e.g. encephalopathy, ascites, jaundice), diazepam may worsen hepatic encephalopathy. In such cases, give short acting benzodiazepines, e.g. oxazepam 15 mg every 2 h to a maximum of 45 mg, then review.

> The diazepam regime for a simple withdrawal should be finished within a week to avoid risk of benzodiazepine dependence. No patient should be discharged with a full script for benzodiazepines.

Fluids and electrolytes: correct dehydration and fluid and electrolyte imbalance particularly hypokalaemia (e.g. with potassium supplements 80–240 mmol/day).

Correct hypomagnesaemia with magnesium aspartate 500 mg orally 2–4 times a day with meals. This is contraindicated in renal failure.

Antipsychotic medication: If the patient remains agitated or has hallucinations administer haloperidol 2.5–5 mg orally and repeat 3–4 times a day if necessary. Alternatively olanzapine 2.5–5 mg may be given orally and repeated three to four times a day. Olanzapine has a lower risk of extrapyramidal side effects.

If there have been periods of prolonged immobility, which may cause rhabdomyolysis and acute renal failure check CPK; rehydrate and monitor fluid balance, turn regularly.

Small doses of clonidine or propranolol may be useful in-patients with uncontrolled hypertension.

Exclude and treat concurrent medical and/or psychiatric conditions.

Alcohol withdrawal seizures

In elective or predicted alcohol withdrawal, early benzodiazepine treatment typically prevents the occurrence of a withdrawal seizure. In well managed medical detoxification units, the prevalence of seizures should be less than 1%.

However, in general alcohol withdrawal, seizures occur in 2–5% of alcohol-dependent individuals approximately 6–48 h after cessation of drinking. Alcohol withdrawal seizures account for 10–25% of adult presentations to an Emergency Department with a seizure.

The seizures are classically single, generalized, grand mal tonic-clonic convulsions without focal features and associated with loss of consciousness during a discrete withdrawal episode. Sometimes there will be a number of seizures over a period of 3–4 days. Rarely, status epilepticus will supervene. Once individuals have experienced a withdrawal seizure they are at increased risk of developing seizures during subsequent episodes of alcohol withdrawal.

The risk for a withdrawal seizure peaks at 12–24 h after the last drink (6–48 h).

The risk of seizures increases in those with a history of withdrawal seizures, idiopathic epilepsy, head injury or concurrent benzodiazepine dependence. The risk of seizure is proportional to the level of alcohol consumption and increases with subsequent episodes of alcohol withdrawal.

The seizure may occur early before the full range of features of alcohol withdrawal becomes apparent. Seizures may herald the onset of delirium tremens, with 22–50% of cases without active treatment going on to develop delirium tremens. Alcohol withdrawal may also lower the seizure

A first or atypical seizure work-up includes

- Routine haematology
- Urea and electrolytes
- Serum calcium and magnesium
- Random blood sugar levels
- Head CT scan or MRI
- EEG
- Plasma and urine drug screen.

threshold in an individual who has seizures from other causes (e.g. post-traumatic epilepsy).

Assessment of alcohol withdrawal seizures

For a first seizure the regular seizure 'work up' is recommended to exclude organic disease or a structural lesion. Investigation is particularly important if seizures are atypical, e.g. multiple or focal seizures.

Management of alcohol withdrawal seizures

Patients with seizures should be admitted for monitoring and treatment, particularly if there is a history of benzodiazepine use.

If seizures are thought to be due to or exacerbated by benzodiazepine withdrawal, higher doses of benzodiazepines may be required and should be followed by a tapering dose regimen [see management of benzodiazepine withdrawal (p. 179)].

Diazepam as described above for the treatment of alcohol withdrawal will also prevent seizure activity.

Long-term prophylactic anticonvulsant therapy (e.g. phenytoin) is ineffective in preventing recurrences of a withdrawal seizure. If a patient is already on phenytoin or another anticonvulsant (e.g. for diagnosed epilepsy), blood levels should be taken to assess patient compliance and the anticonvulsant continued in the usual dose during the withdrawal period, and reviewed subsequently.

There is an increased risk of future withdrawal seizures if drinking continues after a first withdrawal seizure, so the patient should be advised that future attempts to stop drinking should be managed in hospital. The issue of safety with driving also should be considered (p. 406).

NB: In some countries, anti-epileptics such as carbamazepine or oxcarbamazepine are used as prophylactic treatments against alcohol withdrawal, particularly if patients are at risk of seizures.

Further reading

Charness ME, Simon RP, Greenberg DA. Ethanol and the nervous system. *New England Journal of Medicine* 1989; **321**(7): 442–454.

Lingford-Hughes AR, Welch S, Nutt DJ. BAP consensus statement on the treatment of addiction. *Journal of Psychopharmacology* 2004; **18**: 2933–2935.

Treatment of suspected Wernicke's encephalopathy

Consider a diagnosis of Wernicke's encephalopathy in any confused alcohol-dependent patient until proven otherwise and always treat with intravenous thiamine. Wernicke's encephalopathy can present during the course of alcohol withdrawal or DTs, or while the individual is still drinking. It does not always present with the classical triad of symptoms, and thus often goes undetected. There should be a low threshold for diagnosis and particular attention should be given to patients presenting with one or more of the following symptoms: ophthalmoplegia; ataxia; acute confusion; memory disturbance; coma/unconsciousness; hypothermia and hypotension.

It is imperative that parenteral thiamine is given before a dextrose drip, as this has the potential to precipitate or exacerbate Wernicke's encephalopathy.

Any patient with a presumptive diagnosis of Wernicke's encephalopathy should receive an adequate dose of parenteral thiamine—100 mg IV tds at a minimum. There is not clear evidence on the optimal dose of thiamine and some centres use considerably higher doses. In the UK the recommendations are for a minimum of two pairs of IV high-potency B-complex vitamins three times daily for two consecutive days. As each pair of ampoules contains 250 mg thiamine, this regime includes 500 mg thiamine tds. If no response to therapy is observed after this time period (unless the patient is comatose, or unconscious, or the diagnosis of Wernicke's encephalopathy is confirmed by other means) the high dose therapy is discontinued. If an objective response is observed, treatment should be continued for another 5 days with one pair of IV or im high-potency B-complex vitamins once daily. For patients with enduring ataxia, polyneuritis or memory disturbance, high-potency vitamins should be given for as long as improvement continues.

Treatment of suspected Wernicke's encephalopathy

- Parenteral thiamine in adequate doses is urgent, e.g. at least thiamine 100 mg tds IV for 5 days

UK guidelines for treatment of suspected Wernicke's
- At least 2 pairs of ampoules (i.e. 4 ampoules) of high-potency B-complex vitamins IV tds for two consecutive days:
  - If no response to therapy is observed after this time, discontinue
  - If a response is observed, continue with 1 pair of IV or im ampoules daily for another 5 days, or longer if improvement continues.
- Parenteral B vitamins given intravenously in 100 ml normal saline over 30 min very rarely cause adverse reactions, but appropriate resuscitation facilities must be available.
- Follow with oral thiamine and multivitamin supplementation thereafter and as an out-patient.

Prevention/prophylaxis of Wernicke's encephalopathy

All patients undergoing in-patient detoxification should be given parenteral thiamine as prophylaxis for Wernicke's encephalopathy (WE). Parenteral administration is recommended as alcohol interferes with thiamine absorption, and in addition there are often medical complications of drinking, e.g. gastritis, vomiting, which may impair absorption. In addition, oral multivitamin preparations should also be given daily.

In Australia thiamine is typically given as 100 mg IM daily for 3–5 days The longer duration of parenteral thiamine should be used in-patients who are malnourished, with vomiting, or with more severe alcohol dependence. This is then followed by daily oral thiamine.

The only parenteral high-potency B-complex vitamin therapy licensed in the UK is Pabrinex®. One pair of IM high-potency Pabrinex® ampoules should be administered once daily for 3–5 days and ideally be followed by oral vitamin B compound.

Clients undergoing community detoxification should also be considered for parenteral prophylaxis with IM thiamine or Pabrinex® because oral thiamine is often not adequately absorbed.

IM thiamine preparations have a lower incidence of anaphylactic reactions than IV preparations, at 1 per 5 million pairs of ampoules of Pabrinex®, which is far lower than many frequently used drugs that carry no special warning. However, this risk has resulted in fears about using parenteral preparations, and the inappropriate use of oral thiamine preparations. Facilities for treating anaphylaxis should be available. This includes the need for staff to be trained in the management of anaphylaxis and administration of adrenaline injection. This is given intramuscularly.

Precautions: There is a small risk of anaphylaxis with intravenous thiamine, therefore, slow intravenous administration and ready access to appropriate resuscitation measures are necessary.

Prevention of Wernicke's encephalopathy

- Thiamine 100 mg IM daily for 3–5 days
  Or (in the UK):
- At least 1 pair of ampoules of high-potency B-complex vitamins (Pabrinex®) IM daily for 3–5 days
- Follow with oral thiamine and multivitamin supplementation thereafter and as an out-patient.

Further reading

Thomson AD, Cook CCH, Touquet R, Henry JA. The Royal College of Physicians report on alcohol: guidelines for managing Wernicke's encephalopathy in the accident and emergency department. *Alcohol and Alcoholism* 2002; **39**(6): 513–521.

Thomson AD, Marshall EJ. The treatment of patients at risk of developing Wernicke's Encephalopathy in the community. *Alcohol and Alcoholism* 2006; **41**(2): 159–167.

Education and follow-up and after alcohol withdrawal in hospital

Prior to discharge from hospital, ensure the patient understands that they have experienced an alcohol withdrawal syndrome. If they are not yet familiar with it, explain the nature of dependence, and why a goal of abstinence is necessary; i.e. that if they drink, it will mean loss of control and rapid reinstatement of heavy drinking.

Discuss ongoing care with the patient and negotiate a plan. Patients can be given the choice of various treatment options for relapse prevention, and to enhance motivation (as described below) and encouraged to access several of these. Most alcohol-dependent patients are offered pharmacotherapies for relapse prevention before they leave hospital (see below).

An important part of a successful treatment regimen involves continued follow-up and support. Typically, a dependent patient is offered an appointment with a specialist drug and alcohol unit where available, and where the management can draw on a multidisciplinary team including medical officer, nurse/nurse specialist, psychologist, and social worker. Wherever possible a member of the team can meet the patient in hospital, to assist with engagement and subsequent attendance at follow-up.

Some general practitioners have considerable experience in managing alcohol dependence, and can link the patient with private or public psychology services. Discuss the management plan with the patient's general practitioner.

Elective alcohol detoxification of a patient seen in an ambulatory setting

Alcohol withdrawal may be managed electively. This is generally referred to as 'detoxification'. Detoxification is a planned process which allows alcohol-dependent patients to cease drinking in the most comfortable and least distressing manner. It can remove a barrier to cessation of drinking and, in the management of alcohol dependence, it is the first step towards a goal of abstinence and recovery. The emphasis is on preventing a withdrawal syndrome developing or if one does develop, to minimize its symptoms and ensure that adverse consequences, especially DTs are avoided.

Detoxification may be medicated or non-medicated depending on the severity of alcohol withdrawal. It can be conducted on an ambulatory or in-patient basis.

Where to manage alcohol withdrawal electively?

Where detoxification takes place depends on the severity of alcohol dependence and past history of withdrawal, the presence or absence of concurrent medical conditions, and also on what local facilities are available.

The severity of the alcohol withdrawal syndrome is increased by older age, greater duration and amount of alcohol consumption, concurrent sedative (especially benzodiazepine) use/dependence, recent anaesthesia, and in malnourished patients or those with severe vomiting or diarrhoea.

Patients who do not fulfil the criteria on p. 22 are best detoxified in a hospital or in a specialist detoxification unit.

Criteria for undertaking home/ambulatory detoxification

Home (ambulatory) detoxification may be attempted if:
- The patient has mild to moderate alcohol dependence
- The doctor and health care worker have easy access to the patient and can review the patient on a daily basis
- The patient lives with a supportive partner or family
- Low risk of complications:
  - No past history of severe withdrawals or delirium tremens
  - No past history of seizures or epilepsy
  - Not on multiple medications
- Not misusing multiple psychoactive substances
- No concurrent medical or psychiatric problems (including suicidal ideation) which may place the patient at risk.
- The patient is not vomiting or malnourished.

Management of alcohol withdrawal in the home/ambulatory setting
- Daily supervision either by nurse or doctor
- Encourage a quiet and safe environment
- Advise patient of likely signs and symptoms of alcohol withdrawals, and when they should seek assistance
- Monitor daily using a withdrawal scale.
  - With treatment, the score on AWS should remain ≤5 or on CIWA-AR should remain ≤10
- Sedation: Benzodiazepines can be used to reduce withdrawal symptoms; however the safety of their use needs to be maximized and the following precautions taken:
  - The patient should be assessed as reliable to use according to directions and should fulfil the criteria for home detoxification
  - Daily dispensing wherever possible. The patient is reviewed, then given that day's medications

Table 4.12 Examples of home/ambulatory benzodiazepine detoxification regimes

Time period	Oral diazepam regime (Australia)	Oral chlordiazepoxide regime (UK)
Days 1 & 2	10 mg every 6 h	15–20 mg every 6 h
Days: 3 & 4	5 mg every 6 h	10 mg every 6 h
Days: 5 & 6	5 mg morning and at night	5 mg every 6 h
Day 7	5 mg at night	5–10 mg at night
Day 8	Cease	Cease

Titrate dose according to the response of the individual patient.

- Patients should be warned about potential risks of benzodiazepines, in particular:
  - Unsteadiness and possible falls. They should not drive while taking benzodiazepines.
  - Sedation: withhold a dose if sedated, and cease benzodiazepines if drinking resumes
  - Dependence with continued benzodiazepine use: benzodiazepines are for short term use only (not more than one week) because of their potential for tolerance and dependence.

Dose of benzodiazepines: Diazepam 5–20 mg 3–4 times a day depending on the severity of withdrawals reducing/day to zero over the next few days.

In the UK other benzodiazepines with long half lives, e.g. chlordiazepoxide are administered. They pose a lower risk of diversion to the black market as they have lower street value than diazepam and have a lower potential for dependence.

- Thiamine 100 mg daily orally for a month, or indefinitely if the patient resumes drinking. An initial parenteral (IM) dose should be considered, particularly if the patient's diet has been suboptimal or in where malabsorption of thiamine is suspected (e.g. vomiting or heavier consumption).
- Oral multivitamins
- Ensure that patient is well hydrated and eats well
- When doubt exists over abstinence, check breath alcohol levels.

When transfer to hospital is required

If the AWS or CIWA score rises rapidly or if the patient develops withdrawal seizures, agitation that is difficult to control, or hallucinations, transfer to hospital.

With the dosage regime below (and if necessary 2 extra 10-mg doses of diazepam on each of the first 2 days) withdrawal symptoms should be controlled, and the withdrawal rating scales should largely stay below the required thresholds. If the rating scales are not able to be maintained below those thresholds, transfer to hospital.

When a 'detox unit' is needed or preferred

Some drinkers find it easier to stop drinking in a 'detox centre' or specialist alcohol treatment unit, where they are provided with a supportive environment, and are away from ready availability of alcohol.

Other drinkers may be unsuitable for home withdrawal management because of severe dependence or unsuitable home environment (see criteria for home detoxification above).

Most detoxification units provide medicated management of alcohol withdrawal and medical supervision. However, some centres do not have sufficient medical staffing to accept individuals expected to have more severe withdrawals or with co-morbid medical or psychiatric conditions. Identifying an appropriate detoxification unit can be easier with the help of a specialist addictions unit. In some regions, phone assistance lines keep details of the type and location of services. For example in the United Kingdom a directory of treatment services/centres can be obtained from the Alcohol Concern website (www.alcoholconcern.org.uk).

Management of alcohol dependence

Alcohol dependence is characterized by lack of control over drinking. Fewer than 5% of dependent drinkers are able to return to controlled drinking. Accordingly, dependent drinkers are advised to abstain from alcohol. They usually need access to significant treatment and support to achieve sustained abstinence and to prevent relapses.

Following a diagnosis of alcohol dependence, the ideal goal of treatment is abstinence. However, this is not always possible or acceptable to the drinker in the short term. Sometimes and interim goal of 1 month's abstinence may be acceptable, after which the patient may have observed enough benefits of abstinence that they may be prepared to extend this period. Continued follow-up with repeated advice incorporating motivational interviewing techniques is important.

Treatment includes a range of steps, for which the clinician and/or patient are responsible. The patient's family and those around can assist in providing appropriate support.

Steps in the management of alcohol dependence

- Information and education. This may include motivational interviewing to increase chance of stopping drinking
- The patient must then reach a point of acceptance of the need to stop drinking and develop commitment to abstinence
- Management of alcohol withdrawal i.e. detoxification, if not already completed; pp. 115; 116; 122
- Pharmacotherapies—to suppress the drive to drink
- Psychological therapies: e.g. cognitive, behavioural, 12-step facilitation
- Management of medical, psychiatric and social complications or co-morbidity
- Support from family and friends (and for family)
- Mutual support groups/12-step fellowship
- Continual care/follow-up (residential rehabilitation in some cases)
- Personal, lifestyle and environmental change.

If the patient continues to relapse after all these steps have been taken, referral to a rehabilitation unit or therapeutic community may be considered.

Pharmacotherapies to suppress the drive to drink

Pharmacotherapies aim to reduce the internal drive to drink. They may do this through reducing craving or reducing the reward of drinking. In the case of disulfiram, pharmacotherapy provides negative reinforcement for any slip-up.

Pharmacotherapies are prescribed for relapse prevention only after acute alcohol withdrawal is over, usually 7 days after the last drink. This helps clarify whether any symptom, such as nausea, is due to alcohol withdrawal or due to the medication.

Regular follow-up is necessary to assist with patient compliance and to provide support.

Opioid antagonists: naltrexone and nalmefene

Mechanism of action: Alcohol is thought to produce a feeling of well being by releasing endorphins in the brain which act on mu opioid receptors. This contributes to the pleasure or 'reward' from drinking alcohol, which reinforces the behaviour and increases the risk of relapse. Naltrexone and nalmefene are specific opioid antagonists, and it is thought they act by blocking the pleasurable effects of alcohol and also reduce craving for alcohol. Double-blind placebo-controlled studies have shown that naltrexone 50 mg/day for 3 months significantly cut relapse rates by up to 50% if used in association with psychological therapies [see below].

Naltrexone is absorbed from the gastrointestinal tract, metabolized in the liver to 6 beta naltrexol and excreted in the urine. Duration of action is up to 24 h. Nalmefene is used as a long-acting injection which offers cover for weeks or months, so improving compliance.

Opiate antagonist treatments are only a means to assist patients to remain alcohol free. For a successful outcome, they must be prescribed in conjunction with a comprehensive treatment programme as described above, e.g. with individual and family counselling, participation in mutual help groups and regular follow-up.

Although opioid antagonists can be taken by patients who are still drinking, studies to date have only demonstrated their effectiveness among patients with at least five days of abstinence. Currently, it is recommended that treatment be initiated after signs and symptoms of withdrawal have subsided. This also allows clearer differentiation of whether symptoms such as nausea are due to withdrawal or are a side effect of the medication.

Naltrexone may be commenced at half dose (25 mg) for the first few days to reduce side effects of nausea or diarrhoea, then increased to the full dose of 50 mg mane.

As antagonists block the effects of opioid analgesia, they should be discontinued for at least 72 h before elective surgery. Patients on naltrexone should carry a card warning that they are on an opioid antagonist in case of need for emergency analgesia. In an emergency, regional anaesthesia, general anaesthesia or non-opioid analgesics can be used for pain relief. When opioids are used in an emergency, greater than normal doses of opioids are required to achieve pain relief. This carries the risk of respiratory depression and bronchoconstriction presumably due to release of histamine. The patient should be closely monitored in a setting equipped and staffed for cardiopulmonary resuscitation.

Alternative analgesics include the non-steroidal ketorolac (Australia) (when not contraindicated) or tramadol, which acts by serotonergic, as well as opioid systems.

Further reading

Srisurapanont M, Jarusuraisin N. Opioid antagonists for alcohol dependence. *Cochrane Database Systematic Review* 2005; **1**: CD001867.

Acamprosate (calcium acetylhomotaurinate)

Mechanism of action: The precise mechanism of action of acamprosate in humans is unknown. It is thought to reduce craving induced by alcohol withdrawal:

- By antagonizing excitatory glutamate at the NMDA receptor
- Possibly also by stimulating inhibitory GABA-ergic transmission.

Acamprosate is slowly absorbed from the gastrointestinal tract over a period of 4 h. Peak concentrations are reached after 5–7 h and steady state levels are achieved after 7 days.

Acamprosate is not metabolized significantly in the liver, and is excreted unchanged in the urine. The elimination half-life of acamprosate is between 13–28 h. Accumulation of acamprosate may occur in patients with renal impairment.

While recent trials in the USA have shown equivocal results, with no treatment effect reported by Project Combine, meta-analyses of trials have shown that oral acamprosate 333 mg 5–6 tablets/day in three divided dose is significantly superior to placebo in increasing periods of abstinence and preventing relapse.

Further reading

Kranzler HR, Van Kirk J. Efficacy of naltrexone and acamprosate for alcoholism treatment: a meta-analysis. *Alcoholism: Clinical & Experimental Research* 2001; **25**: 1335–1341.

Mason B, Ownby R. Acamprosate for the treatment of alcohol dependence: a review of double-blind, placebo-controlled trials. *CNS Spectrums* 2000; **5**(2): 58–69.

Disulfiram

Mechanism of action: Disulfiram inhibits aldehyde dehydrogenase and leads to accumulation of acetaldehyde after drinking even a few sips of alcohol. Acetaldehyde is a noxious compound and this unpleasant reaction acts as a psychological deterrent to drinking. Inhibition of enzyme activity occurs within 12 h and lasts 5–6 days.

The reaction includes flushing, headache, palpitations, dyspnoea, nausea, hypotension and prostration. It varies in intensity between individuals and usually occurs within 10 min of taking and peaks at 20–30 min, and lasts for 1–2 h. The reaction can be caused even by small amounts of alcohol inadvertently taken in cough mixtures, sauces or dressings of food, etc. The reaction is severe enough to have the individual bed-bound while it lasts.

This form of aversive therapy is effective in motivated and reliable patients who are well supported and who participate in a comprehensive treatment programme, and where dosing of disulfiram is under close supervision. The patient must be able to understand and consent to the use of the medication and be able to remember what will happen if he or she drinks alcohol. Supervised daily dosing by a clinic, pharmacy or family member can play an important role in motivated individuals.

Contraindications: Psychosis, ischaemic heart disease, severe renal or hepatic disease, and hypersensitivity to thiuram derivatives (pesticides; rubber); cognitive impairment, which impedes understanding of or recall of the medication's effects.

Precautions: Patients need to abstain from alcohol for at least 1 day before administration of disulfiram and for at least 1 week after cessation of treatment.

Disulfiram is currently available as 200 mg tablets. Dose is initially 100 mg/day for 1–2 weeks increasing to 200 mg/day for 6 weeks to 6 months (maximum dose 300 mg, i.e. one and a half tablets). Duration of treatment is determined by its degree of success and patient preference. Some patients decide to stay on lifelong treatment.

Other medications under study

Baclofen: A GABA-B receptor agonist, which is currently prescribed to treat involuntary muscle spasm, has shown considerable promise for reduction in alcohol withdrawal symptoms and for reduction of craving in alcohol dependence. A recent randomized controlled trial showed a significant and marked improved in ability to maintain abstinence in dependent drinkers with cirrhosis receiving baclofen.

Ondansetron: A 5HT3 antagonist, licensed as an anti-emetic, was shown in one study to reduce alcohol consumption in early onset alcohol-dependent males. Further studies are required.

Topiramate: This is a relatively new anticonvulsant that has been subject to several controlled trials in alcohol dependence with a degree of success, although is not yet broadly available. The mode of action is unclear but it may reduce glutamatergic function. The adverse effect burden can be quite high with sedation and unsteadiness often problematic. Topiramate is unusual in that it leads to weight loss, which may be beneficial or not depending on the patient's pretreatment medical state.

SSRIs are useful for the treatment of co-morbid depression in cases where an antidepressant is needed. There is no evidence that they have effects on drinking alcohol in dependent patients who are not depressed.

Further reading

Addolorato G, Leggio L, Agabio. R, Colombo G, Gasbarrini G. Baclofen a new drug for the treatment of alcohol dependence. *International Journal of Clinical Practice.* 2006; **60(8)**: 1003–1008.

Johnson BA, Ait-Daoud N, Bowden CL, DiClemente CC, Roache JD, Lawson K, Javors MA, Ma JZ. Oral topiramate for treatment of alcohol dependence: a randomized controlled trial. *Lancet* 2003; **361**: 1677–1685.

Law FD, Nutt DJ. Drugs used in the treatment of the addictions. *New Oxford Textbook of Psychiatry,* 2nd edn [in press, 2008].

Table 4.13 A comparison of the clinical use of naltrexone, acamprosate and disulfiram in treatment of alcohol dependence

	Naltrexone/nalmefene	Acamprosate	Disulfiram
Mechanism of action	Inhibits effects of endogenous opioids at mu receptor sites Anti-craving agent: Useful for the 'reward drinker'*†	Inhibits excitatory glutamates at NMDA receptor. Anti craving agent—useful for the 'relief drinker'*†	Inhibits aldehyde dehydrogenase Aversive therapy—as a deterrent to drinking
Mode of administration	50 mg once daily, can start on half dose for up to one week	Two tablets (333 mg each) tds with meals (omit 1 lunchtime tablet if <60 kg body weight)	One tablet (200 mg) daily. May increase to maximum 300 mg daily—requires close supervision.
When to commence	One week after the last drink (or when withdrawal complete)	One week after the last drink (or when withdrawal complete)	At least 1 day after the last drink
Adverse effects	Nausea, diarrhoea, fatigue headache Hepatotoxicity (dose-related)	Diarrhoea Skin eruptions Mild sedation is occasionally reported	Alcohol/disulfiram interactions: avoid cooking or medicines containing alcohol; wait at least 2 weeks after ceasing disulfiram before drinking alcohol Drowsiness Psychotic reactions Peripheral neuropathy Optic neuritis Hepatitis Impotence Dermatitis Cardiovascular events in susceptible individuals

Contraindications	Acute hepatitis; advanced liver disease;		Advanced liver disease
			Hypersensitivity to thiuram derivatives (rubber); Severe myocardial disease/ischaemic heart disease, psychotic states;
			Drinking in the last 24 h: may precipitate a Disulfiram-alcohol; interaction
	Need for opioid analgesia (e.g. chronic pain)		
	Opioid dependence (may precipitate severe opioid withdrawals)		
	Advanced renal disease	Severe renal impairment	Renal disease
	Pregnancy	Pregnancy	Pregnancy
	Suicidality		
Precautions	Monitor liver function	Monitor renal function	Monitor liver function. If drinking continues check supervision. If drinking then persists, cease.
Drug Interactions	Opioid analgesics—blocked; Illicit opioids—precipitated withdrawal in opioid dependence		Metronidazole Isoniazid Phenytoin Anticoagulants

† Some drinkers consume alcohol primarily for the pleasurable effects—'reward drinkers'. Others drink primarily to relieve symptoms of protracted withdrawal, such as 'relief drinkers'. There is a spectrum of behaviour in between the two extremes, and considerable overlap.

Choosing and combining medications

There are no currently available evidence-based guidelines on which medication to choose and when to combine them.

Naltrexone offers the advantage of once a day dosing, although it may have gastrointestinal side effects. Studies comparing it with acamprosate suggest that it is at least as effective, if not more so. Naltrexone may also offer particular advantages for dependent drinkers who drink episodically, or in binges, as it reduces the reward of drinking, and helps prevent a slip progressing to a full relapse.

Acamprosate tends to have fewer gastrointestinal side effects, and can be used in those who need to take opioid analgesia. However, patient compliance with treatment may be a problem because of the three times a day dosing. For those drinkers who have a persistent low grade anxiety or insomnia after alcohol withdrawal, acamprosate offers the advantage of reducing NMDA activity.

Combination of acamprosate with naltrexone can be used, particularly in patients with severe dependence or severe medical or social complications, or where monotherapy has failed. Either or both of these can also be combined with disulfiram.

Pharmacotherapy should always be instituted as part of a comprehensive treatment programme including approaches to assist patient adherence to the medication regime (see psychosocial interventions, p. 134).

There are no good data on how long medication should be continued. As risk of relapse is greatest for the first 3 months, then gradually reduces over 12 months, most clinicians would suggest continuing for up to 12 months if there is suggestion of benefit. If the client reports significant benefit, or shows sustained good outcomes with few side effects, many clinicians would advise continuing the medication indefinitely. Further research is needed into any potential risks from long- term use of these medications.

Management of medical complications of alcohol use disorders

Alcohol-related liver disease

For every type of alcohol-related liver disease, abstinence is the starting point for any management strategy. Unless alcohol intake is suspended, liver disease can and will progress in most patients.

With fatty liver little else is required other than abstinence, as the liver is not usually inflamed. Liver enzymes should be monitored regularly to confirm that abstinence over a period of 4–6 weeks has led to normalization of liver function tests.

There are no drugs clearly documented as having a major benefit in acute alcoholic hepatitis. Consulting with a gastroenterologist or other physician is indicated, and in some cases intensive care services are required.

The most important part of management of alcoholic cirrhosis is assisting the patient to stop drinking. The remainder of treatment is directed towards the complications of cirrhosis. Prophylactic beta blockade and/or variceal banding in those with portal hypertension should be implemented. Where beta blockade is contraindicated, use of nitrates can be considered as they also lower portal pressure and reduce the risk of bleeding varices. Ascites, portal systemic encephalopathy, infections and other complications of other chronic liver disease are managed in their own right.

Patients with cirrhosis should be monitored twice yearly with αFP and abdominal ultrasound advised, and referred to a gastroenterologist if AFP becomes elevated or if there is evidence of a mass on ultrasound or CT scan.

Management of other liver disease, complicated by alcohol use

Injecting drug users are at markedly increased risk of contracting hepatitis C, B, and D, and they are also at risk of direct drug-related toxicity. Alcohol consumed at hazardous levels will increase the rate of progression of liver disease in patients with hepatitis C and B. It appears to encourage hepatitis C viral replication, as well as causing additive harm to the liver. Patients need to be warned of these potential additive harmful effects and advised to cut back, and to have alcohol free days and, where possible, abstain completely from alcohol. Monitoring the effects of alcohol ingestion on liver function tests is perhaps the most appropriate way of determining with patients how much they should drink.

Cardiovascular disease.

Alcohol related hypertension: Patients must be advised that hypertension does not respond to antihypertensive agents if the patient continues to drink excessively but generally improves with abstinence or when alcohol is markedly reduced.

Alcoholic cardiomyopathy: Abstention from alcohol is mandatory, as with continued heavy drinking 80% are dead within 3 years. Therapy for heart failure and atrial fibrillation (digoxin, diuretics, ACE-inhibitors, anticoagulants)

Other gastrointestinal

Acute pancreatitis

- Treat shock and respiratory failure
- Pain relief with intravenous pethidine 75–100 mg intramuscularly (morphine causes spasm of the sphincter of Oddi)
- Nil by mouth
- Refer urgently to gastroenterologists and/or surgeons.

Chronic pancreatitis

- Abstinence from alcohol to prevent painful relapses (though this may not necessarily arrest progressive pancreatic damage)
- Opiates for pain relief—be aware of risk of opioid dependence
- Management of pancreatic insufficiency with pancreatic extracts.

Diabetes complicated by alcohol misuse

Diabetic patients should exercise caution when drinking alcohol particularly those on insulin (regular heavy drinking reversibly increases insulin resistance) and oral hypoglycaemic agents (risk of hypoglycaemia), biguanides (risk of lactic acidosis). Patients on sulphonylureas may experience unpleasant disulfiram-like reactions when they drink alcohol.

Rhabdomyolysis and myoglobinuria
- Rehydration
- Renal dialysis where appropriate.

Neuropsychiatric
Acute Wernicke's encephalopathy
(pp. 119, 120 for management)

Chronic alcohol-related brain damage
Includes Korsakoff's syndrome, frontal lobe syndrome, reversible alcohol cognitive deterioration, cerebrocortical degeneration, cortical atrophy and alcoholic dementia. It is important to define type of brain damage and exclude other treatable causes of dementia.

The degree of brain damage can be assessed by referring to a neuropsychologist. Patients with marked alcohol-related brain damage (or those with co-existing severe psychiatric or medical problems) may be unable to care for themselves and require long term care or supervision or placement in a residential unit, nursing home or dementia unit. In milder cases, support either at home or in a community location by community health services is possible. Provision of information and support to carers is important.

It can be very challenging finding a satisfactory placement for individuals. Assistance from the social work team, specialist addiction services, or psychiatric, geriatric, and neurology teams may be valuable.

Abstinence from alcohol is important to preserve residual cognitive function, but can be challenging to achieve. Ensuring adequate nutrition and supplementing with thiamine 100 mg daily is recommended plus multivitamins orally daily

Memory retraining techniques—resource books for carers, memory books, memory joggers can be used. Where facilities are available, memory retraining in an appropriate environment and familiar surroundings can be attempted, though the degree of recovery is likely to be small. A structured environment with lifelong support or supervision may be required.

In some cases a guardianship order or inebriates Act may need to be invoked to assist with controlling finances (see Chapter 15, pp. 414, 415)

Psychiatric complications of alcohol misuse

Alcoholic hallucinosis and alcoholic paranoia: Both disorders can develop during a drinking bout, can begin during alcohol withdrawal or can occur within several weeks of the cessation of drinking. They occur in a state of clear consciousness (i.e. the patient is not delirious). These disorders are likely to completely resolve without medication, within a few days or several weeks if alcohol is discontinued. However, the patient may need admission and short-term antipsychotic medication if there are high levels of distress or concerns about safety.

Alcoholic dementia: Abstinence from alcohol will arrest the progression of alcoholic dementia and may lead to gradual improvement in some neuropsychiatric functions and brain scan results.

Depression: With prolonged heavy drinking, around to 80% of individuals will develop depressive symptoms, and around 30–40% of individuals will have symptoms resembling a major depressive episode. In most cases, the depressive symptoms will improve significantly during the first few weeks of abstinence, even without antidepressant medication.

In around 5% of men and 10% of women, the depression will not be alcohol-induced and will require treatment with antidepressant medication. Key indicators that the depression may not be alcohol-induced are when:

• The patient has had symptoms of major depression during significant periods of abstinence in the past (at least 4 weeks or more)
• The initial onset of depression clearly occurred before the onset of heavy drinking
• There is a strong family history of mood disorder
• The patient is still clinically depressed after 4 weeks or more of abstinence.

Studies indicate that patients with ongoing untreated depressive symptoms are more likely to relapse after treatment for their alcohol problem, therefore, concomitant treatment of both disorders is required. Treatment for depression can include counselling to address lifestyle problems (including relationship problems, unemployment, bereavement, or other losses), cognitive behaviour therapy and antidepressant medication if the depression is moderate to severe.

Antidepressant medication should be selected, which is unlikely to potentiate the effects of alcohol, such as the Selective Serotonin Reuptake Inhibitors (SSRIs), venlafaxine, moclobemide or reboxetine. The patient should be reminded that medication is unlikely to be effective if they continue to drink alcohol heavily. With continued drinking the patient may need to consider medication to reduce the cravings for alcohol, such as acamprosate. While naltrexone also reduces cravings to drink, it can sometimes exacerbate depression and should be used cautiously, ensuring the patient's mental state is monitored closely.

Anxiety: Symptoms of uncomplicated alcohol withdrawal symptoms can mimic anxiety and panic disorder. Withdrawal anxiety and its associated symptoms respond to short-term treatment with diazepam, as well as supportive care.

Once detoxification from alcohol is completed, many individuals will experience a protracted post-withdrawal phase. This may last for some months and symptoms may look like an anxiety disorder. Almost any form of anxiety can occur for 3–12 months after drinking has ceased, including generalized anxiety, panic attacks, and social anxiety. The patient should be reassured that the symptoms are likely to abate or reduce over time without treatment. Cognitive behavioural techniques may be helpful in managing the symptoms. However, a small number of patients will have a history of an anxiety disorder preceding heavy drinking, and may need medication for this during recovery. Ideally treatment of the anxiety disorder should be started after drinking has stopped but in many cases this is not possible. Initiation of an effective anti-anxiety treatment, especially an SSRI, can help get the anxiety under control, thus allowing drinking cessation. Benzodiazepines may have a place but only in specialist settings for the risk of misuse of dependence on them is high (see BAP treatment guidelines, p. 184).

Psychosocial interventions to prevent relapse

It is important to remember that remission from alcohol dependence without treatment is well described. Alcohol abstinence is usually the preferred goal, but there are numerous alcohol-dependent individuals who do not accept this, at least initially, and negotiate controlled drinking programmes with the clinician. Patients typically come to the realization that even with limit setting, moderated drinking cannot be satisfactorily achieved or sustained, and abstinence will come to be the accepted goal. Alcohol dependence is a chronic relapsing disorder and long-term goals include sustaining social functioning, and optimizing physical and mental health. Treatment goals include not only abstinence and relapse prevention, but within a 'harm-reduction' model can also include numbers of abstinence days achieved, reduced use of alcohol on drinking days and reduction of discomfort from craving.

Counselling

Much of the out-patient alcohol treatment unit's work involves one-to-one counselling, which may be described as generally supportive, but is increasingly tailored to more specific behavioural treatments. Over the years there has been an array of behavioural treatments, but at the current time the best evidence suggests:

Brief interventions
(p. 91)

Cognitive behavioural coping skills therapy

This psychological approach concentrates on coping and social skills training, emphasizing lifestyle changes in order to reduce the likelihood of relapse. The alcoholic (and family) come to recognize and avoid at-risk situations that trigger drinking, and promote methods to cope with craving. Lifestyle changes are promoted that avoid drinking situations and positive alternatives are developed.

Motivational enhancement therapy

This is a specific approach whereby the therapist style assists the client to focus on their drinking problems, and facilitate change through in depth discussion of the individual situation. Behavioural interaction is facilitated by motivational interviewing techniques developed by Miller and Rollnick. The principles include expressing empathy, deploying discrepancy, avoiding arguments, rolling with resistance and supporting self-efficacy. Stages of this treatment include building motivation and strengthening commitment to change through a series of specific strategies. (see p. 62, section on motivational enhancement.)

Cue exposure therapy

Cue exposure therapy was introduced on the basis that alcohol-related cues lead to craving for alcohol, and that this is a significant precipitant of relapse. Together with coping skills, cue exposure therapy has been shown to reduce cravings for alcohol. The addition of naltrexone to cue exposure and coping skills can result in greater reduction in cravings. Whether cue exposure leads to improved clinical outcomes in terms of abstinence and reduction in alcohol-related harm has been questioned by some recent studies. It remains therefore an experimental therapy.

Community reinforcement approaches

This approach has had positive evaluations, but is not yet widely accepted in regular clinical practice. It is a type of contingency management which involves the client's family, social, community, leisure and vocational contacts through systems of incentives and reinforcements to alter drinking behaviour.

Family involvement

Although family therapies (systems theory, problem-solving, marital therapy) have been used in alcoholism treatment, the important factor is the involvement of significant others in recovery which can enhance treatment outcomes.

Conversely, alcohol dependence is a disorder that affects family members who may themselves develop social or psychological problems needing treatment. These issues include self-blame, guilt, covering up, facilitating drinking behaviour (co-dependence), inability to focus on individual family members' needs and pre-occupation with being responsible for the dependent drinker.

Thus, a joint interview with partners and family should be sought as soon as possible if in the treatment process. There may be particular cultural reasons that put greater emphasis on family involvement from the start of treatment interventions, e.g. Indigenous populations (see Chapter 12, p. 345).

Residential or in-patient treatment (excluding detoxification)

The appropriateness of residential treatment (excluding detoxification) programmes has been subject to increasing scrutiny over the last decade. Issues have included cost effectiveness, the duration of treatment and selection criteria for residential treatment. Clearly, there are some dependent drinkers who require residential treatment, and indeed there are a variety of residential treatment services. Most of the debate is centred on the intensive therapeutic programmes, rather than other issues such as accommodation support services.

Usually in the public arena referral to residential treatment is orchestrated by an out-patient alcohol treatment unit, rather than directly from primary care. However, some centres will accept self-referred clients. In some regions phone services are available to advise members of the public where they can find appropriate residential (or out-patient) services.

Suggested criteria for residential treatment

- Completion of comprehensive assessment and diagnosis
- Failure to respond to out-patient treatment or unable to comply with this treatment
- Lack of social support including homeless, unstable living environment, surrounded by other heavy drinkers
- Co-morbid psychiatric or medical complications, or malnutrition
- Rural domicile with no out-patient services
- Severe life crises
- Co-existing severe drug dependence.

Exclusion criteria for intensive in-patient programmes include impaired cognitive function and a record of disruptive behaviour, e.g. through severe personality disorder.

Support and self-help approaches

Self-help (Mutual-help) organizations

Alcoholic Anonymous (AA)

This organization has operated internationally for more than 60 years and, although not a 'treatment' per se, is a mainstay of alcohol dependence treatment programmes. It has an estimated membership of more than 1 million, and has been a major factor in shaping public attitudes towards accepting the illness concept of alcohol dependence. AA is based on the principle that alcoholism is a physical, mental and spiritual disease which requires lifelong abstinence and participation in a recovery programme. The programme includes regular meetings based around the fundamentals of the 12-steps and 12 traditions (see Appendix, p. 446). The programme also includes a 'buddy system', fellowship, and a potential new social structure involving non-drinkers.

Recently, the effectiveness of the 12-step approach has been evaluated with findings that subjects perform similarly with 12-step treatments as with cognitive behavioural therapy. A factor not to be discounted is treatment cost savings if patients become involved in AA.

All patients attending health professionals should be offered encouragement to attend AA. Ideally, therapists should have contact with appropriate local AA members who could introduce patients to meetings, and an insight into which local meetings may best fit a client, e.g. women, young people, or specific cultural or language groups.

AA is one of several '12-step' self-help groups that teach that alcoholism is a disease and that those affected by it are powerless over the effects of alcohol. It resolutely promotes abstinence as the goal for all its members. AA groups provide a social network, a highly structured approach and clear goals and corresponding steps to recovery.

At AA meetings discussions take place after patients introduce themselves by their first name, acknowledge that they are 'alcoholic' and give a history of their alcohol problems, treatment and recovery.

The AA approach does not suit all and it may have a lower acceptance amongst women. Clearly, involvement of a patient in AA does not preclude the need for comprehensive assessment and the need to address co-existing disorders or provide other concomitant treatments.

There are several groups aligned to AA. Al-Anon is a mutual-help group for partners and relatives of alcohol-dependent people and Al-Ateen aims to support the teenage children of alcohol-dependent people.

Continuing care and rehabilitation

Alcohol dependence responds to persistent and consistent treatment, which is delivered with understanding and enthusiasm. It is inappropriate to consider treatment as consisting only of intensive 2–3-week periods of hospital (residential) therapy, without attention to the future.

At an early stage of treatment, it is important to explain to the patient that alcohol dependence is an enduring disorder, which, if treatment is suspended, is likely to show a chronic relapsing course. The relationship between the treatment service and the patient needs to be maintained over the long term. Alcohol-dependent patients should be advised that if they drink, it nearly always means loss of control and return to heavy drinking, and a progressive downhill course. Accordingly, the clear goal of treatment should be abstinence from alcohol.

Aftercare is essential. The nature of the continuing care will vary widely from person to person. It may consist of:

- Attending a programme of continuing therapy on, say, a weekly out-patient basis
- Regular follow-up by the patient's general medical practitioner, primary care nurse, psychologist or counsellor
- Regular follow-up by a medical or other specialist on alcohol treatment or addiction medicine
- Regular participation in group and counselling programmes of a specialist alcohol problems agency
- Participation in the 12-step fellowship of AA
- Pharmacotherapy, using for example naltrexone or acamprosate for 1–2 years, and regular follow-up with a medical practitioner, often in conjunction with a psychologist or other clinical colleague.

The patient's general practitioner should be made aware of the follow-up arrangements. Referral to a specialist Drug and Alcohol Unit, if available, is recommended. For maximum benefit, pharmacotherapy should always be instituted in conjunction with a comprehensive rehabilitation programme and steps to assist and monitor patients' compliance with medication.

Longer-term residential rehabilitation programmes

The cost-effectiveness of residential treatment against a community-based out-patient therapeutic programme has been debated. However, for some patients with severe alcohol dependence who have repeatedly relapsed despite comprehensive out-patient treatment/rehabilitation, a more intensive in-patient residential treatment programme lasting several weeks or months may be necessary. Residential in-patient rehabilitation is also recommended for patients what have been appropriately assessed and diagnosed:

• As malnourished and homeless without adequate social support or who live in unstable environments with a high risk of relapse (see medical officer/social worker)
• With alcohol related brain damage (e.g. Korsakoff's syndrome—neuropsychologist)
• With co-existing psychiatric disorders (e.g. depression, schizophrenia—psychiatrist)
• With co-existing other medical disorders.

Residential treatment programmes address the same issues and many use a similar use a range of treatment approaches to community based treatment programmes, including pharmacotherapies, psychological therapies, psychosocial interventions and self-help, 12-step, or other therapeutic approaches. There remain some centres that have kept their traditional focus almost exclusively on 12-step facilitation and fellowship.

In addition to providing food and shelter and some 'time out' in a safer environment, residential treatment programmes provide a structured daily routine, and staff-directed programmes and daily activities. Ideally, the programmes should be tailored according to the needs of individual patients.

Drinkers with major psychiatric or medical problems or with alcohol-related brain damage who are unable to look after themselves may require longer term care either in residential facilities or in a nursing home (also see section on guardianship, p. 414).

Harm reduction/palliation in alcohol use disorders

In some cases a dependent drinker cannot or will not cease drinking. In these cases the clinician should consider what can be done to reduce the harms to the drinker and their family and community.

Thiamine can be taken daily to reduce the risk of neurocognitive impairment, though the patient should not be lulled into a false sense of security by believing it eliminates the risk. In those with established cognitive impairment, long-term supervision may need to be organized (see Chapter 15, p. 414).

The clinician has a duty of care to consider the safety of any children who are in the care of the drinker, and to consider their safety on the road or in the workplace (Chapter 15, p. 411).

Some heavy drinkers will agree to limit the risk associated with their drinking, e.g. by leaving their car keys at home, or only drinking when their children are in the care of a responsible adult for the night. Others are unable to achieve this control. The safety of the drinker in relation to driving should be assessed and action taken if the risk of repeated drink driving seems high (see chapter on drink driving, p. 400). It is the responsibility of the treating clinician to consider the safety of any children under the care of the drinker (p. 407).

Living with a dependent drinker can be an extremely difficult experience. Several agencies offer support to the spouses and children of dependent drinkers. Mutual support is available through AA (for adult family members) and Al Ateen (for teenagers).

Prevention of alcohol use disorders and associated harms

A range of preventive measures have been successfully employed to reduce the risk of alcohol use disorders and alcohol-related harm.

Supply control, through taxation, limiting opening hours and density of licensed premises, policing responsible service of alcohol, and limiting sale of alcohol to young people, have all demonstrated effectiveness. Community-wide efforts such as mass media campaigns and school education campaigns have varying levels of success, and public policy needs to be regularly reviewed and informed by the evidence base. More recently, preventive initiatives have examined the effectiveness of increasing a young person's sense of connectedness with family, school or other group.

In Australia and elsewhere, random breath testing has significantly reduced alcohol-related road traffic accidents and mortality. In addition to educational and treatment programmes for drink drive offenders, ignition interlock devices have been successfully employed to reduce recidivism. These prevent the vehicle starting if the driver's breath alcohol exceeds a pre-set limit. They appear to work best when combined with treatment measures.

Health professionals have an important role in preventing alcohol-related harms by informing their patients about responsible drinking levels, and providing brief screening and, where necessary, intervention for all their patients.

Alcohol drug interactions

When prescribing any medication to a person with an alcohol use disorder, potential impacts of their drinking must be considered.

Acute alcohol consumption may inhibit a drug's metabolism by competing with the drug for the metabolizing enzymes, thereby prolonging and enhancing the drug's availability, and increasing the risk of side effects. Chronic alcohol consumption may induce drug metabolizing systems, thus decreasing the drug's blood level.

Alcohol's sedative effects can add to the sedative effects of another drug. Great caution and adequate safeguards must be employed when prescribing a potentially addictive drug such as benzodiazepines to an out-patient who has been alcohol dependent.

Table 4.14 Alcohol drug interactions

Medication	Type of interaction
CNS depressants: • Benzodiazepines • Barbiturates • Phenothiazines • Tricyclic antidepressants • Antihistamines • Opiates • Anaesthetic agents	Acute alcohol consumption potentiates the sedative effects of CNS depressants, particularly in the elderly.
Oral hypoglycaemic agents: • Sulfonylurea compounds	Diabetics on sulfonylureas should be advised not to drink. Acute alcohol ingestion prolongs availability of hypoglycaemic agents leading to hypoglycaemia. Hypoglycaemia may also occur if there is malnutrition or depletion of glycogen stores Chronic alcohol administration decreases the availability of hypoglycaemic agents with risk of hyperglycaemia
Antipsychotic medication: • Phenothiazines	Acute alcohol consumption increases sedative effects, impairs co-ordination and may result in liver impairment
Anticonvulsants: • Phenytoin	Acute alcohol ingestion cause side effects Chronic alcohol ingestion increases risk of withdrawal seizures

Table 4.14 (*Contd.*)

Medication	Type of interaction
Inhibitors of gastric alcohol dehydrogenase: • Cimetidine	Raise BAC—at low doses of alcohol [uncertain clinical significance at higher doses].
Oral anticoagulants: • Warfarin	Acute alcohol ingestion increases risk of haemorrhage. Chronic alcohol consumption decreases anticoagulant effects.
Non narcotic analgesics: • Aspirin, NSAIDs • Paracetamol	Increased risk of GI bleeding. Chronic alcohol consumption increases risk of liver damage with paracetamol overdose.

Further reading

Anton RF, Swift RM. Current pharmacotherapies of alcoholism: A US perspective. *American Journal on Addictions* 2003; **12**: S53–S68.

Edwards G, Marshall EJ, Cook CCH. The treatment of drinking problems, 4th edition. Cambridge: Cambridge University Press, 2003.

Lingford-Hughes AR, Welch S, Nutt D. Evidence based guidelines for the pharmacological management of substance misuse, addiction and co-morbidity: recommendations from the British Association for Psychopharmacology. *Journal of Psychopharmacology* 2004; **18**(3): 293–335.

Loxley W, Toumbourou J, Stockwell T, *et al. The prevention of substance use, risk and harm in Australia: a review of the evidence.* Canberra: The National Drug Research Centre and the Centre for Adolescent Health, 2004.

McCaul ME, Petry NM. The role of psychosocial treatments in pharmacotherapy for alcoholism. *American Journal on Addictions* 2003; **12**: S41–S52.

Raistrick D, Heather N, Godfrey C. Review of the effectiveness of treatment for alcohol problems. London: National Treatment Agency for Substance Misuse, 2006.

Scottish Intercollegiate Guidelines Network, Royal College of Physicians, Edinburgh. *The management of harmful drinking and alcohol dependence in primary care—National clinical guidelines 2003.* Available at: www.sign.ac.uk

Soyka M, Chick J. Use of acamprosate and opioid antagonists in the treatment of alcohol dependence: a European perspective. *American Journal on Addictions* 2003; **12**: S69–80.

Tobacco

Epidemiology

Cigarette smoking peaked in many western countries in 1940s and 1950s, when 75% of men and 30% of women smoked cigarettes. It has since declined greatly in response to concerted public health campaigns and legislation; for example in Australia and some Scandinavian countries the prevalence is now 16–20% of both men and women. Elsewhere in Europe the prevalence of cigarette smoking reaches approx 50%, and in South East Asia and East Asia the prevalence has risen hugely, more in males, but increasingly also in females over the past 2–3 decades, while Asia is an unashamed marketing target of the tobacco industry. More than 50% of males in Asia still smoke today and one in every three cigarettes smoked in the world today is smoked in China, where there are said to be 1000 cigarette brands. Lower socio-economic status is the major risk factor for continuing smoking in the developed countries. Even in Australia, with a low overall prevalence of smoking, some isolated and disadvantaged Indigenous communities have smoking rates of up to 80%.

The international Framework of Tobacco Control formulated by the World Health Organization clearly sets out targets that individual countries can achieve in order to reduce tobacco promotion and use. To date, more than 150 countries around the world are signatories to this document.

In many developed countries the decline in prevalence has followed anti-smoking media campaigns, tobacco price increases, bans on promotion of tobacco, restricted smoking in the workplace and public venues, and the advent of pharmacotherapies to aid in smoking cessation.

As well as the aforementioned tobacco control interventions used to reduce the level of smoking, there needs to be a better understanding of the complex nature of tobacco smoking itself so that doctors and other health care professionals can more effectively intervene to reduce the prevalence.

Impact of smoking

The World Health Organization estimates that smoking is the cause of 4% of the global burden of disease. It is a well recognized risk factor for lung cancer, aerodigestive and other cancers, chronic obstructive pulmonary disease, other respiratory diseases, and cardiovascular and peripheral vascular diseases. It is also a risk factor for type 2 diabetes and for renal disease.

Antecedents

Although initiation into smoking, that is, the first cigarette(s) ever smoked, is ruled by a multiplicity of factors including peer pressure, bravado, rebellion, advertising, weight control and curiosity, the evidence points to biological predisposition to 'responsiveness' to nicotine in the brain in some smokers and greater ability to metabolize nicotine in the liver. These predispositions are likely to lead to strong neurological rewards from smoking, and a predisposition to repeated use of cigarettes, which may initiate a lifelong 'relationship' with smoking.

There is growing evidence of differences in liver metabolism of nicotine. Poor metabolizers are reported to smoke less and find quitting easier than fast metabolizers. Racial origin can also impact on nicotine metabolism.

Some researchers believe that the reactions to the very first cigarettes smoked are a clue as to whether a person will go on to smoke continuously. The more sensitive (or responsive) the first-time smoker is to nicotine the more likely he or she is to go on to become a regular, daily smoker. Studies have shown that identical twins separated from their parents and each other at birth are both likely to be dependent smokers if their biological parents were dependent smokers, irrespective of personal histories of exposure or non-exposure, or environmental and cultural circumstances.

Many smokers have discovered nicotine is anxiolytic and that it may have an anti-depressant effect. They may 'self-medicate' with smoking tobacco to counteract anxiety or a depressed mood.

Pharmacology

Nicotine is a fast-acting drug with a short activity (half-life of 20–40 min). The most effective means of delivering nicotine to the brain is through smoking. Nicotine encourages the expression of a vast array of neurotransmitter substances in the brain, all of which have positive neurological effects in some people. In general, smokers report relaxation and stimulation, as well as anxiolytic effects. With as little as one inhalation from a cigarette, dependent smokers immediately feel less anxious, less moody, less distressed, less hungry, and less aggressive, are able to concentrate more effectively, and are relieved of strong urges to smoke. These positively reinforcing effects that occur very quickly are the bases for nicotine dependence.

There are potential nicotine receptor sites throughout the brain. However, there is evidence that individuals have different numbers of accessible receptor sites and this may be genetically predetermined. Neuronal nicotinic acetylcholine receptors have acetylcholine as their natural ligand on the $\alpha_4\beta_2$ subunit. It seems that nicotine can act very effectively at these subunit sites (and possibly others) and elicit the expression of dopamine, serotonin, β endorphin, noradrenaline, vasopressin, acetylcholine and many other hormones into the interstitial spaces between neurones. When this occurs at sites such as the hippocampus and nucleus accumbens then mood, memory, and cognitive ability may be enhanced.

Nicotine causes mild increases in blood pressure and pulse, particularly in naïve smokers.

There are complex metabolic interactions between nicotine and many substances that people use. The most common interaction studied is that between nicotine and caffeine.

Interactions between smoking and medications or psychoactive substances

These medications may require a DECREASE in dose on cessation of nicotine use as CYP1A2 plasma levels are increased with smoking, leading to higher rates of metabolism of these drugs.

Medications that may require a reduction in dose on smoking cessation:

- Paracetamol
- Caffeine
- Oestrogens
- Imipramine
- Lidocaine
- Oxazepam
- Pentazocine
- Propranolol
- Theophylline
- Warfarin
- Insulin
- Prazosin
- Clozapine.

These medications may require an INCREASE in dose on cessation of smoking, as nicotine reduces their rate of metabolism.

- Isoprenaline
- Phenylephrine.

Pathophysiology

It is estimated that one in two smokers dies prematurely from smoking related diseases. It is unclear why certain individuals are more susceptible to the adverse effects of smoking than others.

While nicotine is the component of tobacco that causes dependence, it is one of the least harmful components in terms of complications. Inhalation of gases, particulate matter, and the estimated 3000 constituents of tobacco smoke are associated with a wide range of adverse consequences.

Pure nicotine delivered slowly and in low doses (unlike from a cigarette, which is in high dose, bolus form) is associated with few medical consequences. In high dose, bolus form (as with smoking), nicotine can cause vasoconstriction, tachycardia, nausea, and headaches in those naive to nicotine.

Respiratory disorders

Smoking impairs the cough reflex, ciliary function, and immune response, and these factors predispose to acute bronchitis. Repeated episodes of acute bronchitis may be followed by chronic bronchitis and chronic obstructive pulmonary disease (COPD) including emphysema. While structural destruction in emphysema is irreversible, smoking cessation leads to improved oxygen transfer capacity and improved ciliary function with improved clearance of particulate matter from the airways. These positive responses begin to occur within days of reduced exposure to the particulate matter and gases inhaled from smoking.

Cardiovascular disorders

The cardiovascular effects from smoking are due both to the acute effects of nicotine boli, and the chronic effects of inhalation of carbon monoxide and other toxins. Acutely smoking impairs endothelium-dependent vasodilatation in both macro- and micro-vascular beds, and enhances platelet aggregation. These effects may in part be due to impaired nitric oxide formation. Chronically, smoking causes endothelial inflammation and promotes atheroma formation. The lipid profile is also altered in smokers with higher serum cholesterol, triglyceride, and low-density lipoprotein (LDL) levels, but lower high-density lipoprotein levels than in non-smokers

These effects lead to increased risk of disease throughout the vascular system in both active and passive smokers, including myocardial infarction, cerebrovascular accidents and peripheral ischaemia.

Many of the effects of smoking on the vascular system are reversible. Reversal begins within days of reduced exposure to the inhaled carbon monoxide and other toxins, and with nicotine delivered in less bolus like manners.

Cancers

Risks of cancers, particularly lung cancer, are very high in smokers and continue to occur many years after quitting smoking. The risk of lung cancer in men who smoke is 22 times higher than for non-smokers. The cause of these cancers is likely to be multifactorial, and more than 20 carcinogens have been documented in tobacco smoke.

Core clinical syndromes

Intoxication

As described above, nicotine use results in relaxation, anxiolysis and improved concentration. In the novice smoker, nicotine may lead to light headedness and nausea (see toxicity p. 158).

Dependence and withdrawal

Nicotine is a strongly addictive substance, which provides reward and reinforcement to the smoker.

Development of tolerance: Unlike most drugs of dependence, smokers do not require increasingly higher nicotine plasma levels to elicit an effect. This is possibly due to the very short active half life of nicotine. Smokers do, however, develop tolerance to the adverse effects of smoking; for example, deep inhalations cause initial light headedness in novice smokers, but not in experienced smokers.

Dependent smokers adjust or titrate their nicotine blood levels by inhaling deeper or longer to affect a higher nicotine level or inhaling more lightly and puffing quicker to lower levels.

Smokers smoke both for the positive rewards of nicotine and the relief of withdrawals.

Nicotine dependence develops with repeated self-administration of nicotine which leads to tolerance of the adverse effects of smoking, withdrawal and compulsive use of nicotine. Nicotine dependence typically involves daily use of nicotine for at least several weeks.

Nicotine withdrawal

Nicotine withdrawal is defined as occurring where abrupt cessation of nicotine use, or reduction in the amount of nicotine used, is followed within 24 h by ≥4 of the following symptoms or signs:

Features of nicotine withdrawal

- Dysphoria (depressed mood)
- Insomnia
- Irritability, frustration or anger
- Anxiety
- Difficulty concentrating
- Restlessness
- Decreased heart rate
- Increased appetite or weight gain.

These symptoms cause clinically significant distress or impairment in social, occupational, or other important areas of function, and are not due to a general medical condition or another mental disorder.

Most smokers show at least some symptoms of nicotine withdrawal. This comprises a combination of anxiety, distress, aggressiveness, urges to smoke, inability to concentrate, increase in appetite, and general moodiness. These acute symptoms occur in some smokers even between cigarettes as nicotine blood levels quickly fall. On stopping smoking, withdrawals can persist for days or weeks.

Longer-term symptoms of withdrawal can include depression and infrequent, but irritating urges to smoke linked to situations of psychological distress and other strong, often negative, triggers. Smokers have learned that these events can be 'cured' by smoking.

Other physical symptoms of withdrawal that may occur within weeks of quitting include mouth ulcers and cough, which ironically may appear for the first time or increase after quitting smoking.

Relief from the acute symptoms of withdrawal usually occurs within the first few puffs of a cigarette. The learning of the 'relief' provided by smoking becomes an insidious factor encouraging further smoking.

Natural history

Smoking, as with any dependence on a psychoactive substance, can be viewed as a chronic illness. This can help understand why some smokers may not be receptive to messages about quitting or find it difficult to quit. Like any chronic illness, some smokers have:

- A long history—they may have been smoking for many decades
- Remissions—they may have been able to occasionally cease smoking
- Relapses—they typically have gone back to smoking many times
- Poor spontaneous recovery—just stopping smoking without any effort is unusual
- Limited treatment outcomes—at best 50% of treatment-seeking smokers are able to quit for good.

Smoking shows convincing evidence of being a compulsive behaviour, rather than a 'bad habit' as:

- 96% of smokers do it daily
- Few smoke less than five per day
- 50% smoke within 30 min of waking
- 48% have not abstained for more than one week in the past five years
- 67% say they wish to quit
- Heavier smokers wish to quit equally
- 80% have tried to quit, 58% more than once
- 75% of self-quitting attempts fail in the first week
- Smokers who attempt to quit many times still want to quit.

Smokers have also 'learned' the pleasurable neurological effects of smoking in combination with other substances, such as alcohol, caffeine and cannabis. Potent, cue-conditioned responses resulting in strong urges to smoke may accompany the use of these substances. Smokers are known to consume at least twice the amount of alcohol and caffeine as non-smokers, and may have lower tolerance to alcohol or caffeine toxicity on quitting smoking.

Some smokers have few symptoms of withdrawal when nicotine deprived; many spontaneously cease smoking without aid and do not relapse, while others self-report formidable and overwhelming withdrawal symptoms on cessation, and though persistently attempt to quit, always relapse.

The experienced relief provided by nicotine for negative symptoms, such as anxiety, means that smoking is used to relieve all types of anxiety states, or negative situations and events, as well as in withdrawal.

There is substantial evidence that most smokers want to quit. Relapse is endemic in smokers who make an unaided quit attempt, with 50–75% relapsing within one week of a concerted quit attempt, and more than 62% within the first 2 weeks, with an ever reducing likelihood of relapsing after 3 months. At best, about 5–15% of smokers committed to quitting on their own are still not smoking one year later. Hence, the first 2 weeks, then the first 3 months are important targets dates for interventions in helping smokers quit.

Assessment of smoking including level of nicotine dependence

Smokers may require an assessment of their level of dependence, history of quitting attempts, their environmental exposure and their medical status in order to recommend suitable individualized treatment.

Level of dependence: Smokers range in levels of nicotine dependence from mild through to severe. Ability to quit smoking has been shown to be directly related to measurable levels of dependence, with multiple attempts to quit unsuccessfully correlated with higher levels of dependence. One simple question from the Fagerström Tolerance Questionnaire (FTQ) can be used to assess level of dependence: How long after you wake do you smoke your first cigarette? A short 'time to first cigarette' within the first half-hour of waking, indicates high levels of dependence. It also correlates with severity of withdrawals and relapse risk. Time to first cigarette (TTFC) should be asked of every current smoker. Once dependence is established, with continued smoking the level of dependence does not change over time.

Note that number of cigarettes smoked, brand of cigarettes (including level of nicotine in the cigarette) or duration of smoking are not related to levels of dependence:

- Length of abstinence with previous cessation attempts—(days, months, years?). The shorter the length of abstinence the more frequent follow-up should be
- Symptoms of withdrawal at last quit attempt—watch for these symptoms in this quit attempt and vigorously treat them
- What is the exposure to other people's smoking—in the home, at work?
- Proximal smoke → increased likelihood of relapse, therefore lowering exposure to passive smoking needs to be discussed
- Concomitant alcohol and caffeine use. Nicotine → reduced potency of both of these substances therefore smokers tend to drink alcohol and caffeine in higher amounts than non-smokers (about double); will need to reduce intake of these by at least half during quit attempt
- Assess other substances smoked, e.g. cannabis (known to increase risk of relapse to tobacco smoking)
- Medical complications and co-morbidities
- Current or previous history of depression or depressive episodes (depression is known to be exacerbated in withdrawals and to increase risk of relapse).

Overview of treatment to assist in smoking cessation

The main approaches to therapy for smoking cessation that are not mutually exclusive are brief intervention and more intensive interventions.

Which treatment to offer?

If the individual has:
- No previous experiences in quitting → Brief Intervention
- Short lived past attempts to quit (less than several days abstinence) or whose past quit attempts have been difficult with or without pharmacotherapy → Intensive Interventions.

Whatever the treatment employed, a smoker should pass through the transition from smoker to non-smoker with minimum withdrawals, either acute or chronic, physical and psychological. The search still continues for this ideal method.

Screening and brief intervention

There is evidence that short recurring comments on smoking status by a primary care health worker can effect a quit rate of about 5% in the smoking community and is therefore a cost-effective intervention that takes little time or training.

A guide to how to conduct brief intervention is the easy to use '5As' (see Box): Address, Assess, Advise, Assist, and Arrange follow-up. Simple health warnings to every smoker every time he/she visits a doctor or health worker is the minimum that should be done. Offering nicotine replacement therapy (NRT) may also be a part of brief intervention.

The core steps of brief intervention can be summarized using the '5 As'	
ADDRESS	The patient's agenda
ASSESS	The reasons for quitting, current status and past attempts
ADVISE	Personalized message-coping strategies
ASSIST	Tips for quitting, medications
ARRANGE	FOLLOW-UP
	Solve projected problems, discuss relapse risks, encourage a repeat attempt

More intensive management of smoking

There are two components to smoking cessation treatment: acutely arresting the activity of smoking and then the maintenance of long-term abstinence. Relapse to smoking is so endemic within the first two weeks of a quit attempt that this period should be the main focus of attention in the first instance when helping a smoker to quit.

There is evidence that some smokers in developed countries around the world who have been exposed to a strong anti-smoking climate are 'harder targets' who require intensive help, pharmacological interventions and relapse prevention advice. They are often smokers who have medical repercussions from smoking but persist and, by definition, show high dependence.

These smokers respond well to frequent counselling and medications. Interventions and time taken in consultations are dose related to successful permanent quitting. This level of intensity is reported to be at least as cost effective in this group of smokers as any other medical intervention might be for any other illness.

At best, with any single pharmacotherapy, about 30% of treatment seeking smokers will remain abstinent from cigarettes one year after treatment. Increasing therapy (combining therapies and increasing doses) and intensive counselling can improve permanent abstinence rates to around 50%. There is a dose relationship between pharmacotherapy and frequency of counselling, as dependence on cigarettes is not solely that of a pharmacological process, but a concomitant psychosocial behaviour.

Commonly used methods to quit smoking

'Cold turkey'

Simply stopping smoking without any medication is the commonest form of a quit attempt (80%). However, most smokers (92%) who attempt 'cold turkey' relapse and multiple attempts over many years are necessary to achieve permanent abstinence. A recent US study has shown that it may take as many as 14 formal attempts to finally stop smoking.

Table 5.1 One-year success rates by intensity of intervention (across all settings)

No action	1 %
Brief advice in primary care	5–8 %
Brief advice plus NRT in primary care	10 %
Intensive professional counselling alone	15–20 %
Intensive professional counselling plus NRT	30–40 %

Pharmacotherapies to assist in smoking cessation
Nicotine replacement therapies (NRT)
One of the most effective and commonly available pharmacotherapies for treating nicotine dependence is nicotine replacement therapy. Some researchers prefer the term 'nicotine reduction therapy' as the peak arterial blood levels these therapies delivered are often only one-fifth of the nicotine derived from cigarettes.

Replacement therapies double the chance of achieving stable remission from smoking compared to an unmedicated quit attempt.

Nicotine gum
Nicotine is absorbed through the oral mucosa quite readily, as tobacco chewers and cigar smokers are aware, and considerable blood levels of nicotine can be obtained through the use of nicotine gum. Nicotine gum shows ample long-term success above placebo in all controlled trials to date. As doses or combination of nicotine products increase outcomes can improve to 40% or more validated abstinence at 12 months.

If a smoker smokes within the first 20 min after waking and smokes more than 20 cigarettes per day, excluding medical contra-indications, they would be appropriate for 4 mg nicotine gum. Others should start with 2 mg gum and increase the frequency or dose if needed.

The nicotine patch
Slow release, low dose nicotine from the transdermal patch delivers nicotine, but the dose is not in a bolus form and, therefore, is less rein-forcing than cigarette smoke and nicotine gum. Craving is the symptom most likely to abate with the use of nicotine patch. Anxiety, irritability, low mood, and concentration all are known to improve with patch.

Smokers who are highly dependent or smoking a large number of ciga-rettes per day may find one patch is not sufficient and may need to add oral NRT or in some cases a further patch (Fig. 5.1).

There is no evidence that weaning to lower doses of nicotine patch enhances long term efficacy. The US Surgeon General's Clinical Practice Guidelines for Smoking Cessation reiterates that there is no need to wean off NRT.

Recommendations for nicotine patch use

- In most cases initiate patch at night prior to sleep—change every night
- Sleep disturbances—particularly vivid dreaming is common, however rarely affects abstinence rates. If serious, transfer to 16-h patch, applied *mane*
- Rotate patch around upper part of the body. Not on the waist-line. Avoid fatty/hairy areas
- Up to 10% of patch wearers can have severe skin irritation. This can be due to either patch adhesive or local high-dose nicotine on skin. Site rotation often prevents this. If not hydrocortisone cream may provide relief.

Combination nicotine therapies

The nicotine dose delivered by the nicotine patch or gum alone may be inadequate for some smokers and they may continue to need to smoke, and/or have withdrawals despite these therapies. Many clinicians supplement nicotine patch therapy with nicotine gum or other forms of oral NRT for 'break-out' smoking. Advantages for combined therapy have been demonstrated. There is scope for the combination of patches, wearing several at once, and the combination of patch and other, perhaps inhaled forms of nicotine (see attached algorithm).

Other forms of nicotine replacement therapies are less widely available, but have shown excellent results.

Nicotine nasal spray

Trials have shown high long-term abstinence rates using nicotine nasal spray. Smokers with higher levels of nicotine dependence were more successful with this than on other types of therapy. However, nasal bleeding occurs in most trial patients. Nasal spray is not readily available.

Nicotine inhaler

Trials have shown good long-term abstinence; however, dependence potential is high as it is a quick reinforcer, and there is a risk that smokers will convert to this 'cleaner' form of nicotine inhalation. However, it can be considered a safer form of nicotine use and should be considered as a form of harm-reduction.

Nicotine lozenge and sublingual tablet

These have varying availability. Smokers commonly under-use these devices. If sufficiently used however they show cessation rates equal to other forms of NRT.

Nicotine delivery devices

In order of speed of delivery, risk of vascular effects and risk of dependence:
- Cigarette
- Nasal spray
- Inhaler
- Sublingual tablet
- Lozenge
- Gum
- Patch

Combination therapies

Many dependent smokers do not respond to a single pharmacotherapy and a combination of therapies may be required. In clinical practice, this is becoming increasingly necessary to effect cessation of smoking. Combinations can be that of several types of NRTs together or for example Bupropion with NRT of any or all types.

Duration of nicotine replacement therapy

In general, a minimum of 7 weeks use of NRT is recommended to reduce risk of relapse. Replacement therapy is a recommended course of treatment rather than an indefinite substitution for smoking behaviour, however very long-term use has shown no evidence of harm. There is no evidence that weaning off these therapies is of greater value that simply abruptly stopping.

A reduction of patch strength to doses such as 21, 14, then 7 mg is not required. Abrupt cessation of 21 mg nicotine patch after approximately 7 weeks of usage will not precipitate withdrawals or relapse.

Contraindications or precautions to the use of nicotine replacement therapy

Coronary artery disease and nicotine replacement therapy: There is no objective evidence for the risk of nicotine toxicity or adverse effects of NRT in ischaemic heart disease. Using any form of NRT is les harmful than smoking. Nicotine replacement therapy is currently contraindicated in the first 48 h of acute myocardial infarct or in the setting of recent onset, unstable angina.

Pregnancy and lactation

It is always preferable that a women stops smoking prior to conception or diagnosis of pregnancy. However, if she continues to smoke it is now considered less harmful to use nicotine-containing products than to continue to smoke. Continuous delivery forms of nicotine, i.e. the patch, are generally not recommended as there is a risk of harmful neuronal effects on the foetus. Pulsatile nicotine, such as gum or lozenge, is recommended, as the foetus has remissions from nicotine between cigarettes.

NRT: common problems

Reluctance to use NRT: Some smokers are reluctant to use NRT, seeing it as a passive activity or a 'crutch' and may be strongly opposed to the use of any substance, particularly a pharmaceutical product that contains nicotine, in helping them to quit smoking.

Underdosing: There are many misconceptions as to the dosage and absorption of nicotine in NRT. Most smokers achieve plasma nicotine levels by smoking tobacco far above those delivered by even the highest doses of NRT—hence, under dosing is a common problem with NRT. 21 mg nicotine patches deliver plasma levels around 10 ng/mL, 2 mg nicotine gum about 7ng/mL and 4mg nicotine gum about 15ng/mL. This compares with plasma nicotine levels after a cigarette of 40 ng/mL. These blood levels are similar with the lozenge and sublingual tablets. Inhaler and nasal spray also deliver less than optimal doses to match smoking.

Evidence of under-dosing may be:
- Concomitant smoking while on patches, gum or other NRT
- Symptoms of nicotine withdrawal while on NRT
- Discontinuation of therapy due to over-assuredness.

Table 5.2 Other common problems with NRT

Problem	Solution
Hiccups or indigestion with gum	Chew less vigorously.
Rash around patch site	Ensure patch site is being rotated. Can use 1% hydrocortisone cream.
Vivid disturbing dreams on patch	Apply new patch prior to sleep or use 16-h patch.
Inhaler seems ineffectual	Breathe in and out from it rather than deep breaths.

Remedies
- High levels of nicotine dependence require higher doses of nicotine replacement therapy. The 4 mg nicotine gum has been shown to be the most effective of all NRTs in heavily dependent smokers
- Frequent daily use of short-acting NRTs, e.g. as many gums as cigarettes smoked per day
- The clinician should note the effect NRTs are having on numbers of cigarettes smoked and titrate the NRT accordingly (Fig. 5.1). For example, if smoker who initially smoked 20 cigarettes per day on a 21 mg nicotine patch has reduced to 10 cigarettes, then the addition of oral nicotine (e.g. gum) or of another whole 21 mg patch may be appropriate. If 5 are now smoked per day then add ½ a patch or less, etc. Nicotine inhaler can also be added in this way if few cigarettes are still smoked, or if there are still strong urges to smoke, even if the smoker has maintained abstinence
- Strongly recommend that patients continue NRT for at least 7 weeks.

Risk of toxicity: Toxic levels of nicotine are very rare in smokers, but are more common in those naïve to smoking. Nausea is the primary symptom of toxicity. Light headedness may also occur. There is little to no risk of toxicity in children as most would not continue to use oral forms of the products. If swallowed there is very little absorption. Patches should, however, be kept out of the reach of children

Other pharmacological interventions
Bupropion hydrochloride
Increases the release of dopamine and noradrenaline, and it is these activities that are believed to be the cause of the positive effects it has in smoking cessation. Bupropion can promote up to 30% quit rates in smokers and is safe to use in most smokers.

Bupropion is commenced while the smoker is still smoking.

One 150 mg bupropion tablet is taken for 3 days then the dose is increased to two 150 mg tablets 8 h apart daily. Smokers may lose a desire to smoke or find smoking unrewarding within a few days after commencement of bupropion. A set quit date is recommended by the manufacturers, but some smokers feel disinclined to smoke and find it distasteful prior to their designated day. Cessation should be encouraged if this occurs.

Contraindications for bupropion
- Seizure or history of seizure disorders
- Central nervous system tumour
- Abrupt alcohol or benzodiazepine withdrawal
- Use of a monoamine oxidase inhibitor in last 14 days
- Eating disorders.

Clinical experience suggests that about one-third of smokers eligible for bupropion will do well and discontinue smoking, one-third will seemingly have no effect, and one-third will reduce their tobacco smoking, but not eliminate it. There is currently no known indicator that best predicts the efficacy of bupropion in smoking cessation pharmacotherapy for any given smoking patient. Choice of nicotine replacement therapy (NRT) and bupropion hydrochloride is made based on medical status; however, patients may find one type of treatment more practical than another.

If no benefit has occurred from bupropion after 2 weeks, discontinue this treatment and attempt use of NRT instead.

If bupropion has impacted on smoking, it should be continued for at least 7 weeks.

If there is a reduction in smoking, but cessation has not occurred, NRT can be added in some form to eliminate smoking.

Adverse side effects
- Seizures—rare
- Insomnia (can be reduced by taking the second dose of bupropion no longer than 8 h after the first)
- Sleep disturbance is a common symptom of withdrawal and may be unrelated to medication.

Varenicline tartrate
A partial agonist at the $\alpha_4\beta_2$ nicotinic acetylcholine receptor, reducing the rewarding effects of nicotine. Dosage is 0.5 mg for the first 3 days, 1 mg (taken as 0.5 mg bd) for the following 3 days and then 1 mg bd until the end of the 12-week treatment. Safe and well tolerated, there are no contraindications to its prescription for smoking cessation. It is used for at least 12 weeks. A quit date is set within 2 weeks of commencement of drug. However, it has been noted that some smokers reduce their smoking prior to this date, but may not completely quit by the set quit date. They should be encouraged to continue varenicline.

Trials have shown good validated long-term abstinence rates comparable to combination NRTs. Continued use beyond the recommended 12 week time period as a maintenance therapy to prevent relapse has been shown in trials to be effective.

Side effects: Nausea most common (30%)

Precaution: Depression and suicidal ideation have been reported as side-effects; however, it is unclear to what extent this reflects pre-existing depression exacerbated by nicotine withdrawals. These symptoms should be closely monitored irrespective of the medication with anyone with a history of depression.

Medications not in widespread use

The medications below have been studied in trials, but currently are not recommended as first line treatment, predominately due to side-effects.

Clonidine: Clonidine hydrochloride is a pre-synaptic agonist reducing sympathetic activity and mimicking a nicotine effect. Clonidine, an anti-hypertensive medication, has been used in the treatment of opioid withdrawals and has shown some efficacy in the treatment of nicotine withdrawals. In tablet form, however, there are considerable side-effects, particularly the lowering of blood pressure and constipation. Transdermal clonidine patch has shown some benefit in acute nicotine withdrawals with fewer side-effects and considerable relief of cravings, anxiety and irritability, although it is not favoured as a treatment in smoking cessation.

Naltrexone's opioid antagonistic effects may be helpful in reducing the positive effects of smoking.

Mecamylamine: Another blocker of the positive effects of nicotine. However, this antagonist has shown poor efficacy due mainly to side effects. Particularly severe constipation may deter the user.

Silver nitrate and silver acetate: Have been used as over-the-counter aversive substances to produce a 'bad taste' while smoking. Not only does lack of compliance interfere with successful abstinence, but continuation to smoke despite the bad taste suggests lack of efficacy of these products.

Nortriptyline: An antidepressant not commonly used for smoking cessation due to the side-effects, mainly cardiovascular, which require intense monitoring. Specialists in smoking cessation have increasingly used this drug successfully, however, in harder-to-treat smokers.

Glucose or dextrose is a recent and simple innovation to assist smoking cessation based on the increased demand for sweet substances that smokers manifest during the withdrawal phase. It is hypothesized that either the satiation effects of glucose dampen a desire to smoke or that glucose directly affects the neuronal systems involved with nicotine. A few trials to date have shown encouraging outcomes. Weight gain in the placebo controlled trials was increased in those on placebo, rather than those on the active dextrose!

Behavioural interventions

As well as pharmacological interventions, behavioural interventions also play an (almost equally) important role in smoking cessation. Many smokers conceive of their smoking as a pleasurable habit that is too difficult to stop, especially after many years. A focus on the sociobehavioural aspects of smoking cessation is needed in order to better prevent relapse.

The initial assessment the smoking (and quitting) history will greatly help provide clues to a patient's needs.

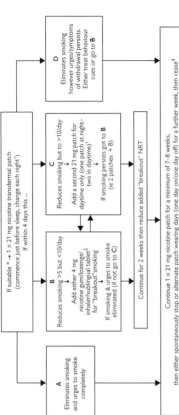

A

Eliminates smoking and urges to smoke completely

B

Reduces smoking >5 but <10/day

Add either 4 mg nicotine gum/lozenge/ inhaler/sublingual tablet[2] for "breakout" smoking

If smoking & urges to smoke eliminated (if not go to **C**)

C

Reduces smoking but to >10/day

Add a second 21 mg patch for daytime only (one patch at night— two in daytime)[3] →

If smoking persists got to **B** (ie 2 patches + B)

D

Eliminates smoking however urges/symptoms of withdrawal persists. Either treat behaviour cues or go to **B**

If suitable * → 1 × 21 mg nicotine transdermal patch (commence just before sleep, change each night[1]) If within 4 days this ...

Continue 1 × 21 mg nicotine patch for a minimum of 7–8 weeks, then either spontaneously stop or alternate patch wearing days (one day on/one day off) for a further week, then cease[4]

Continue for 2 weeks then reduce added "breakout" NRT

* CONTRAINDICATIONS: 1) PREGNANCY OR LIKELIHOOD (other NRT OK but not Patch)
2) RECENT CARDIOVASCULAR EVENT (48hrs)

1. Applying patch last thing before sleep allows a slow rise of nicotine overnight—the likelihood of 1st cigarette of the day "urge" is diminished.
2. Either 4 mg nicotine gum or lozenge depending on patient choice. Inhaler or sublingual tablet can be used if patient needs faster reinforcement.
3. No evidence in our experience of toxicity. Consider reducing dose if nausea occurs.
4. No evidence for weaning (or reduction) of patch strengths.

Fig. 5.1 Combination nicotine replacement therapy algorithm for hard-to-treat smokers.

Adapted from : Renee Bittoun. A combination nicotine replacement therapy (NRT) algorithm for hard-to-treat smokers. *Journal of Smoking Cessation* 2006; **1**: 3–7.

Some aspects of behavioural changes that need to take place to effect permanent abstinence are:
- Educate the patient on the nature of nicotine dependence
- Educate about withdrawal symptoms and the time-course of withdrawals
- Encourage and provide evidence based 'tips' that will help (Fig. 5.2)
- Arrange frequent follow-ups

Adjust or change pharmacotherapy when needed.

What 'tips' are useful and which may be counterproductive?
Tips that have NOT been demonstrated to be helpful:
- There is no evidence that drinking water alleviates withdrawals, flushes the system of nicotine or is valuable as a distraction technique
- Should we recommend total changes in social and environmental contexts? Changes in habits do not necessarily help. Just as treatment for phobias involve the repeated exposure to the cause, cue exposure (the repeated exposure to triggers) has been shown to diminish responses and urges to use. Thus smokers should not avoid situations that may trigger an urge to smoke, such as using the telephone, driving a car, arguments or even going to a bar or club. Only where there is a significant impact of another drug itself should that behaviour be avoided, e.g. alcohol or cannabis use and exposure to someone else's tobacco smoke
- Do not recommend cutting down or nicotine 'fading' (weaker cigarettes) as dependent smokers tend to compensate by inhaling deeper and extracting as much or more nicotine, and particulate matter than through stronger or more numbers of cigarettes.

Social context
Cue conditioning often leads to cravings and strong urges to smoke in situations where smokers have often smoked and are free to do so.

Well-established smoking environments are often in the home and it is there that smokers are strongly affected by cues that create urges to smoke. Eliminating their own smoking from the home surroundings is the first step towards extinguishment of cravings in a smoker's personal surrounds.

Relapse prevention
Refer to assessment of smoking history to identify potential triggers for relapse.

Note that lapses (even a single puff) become full relapses in 95% of cases so that patients must be warned about the temptation to limit their smoking to 'the odd puff'.

Three main risk factors for relapse in the initial quitting phases are:
- overwhelming withdrawals
- close proximal smoking by others
- increased alcohol consumption.

Longer-term risks are poor responses to negative life events.

Follow-up: Implicit in relapse prevention is the scheduling of follow-up visits. There is evidence that scheduled, consistent and frequent enquiries into smoking status and efficacy of treatments for the weeks immediately post quitting with continuing enquiries for the first three months will help smokers maintain abstinence.

Methods for smoking cessation with little evidence for efficacy

There are many alternative remedies, including creams, teas, drops and so-called 'wonder cures' that are currently available that have never been subjected to proper clinical trials and those that have, have shown poor efficacy.

Hypnotherapy and acupuncture: There is much anecdotal evidence that both of these therapies have helped many smokers quit smoking; however few trials have ever demonstrated positive outcomes. Some studies have shown both real and sham acupuncture points elicit the same results, and there is no evidence that acupuncture has any effect on nicotine withdrawals.

Weaning off nicotine by reduction of numbers of cigarettes or nicotine content: Many smokers have felt comforted by the notion that by reducing the number of cigarettes they smoke per day or reducing the intake of nicotine by smoking the so-called 'milder' cigarettes would assist them in quitting smoking. A dependent smoker is most likely to titrate the nicotine content required so that either more cigarettes are smoked when the concentration of nicotine is lowered, or deeper inhalations are made as compensation for reducing the number of daily cigarettes smoked, raising blood carbon monoxide levels. However, if strict smoking criteria are adhered to, that is a regimented daily reduction, this method may have some positive outcome.

Harm reduction/palliation

As smoked nicotine intake is suppressed when on NRT and, correspondingly, particulate matter and harmful carbon monoxide intake is reduced, harm-reduction is a reasonable and safe option to consider in smokers unwilling or unable to quit. It is less harmful to smoke while using NRT than smoking without it. Reducing smoking in this manner may also be a gateway to quitting. Temporary abstinence is common where smokers use NRTs in situations where smoking is banned, e.g. airports, workplaces. This is safe and should be encouraged as a harm-reduction strategy. Health groups around the world advocate 'a cutting down to quit' regimen that involves daily alternating smoking a cigarette with any form of NRT such as gum, lozenge, sublingual tablet or inhaler. The formula called NARS (Nicotine Assisted Reduction to Stop) has shown good unintentional long-term quitting rates.

> **Benefits of using NRT for temporary abstinence**
>
> • Relieves cravings and other withdrawal symptoms
> • Reduces cigarette consumption and prevents compensatory smoking
> • Smokers may learn that they can manage without tobacco for several hours, which may increase motivation and confidence to quit altogether.

Prevention

The international Framework of Tobacco Control (FTC) formulated by the World Health Organization clearly sets out targets that individual countries can achieve in order to reduce tobacco promotion and use. To date, more than 150 countries around the world are signatories to this document.

In many developed countries the decline in prevalence of smoking has followed anti-smoking media campaigns, tobacco price increases, bans on promotion of tobacco, restricted smoking in the workplace and the advent of pharmacotherapies to aid in smoking cessation.

As well as the aforementioned tobacco control interventions used to reduce the level of smoking, there needs to be a better understanding of the complex nature of tobacco smoking itself so that doctors and other health care professionals can more effectively intervene to reduce the prevalence.

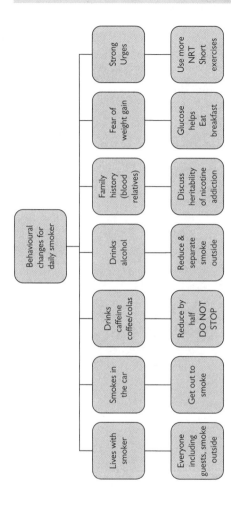

Fig. 5.2 Tactics to assist quitting.

Conclusion

There are no longer any grounds for doctors and other health care workers to ignore the management of smoking. With care and diligence to the ever-increasing treatments available, we can look forward to expecting many smokers to quit permanently or at least to reduce the harm caused by smoking.

Further reading

Treating tobacco use and dependence. Clinical practice guideline. U.S. Department of Health and Human Services. June 2000. Full text available at: www.surgeongeneral.gov/tobacco/default.htm

Sedative hypnotics

Sedative hypnotics are central nervous system depressants that act on the GABA-A receptor system, the main inhibitory system in the brain. Numerous sedative hypnotic drugs are available on prescription, or in some countries can be purchased in pharmacies or (illegally) on the streets or over the internet.

Sedative hypnotics include:
- Benzodiazepines
- Zolpidem, zopiclone and zaleplon ('Z' drugs)
- Barbiturates.

Benzodiazepines

The most commonly used sedative hypnotics are the benzodiazepines, which were first introduced into clinical practice in the 1960s. Prior to the introduction of benzodiazepines, the most commonly available sedative hypnotics were the barbiturates and non-barbiturate drugs, such as methaqualone and chloral hydrate. Benzodiazepines, marketed as a safer alternative to barbiturates, is now one of the most prescribed drugs on the market. The last decade has seen the introduction of the so called 'z drugs', which include zolpidem and zopiclone, as hypnotics.

Epidemiology

In Western societies, it is estimated that 10–20% of adults regularly take benzodiazepines. Although in the past decade there has been a relative reduction of prescriptions for day-time use in anxiety treatment, hypnotic use remains quite stable. Self-medication with benzodiazepines is also common, particularly by people who are alcohol or opioid dependent, or who misuse psychostimulants. 35.5% of the total PBS medicines obtained by doctor shoppers in Australia are for benzodiazepines.

Pharmacology

Benzodiazepines have sedative/hypnotic, anxiolytic, anti-convulsant, and muscle relaxant properties.

They increase gamma aminobutyric acid (GABA) inhibition by acting as indirect modulators on the GABA A receptor, which has specific binding sites for these drug—the so-called benzodiazepine receptor. There are a number of different subtypes of the GABA-A receptor that are thought to mediate the various actions of benzodiazepines. For instance the alpha 1-GABA A receptors mediate sedation/ataxia, some anterograde amnesia and some seizure protection; alpha 2 and 3–GABA-A subunits mediates anxiolysis, and some anticonvulsant and skeletal muscle relaxation. Alpha 5 units are highly localized in hippocampus and contribute to the amnestic actions.

Benzodiazepines are well absorbed after oral use. A number of long-acting benzodiazepines, e.g. diazepam, are metabolized in the liver to active metabolites, e.g. nordiazepam, and excreted in the urine. In a setting of illicit drug use, oral benzodiazepines may be crushed or otherwise prepared for injecting. Very lipophilic benzodiazepines, such as flunitrazepam, are sometimes crushed and snorted.

The duration of action of benzodiazepines depends on the half life of the parent drug and its active metabolite (see table 6.1). Because of long half- lives, urine drug screens of long-acting benzodiazepines may test positive for up to several weeks after use.

Side effects of benzodiazepines

- Drowsiness, dizziness
- Tiredness
- Dysarthria
- Ataxia, risk of falls (particularly the elderly)
- Impaired psychomotor performance and reaction time (increased risk of accidents)
- Poor memory and concentration
- Anterograde amnesia (occurs after taking the drug)
- Emotional blunting
- Rarely, paradoxical excitement and disinhibition (particularly in children and the elderly).

There is no current evidence to indicate that benzodiazepine use or withdrawal results in permanent structural or functional brain damage.

Clinical indications

- Insomnia—short-term use only, less than 2 weeks, or tolerance and dependence may develop*
- Anxiety/panic attacks—short term use only, while other appropriate medications (e.g. antidepressants) are initiated. Sometimes used for breakthrough acute anxiety symptoms which are not well controlled by other means
- Pre-anaesthetic medication
- Seizures/epilepsy—acute use especially to cease seizure activity p. 118
- Skeletal muscle relaxation (muscle spasms, e.g. acute back pain)
- Withdrawal syndromes:
  - Benzodiazepine withdrawal (p. 180)
  - Alcohol withdrawal (pp. 115, 116, 389)
  - Opioid withdrawal (p. 216)
  - Cannabis withdrawal (p. 196)
- Certain other psychiatric illnesses, e.g. mania, psychotic states including drug-induced psychosis, where benzodiazepines are often used combination with antipsychotic medication in short term management of acute psychosis (pp. 260, 266).

---

* Controlled trial data for eszopiclone (the active enantiomer of zopiclone) have shown efficacy for over six months and it now has a license for long-term treatment of insomnia in the USA.

Table 6.1 Benzodiazepine half life and conversion table

Form of benzodiazepine	The dose of that benzodiazepine which is approximately equivalent to diazepam (5 mg)	Approximate $t_{1/2}$ (hours)
Ultra-short acting benzodiazepines ($t_{1/2}$ < 4 hrs)		
Trizolam	0.25 mg	1–3 hrs
Midazolam	15 mg	1–3 hrs
Short to intermediate acting benzodiazepines		
Oxazepam	15 mg	4–15 hrs
Lorazepam	1 mg	12–16 hrs
Temazepam	10 mg	5–15 hrs (10 hrs)
Bromazepam	3 mg	20 hrs
Alprazolam	0.5 mg	6–25 hrs
Flunitrazepam	1 mg	20–30 hrs
Clobazam	10 mg	17–49 hrs
Nitrazepam	5 mg	16–48 hrs
Long acting benzodiazepines includes effects of active metabolites:		
Clonazepam	0.5 mg	22–54 hrs
Diazepam	5 mg	20–80 hrs
Chlordiazepoxide	10 mg	>50 hrs
Flurazepam	15 mg	>50 hrs
Chlorazepate	10 mg	>50 hrs
'Z' drugs		
Zolpidem	10 mg	2.4 hrs
Zopiclone	7.5 mg	5.2 hrs
Zaleplon	10 mg	1.5 hrs

NB: Benzodiazepines with long half lives should be avoided in patients with hepatic or renal decompensation. Adapted from NSW Drug & Alcohol Withdrawal Guidelines & Guidelines for the prevention and management of benzodiazepine dependence. Monograph Series no 3, NHMRC, 1991, MIMS Australia.

Short half-life drugs have a higher risk of withdrawal problems with inter-dose and early morning anxiety. Long half-life preparations have more residual day time drowsiness and cognitive impairment.

Core clinical syndromes

Benzodiazepine overdose/intoxication

- Drowsiness, confusion
- Dysarthria, ataxia
- Impaired co-ordination and concentration (increased risk of accidents)
- Coma
- Respiratory depression (use with care in-patients whose respiratory system is compromised)
- Death (particularly if used in combination with other CNS depressants such as alcohol, opioids).

Non-dependent benzodiazepine misuse

Benzodiazepine misuse/hazardous use: A person may misuse benzodiazepines, e.g. purchase them from the street, use intermittently in supratherapeutic doses, or dissolve oral preparations for use in the intravenous route, but may not yet have clear adverse effects or dependence.

Harmful benzodiazepine use (ICD): An individual may experience physical harms from their use of benzodiazepines (e.g. falls in the elderly, accidents, or other complications of injecting benzodiazepines).

Benzodiazepine abuse (DSM): Benzodiazepine abuse occurs when recurring benzodiazepine misuse results in repeated adverse social impacts, but the individual is not dependent on benzodiazepines. For example, their benzodiazepine use may result from a conscious desire to intermittently use benzodiazepines as 'downers' to overcome excitatory effects of psychostimulants, for the relief of alcohol or opioid withdrawal symptoms, or to relieve insomnia, stress or anxiety.

> ### Patients at increased risk of benzodiazepine abuse/dependence
>
> - Insomniacs (particularly the elderly)
> - Patients with chronic pain (prescribed benzodiazepines for muscle relaxation, insomnia, anxiety)
> - Patients with:
>   - Alcohol dependence (for alleviation of withdrawal symptoms—see pp. 115, 116, 122, 123)
>   - Opioid dependence for alleviation of withdrawal symptoms (includes those on methadone or buprenorphine maintenance programs- see p. 216)
>   - Psychostimulant abuse/dependence (as a 'downer'—see p. 260)
> - Psychiatric illnesses:
>   - Generalized anxiety disorders
>   - Panic attacks
>   - Agoraphobia
>   - Psychotic states
>   - Depression
>   - Anti-social personality disorders
> - Polysubstance users (see p. 283).

A high level of awareness of potential benzodiazepine use or misuse is necessary.

Benzodiazepine dependence

Dependence on benzodiazepines may occur after regular, daily use for more than 4–6 weeks, even at therapeutic doses. When a person is dependent on benzodiazepines, they will typically experience withdrawal symptoms on cessation or marked reduction in dose (see below), they become tolerant to the hypnotic and sedative effects. In some cases, usually where use has been at supratherapeutic doses, they may have impaired control over use (e.g. be unable to stop use when they want to) or be aware of a strong desire to use benzodiazepines, and may continue to use despite evidence of harms (e.g. falls, accidents, injuries). Once benzodiazepine dependence has developed it is difficult to successfully discontinue use.

The benzodiazepine withdrawal syndrome

The benzodiazepine withdrawal syndrome is a cluster of somatic, psychological and behavioural symptoms, which arise on abrupt discontinuation or dose reduction of benzodiazepines in a benzodiazepine dependent individual.

Abrupt discontinuation of benzodiazepines, or tapering off benzodiazepines too quickly, when it is prescribed for insomnia, generalized anxiety disorders, panic attacks, or agoraphobia, may result in either recurrence of the underlying disorder, a rebound of symptoms or a benzodiazepine withdrawal syndrome. These are difficult to distinguish in clinical practice as they may occur simultaneously or sequentially.

The time course of benzodiazepine withdrawal depends on the half life of the benzodiazepine used. For short-acting benzodiazepines (oxazepam, temazepam, lorazepam), onset of withdrawal symptoms occur 1–2 days after the last dose, peaks at 2–5 days and lasts 2–4 weeks or more. For longer-acting preparations (diazepam; chlordiazepoxide), onset of withdrawal symptoms occur later, peak at 7–10 days and last for 8 weeks or longer (see below). In some cases, a protracted withdrawal phase may last up to 12 months.

The risk of benzodiazepine withdrawal and the severity of the withdrawal syndrome is increased with shorter half- life of the drug, higher doses, the rapidity of withdrawal, the underlying personality of the patient, and co-existing medical, alcohol and other drug problems. Two-thirds of benzodiazepine dependent patients are women. Benzodiazepine withdrawal seizures are serious and life threatening.

Benzodiazepine withdrawal syndrome—clinical features

Somatic symptoms and signs
- Sweating
- Tremor, fasciculations
- Muscle pain, stiffness and aches (limbs, back, neck, jaw)
- Dizziness, light-headedness
- Parasthesia, shooting pains in neck and spine
- Palpitations
- Visual disturbances (blurred vision, diplopia, photophobia, vision lags behind eye movements)
- Tinnitus, headache
- Gastro-intestinal symptoms: nausea, anorexia, weight loss, diarrhoea (may resemble irritable bowel syndrome). Weight loss is prominent in the long term.
- Faintness and dizziness; sense of unsteadiness
- Menorrhagia and breast pain
- Spontaneous orgasms.

Psychological symptoms
- Rebound insomnia, nightmares
- Anxiety, panic attacks
- Irritability, restlessness, agitation
- Poor memory and concentration
- Perceptual distortions—sensory hypersensitivity (light, sound, touch, taste); abnormal sensations, e.g. 'cotton wool' sensations
- Metallic taste
- Distortions of body image
- Feelings of unreality, depersonalization, derealization
- Depression, dysphoria.

Acute Brain Syndrome
- Confusion; disorientation (may be intermittent). A common cause of confusion in the elderly.
- Delirium (in the absence of autonomic hyperactivity)—particularly in the elderly
- Delusions, paranoia
- Hallucinations (visual, auditory)
- Grand mal seizures—occur 1–12 days after discontinuing benzodiazepines. Patients taking high doses (>50 mg diazepam equivalence) are at increased risk of seizures

Consider benzodiazepine withdrawals in unexplained seizures in an adult.

Grand mal seizures and delirium constitute serious and potentially life threatening withdrawal symptoms.

Complications of benzodiazepine use

Physical complications of benzodiazepine use

- Overdose/intoxication (accidental or suicidal)
- Accidents, injuries.
- Benzodiazepine dependence and withdrawal (by far the most important)
- Complications of injecting oral preparations: As well as the usual risks of injecting drug use (see p. 367), there are added risks when powders or gels intended for oral use are prepared for and used intravenously, e.g. local vascular irritation, and as veins become less accessible, users may deliberately, or accidentally inject into arteries. This may result in particulate matter lodging in peripheral vasculature, resulting in ischaemia and gangrene, and diffuse lung disease.

Neuropsychiatric complications of benzodiazepine use/co-morbidity

Memory impairment/anterograde amnesia: Impairment of ability to learn new information. However, the recall of information learned prior to taking the drug is not affected (indeed, can even be enhanced). This memory impairment is more likely with intravenous administration or high oral doses; when other sedative agents are used (e.g. alcohol); and with short half-life, high potency benzodiazepines (e.g. triazolam). The sedative and amnestic effects are sometimes used preoperatively or to subdue a victim, and erase the victim's memory of the crime. For example, flunitrazepam has been termed the 'date rape' drug when slipped into the victim's drink (though in the majority of such cases alcohol is the sole or primary intoxicant).

The amnesic effect of high dose benzodiazepines is more commonly an undesired side effect of misuse. Individuals using high doses (e.g. up to 25 tablets as a handful), may commit crimes, while disinhibited, e.g. assault or shoplifting, then not remember this the next day.

With long-term use of benzodiazepines, even with therapeutic doses, the problem is with consolidation of memory, i.e. information of interest is noted and can be recalled immediately, but is not transferred into long-term memory. However, recall of information learned prior to benzodiazepine intake is not affected. This is more likely in the elderly where it may resemble dementia.

Anxiety: During benzodiazepine withdrawal, a number of symptoms that resemble an anxiety disorder, can occur including social phobia, generalized anxiety disorder, obsessive-compulsive disorder, and panic disorder (see p. 173). It is difficult to distinguish whether these symptoms represent a recurrence of the underlying anxiety disorder currently being treated, or a rebound of symptoms during the benzodiazepine withdrawal. However, withdrawal-related anxiety symptoms are time-limited, improving significantly within a month and disappearing altogether within several months. If the symptoms represent re-emergence of a pre-existing anxiety disorder, they are likely to persist and worsen during the first month post-withdrawal.

Depression: While not common, benzodiazepines have been reported to cause depression or exacerbate existing symptoms of depression. Depression may emerge during benzodiazepine withdrawal and can lead to relapse.

Paradoxical disinhibition: Rarely, instead of having the expected calming, sedating effect, benzodiazepines may cause irritability, restlessness, hostility, aggressiveness and violence, and resemble hypomania or psychosis.

Psychosis: Psychotic symptoms in a state of clear consciousness may develop during benzodiazepine withdrawal. These include agitation, aggression, persecutory delusions, and hallucinations (mainly visual) in association with other symptoms of benzodiazepine withdrawal (see p. 173).

Delirium: May occur during:
- **Benzodiazepine withdrawal:** with confusion, delusions, hallucinations in association with other symptoms of benzodiazepine withdrawal (see p. 173) or
- **Benzodiazepine overdose:** with disorientation, confusion, memory impairment in association with reduced level of consciousness, and other signs of benzodiazepine overdose.

Social complications of benzodiazepine use

The above physical and neuropsychiatric complications of benzodiazepine use have the potential to impact on family, work, financial, relationships, and other social factors.

Natural history of benzodiazepine dependence

Most use of benzodiazepines is short term or confined to use to induce sleep. Approximately 30% of people who start taking benzodiazepine develop dependence on these drugs and this is well described as occurring at therapeutic doses of people taking the equivalent of 15 mg diazepam daily for 3 months. Forty per cent will experience a withdrawal syndrome when the drug is discontinued under double blind conditions; this increases to 70% after 6 months' administration. The risk of dependence increases as the dose extends into supra-therapeutic ranges. There is relatively little information on the natural history of benzodiazepine dependence, except that, without intervention, it tends to be long-term and there is a tendency to relapse after a period of non-use. Continuing use is characterized by increased dependence, in common with the ever-present risk of the withdrawal syndrome when supply is interrupted. The natural history in treated populations varies widely, with abstinence rates of 70% at 1 year being reported in the people prescribed benzodiazepines legitimately, and also in elderly populations and ranging down to 20% in other studies, and below in street users of these drugs.

Screening and opportunistic intervention

• Routinely inquire whether benzodiazepines are taken for insomnia, stress, anxiety, etc.
• How much is taken, whether daily or intermittently, and for how long.
• Determine whether the patient is using benzodiazepines hazardously or harmfully, or whether the patient is dependent on benzodiazepines.

If the patient is not dependent, but using benzodiazepines hazardously/harmfully, the principles of brief intervention can be applied, as described by the FLAGS acronym, i.e.

F—Feedback on problems experienced or likely to be experienced
L—Listen to readiness to change
A—Advise patient about the potential risks associated with continued benzodiazepine use, in particular benzodiazepine dependence and withdrawals and recommend change in pattern of use
G—Negotiate goals
S—Set strategies.

If the patient is benzodiazepine dependent, follow the 10-step management of benzodiazepine dependence (p. 183).

Assessment and management of benzodiazepine overdose/intoxication

History Where history is possible (from patient, or collateral sources), try to identify:
- How much benzodiazepine was taken and the time it was taken
- Usual benzodiazepine dose, its frequency (whether daily or intermittently) and duration—to assess likelihood of dependence and subsequent risk of benzodiazepine withdrawal
- What other substances were taken concurrently (including alcohol, prescribed and illicit drugs, especially other respiratory suppressants such as opioids)
- Any major co-existing medical conditions
- Any major psychiatric co-morbidity, e.g. depression. Was the overdose suicidal or accidental?
- When the patient is stabilized, a fuller assessment can be completed (p. 36).

Clinical examination Patient may be:
- Drowsy
- Confused
- Slow, slurred speech
- Ataxic, poor co-ordination of movements
- Comatose.

Death is due to respiratory depression (particularly when taken in combination with alcohol and other CNS depressants). Look for signs of head injury or other injuries.

Investigations Routine baseline investigations:
- FBC
- Urea and electrolytes
- LFTs
- Blood sugar levels
- Arterial blood gases (if indicated)
- Blood alcohol concentrations
- Plasma or urine drug screens: will determine if there is polysubstance use
- CT head or MRI (if head injury is suspected).

Management of benzodiazepine overdose/intoxication

Simple benzodiazepine overdose is rarely life-threatening, general supportive measures are all that is required. Overdose may be more dangerous when benzodiazepines are used in combination with other CNS depressants (e.g. alcohol, opioids).
- General supportive measures: maintain airways, breathing, circulation. (May require assisted ventilation, in mixed overdose with alcohol, opioids and other CNS depressants.)

- If gastric lavage and activated charcoal is considered necessary, take necessary precautions to avoid aspiration.
- In rare cases the specific benzodiazepine antagonist flumazenil may be given 1–2 mg slow IV infusion over several minutes as this often leads to rapid return to consciousness within a few minutes. As the duration of action is brief and shorter than the benzodiazepine agonists used in the overdose, repeat doses may be required after 1–2 h, so continuous monitoring is also required.

Warning—Flumazenil may precipitate a withdrawal syndrome including seizures in-patients with benzodiazepine dependence. This risk is increased if other pro-convulsant drugs (e.g. tricyclic antidepressants) have also been taken. It can also precipitate panic attacks.

- Administer parenteral thiamine, particularly if the patient has a concurrent alcohol problem (before glucose is given; see p. 114).
- If concurrent opioid overdose is suspected, administer naloxone (see p. 212)
- Exclude other causes of coma.

Assessment and management of the benzodiazepine withdrawal syndrome

Identify the problem early by taking a comprehensive drug and alcohol history and psychiatric history (pp. 37–41).

It is important that a routine history of benzodiazepine use be taken. Once a diagnosis of benzodiazepine dependence is made the time frame of benzodiazepine withdrawals can be predicted by the preparation taken (whether long- or short-acting) and the time of the last dose. (See p. 172).

History taking should include:
- Co-existing substance use or dependence, particularly alcohol, opioids and psychostimulants
- Psychiatric history and medication taken for the treatment of anxiety, generalized anxiety disorder, panic attacks, agoraphobia, psychosis.

Conduct an appropriate *clinical examination* including a thorough mental state examination.

Routine investigations, as well as blood alcohol concentrations, and plasma or urine drug screens maybe helpful, particularly in cases of polysubstance use.

Hospital in-patient treatment
Moderate benzodiazepine withdrawals
- Reassurance and support
- General supportive care, monitor vital signs and mental state every 4–8 h
- If the patient has been taking a short-acting benzodiazepine preparation, switch to a long-acting preparation, such as diazepam orally.
  Refer to equivalence table to convert the dose to diazepam. A general rule of thumb is that the smallest dose form of another form of benzodiazepine is equivalent to 5 mg diazepam.

Day 1: Administer 40% of the stated usual daily dose as the diazepam equivalent (If you are certain of the patient's dose it is permissible to prescribe 80% of it). Administer in divided doses for the next 3 days until the patient is stabilized and not showing signs of overt withdrawal.

Day 5 onwards: Gradual step wise reduction by 10% of the initial daily dose. Titrate dose and speed of reduction according to the individual response every few days.

If significant withdrawal symptoms recur, either slow the reduction or return to the previous dose until patient is stable, then reduce more slowly (e.g. by 2.5–5 mg every 7 days), according to the patient's response, until the drug is ceased.

When the need for in-patient admission is over, dose reduction may continue as an out-patient (see below). This allows for very gentle and slow weaning off benzodiazepines (see below). However, it is important that limited amounts of benzodiazepines are dispensed, preferably on a day-by-day basis.

Clinical example

A patient presents for in-patient benzodiazepine withdrawal management, having been taking 20 × oxazepam 30 mg tablets every day for 3 months:
- Calculate each oxazepam 30 mg tablet is equivalent to 2 diazepam 5 mg tablets, so the patient is taking the equivalent of 40 × diazepam 5 mg tablets daily, or 200 mg diazepam
- Reduce this outside dose to a starting dose of 40% on day 1, i.e. 16 diazepam tablets daily (80 mg). This is given as 20 mg four times daily
- Once stable (no tremor, sleeping at night), commence reductions of 10%. This can be titrated slowly according to the patient's response.

Severe benzodiazepine withdrawals (with delirium or seizures)
May require transfer to a high dependency unit or intensive care unit. Seek specialist advice:
- Administer diazepam 10 mg by slow IV injection; repeat after 30 min if necessary. Alternatively, IV midazolam may be administered
- Consider other potential causes of delirium or seizures, especially alcohol withdrawal, infections. (See p. 112, Table 4.10)
- If hallucinations are present, administer haloperidol 2.5–5 mg intramuscularly or orally. Repeat every 4–6 h if necessary. Alternatively, administer olanzapine (5–10 mg orally).

Once the acute phase is over:
- Monitor withdrawal symptoms and continue with oral diazepam, generally 40–80 mg daily in three or four divided doses for 2–3 days.
- **Tapering regimen:** once patient is stable, reduce the dose of diazepam by 10% as described above until the dose reaches 20–40 mg/day.

(Care should be taken in treatment of benzodiazepine withdrawal in the elderly and return to oral administration of diazepam as soon as feasible).

Post-discharge management
If the patient is still on diazepam at the time of discharge, arrangements need to be made for continuing its gradual dose reduction as an outpatient. With the patient's consent, and following privacy release guidelines, involve the GP in the ongoing management. The GP, (or specialist), continues the dose reduction of diazepam and monitors the patient at daily to weekly or fortnightly intervals as required. The patient is gently weaned off diazepam (see below for *out-patient tapering benzodiazepine regimen.*). Ideally, organize daily or weekly dispensing of diazepam via a pharmacy or clinic before the patient leaves hospital.

Psychological treatments are equally important adjuncts to the management during this phase (See below, p. 182).

Ambulatory benzodiazepine withdrawal management (detoxification)
Suitability for out-patient benzodiazepine withdrawal management
Outpatient benzodiazepine withdrawal management is appropriate for patients with mild benzodiazepine withdrawal who do not have a history of seizures, who are not concurrently dependent on alcohol or other

substances and who do not have significant concurrent physical or mental illnesses.

Wherever possible, the starting dose of diazepam should not exceed 40 mg diazepam/day. Any patient who requires a higher starting dose should have their benzodiazepine reduction commenced by a specialist or as an in-patient. They can then be discharged to an out-patient regime when the diazepam dose has fallen to 40 mg.

Ambulatory detoxification requires the patient's commitment and close liaison between the medical officer, general practitioner and psychologist/counsellor.

Reassure and support the patient and draw up an agreed treatment plan. Clarify the patient's understanding of the treatment plan. Some doctors seek verbal agreement while others prefer a signed written agreement of the plan. Patients generally agree to the nature of regulated dispensing, the need for random urine drug screens and not to doctor shop or seek benzodiazepines from other sources.

In Australia a patient can sign a voluntary release of information, to allow the Health Insurance Commission to regularly post to the doctor a listing of any publicly subsidized scripts dispensed for psychoactive substances. This helps to ensure that the treating doctor is the only source of benzodiazepines.

Diazepam dose regime
Convert the patient's reported usual dose of benzodiazepine to the diazepam equivalent using the equivalence table (p. 170). Patients often exaggerate their dose so commence the patient on 40% of their usual benzodiazepine dose in diazepam equivalents.

Tapering regimen: Once the patient is stable and free from withdrawal, gradually reduce the diazepam dose in a stepwise fashion e.g. by 5 mg or by 5% every 1–2 weeks. Titrate dose reduction according to the patient's response, taking into consideration anxiety, the quality of sleep and presence of tremor. If, on reduction, withdrawal symptoms recur, maintain at the previous dose until the patient is stable and then continue tapering with smaller dose decrements at longer time intervals, e.g. by 2.5 mg every fortnight. The patient has to be comfortable with, and agree to, the rate of reduction.

Final dose reduction: Typically, the final dose reduction, e.g. from below 20 mg/day is the most challenging for the patient.

Reassure the patient that the diazepam dose regimen and dose reductions are prescribed at a rate that minimizes discomfort. The medication should be taken 'by the clock' at agreed regular intervals rather than on a prn basis in response to insomnia or anxiety. This breaks the pattern of using a chemical solution to stressors.

Fully weaning off benzodiazepines varies greatly and may take weeks to months. In some severe cases, this may extend to more than a year.

Psychological treatments are mandatory for a successful outcome (see below, p. 182).

Other countries use similar regimes—see section in Lingford-Hughes *et al.* (2004).

Patient education and information
- Fully inform the patient about the potential side effects of benzodiazepines:
  - Falls (particularly in the elderly)
  - Danger of driving or operating machinery because of risk of accidents, injuries
  - Warn of the risks associated with concurrent use of alcohol, opioids and other CNS depressants
  - Pregnant women should avoid chronic use of benzodiazepines because of the risk of the neonatal withdrawal syndrome
- Patients should be advised not to take benzodiazepines on a regular basis for more than a few weeks because of the risk of dependence
- Benzodiazepine dependent patients should not suddenly stop their medication, or reduce their doses too quickly. In general, the withdrawal may be more distressing and life-threatening than continued use
- Inform the patient fully about the signs and symptoms of benzodiazepine withdrawal
- Psychological treatments are very important.

Psychological treatments
- Practical advice can be provided on good sleep hygiene, such as avoiding caffeine-containing drinks within 6 h of bedtime, plenty of daytime exercise, avoiding daytime naps, and a relaxing evening routine
- Explore alternative methods of coping with stress, anxiety, panic attacks or insomnia, e.g.
  - Relaxation therapy
  - Stress management
  - Meditation
  - Group therapy
- Explore alternative or adjunctive treatment options:
  - Cognitive behavioural therapy
  - Psychotherapy—has a useful role during benzodiazepine dose reduction, and the psychologist or other counselling staff can provide training in relaxation techniques, as well as increase the patient's awareness of triggers to benzodiazepine use and alternative ways of coping with these.

Management of benzodiazepine dependence

Management of benzodiazepine dependence

- Patient information and education
- The patient must reach a point of acceptance of the need to stop and develop a commitment to stop
- Management of benzodiazepine withdrawal: detoxification is the first step
- Pharmacotherapies: Substitution with a long-acting benzodiazepine preparation, e.g. diazepam for treatment of withdrawal (see above)
- Psychological therapies: a very important aspect of treatment, includes counselling, CBT, psychotherapy, etc.
- Treatment of underlying medical and psychiatric co-morbidity (see below)
- Support of and from family and friends
- Mutual support groups: AA, 12-step fellowships, anti-benzodiazepine groups, etc.
- After care/continual care/follow-up rehabilitation
- Personal life style and environmental changes: simple measures, such as increased exercise, getting out of the house, looking to other relaxing activities, such as music, meditation or yoga.

Treatment of co-morbidities

Referral to a psychiatrist for assessment and treatment of concurrent depression or anxiety may be required. Psychiatric assessment is much easier once any severe benzodiazepine abuse or dependence is under control, but in some cases concurrent treatment may be necessary.

Anxiety: Pre-existing anxiety disorders will need treatment and stabilization to facilitate benzodiazepine withdrawal, e.g. with SSRIs. Maintenance therapy with benzodiazepines may be helpful in some highly selected patients with a pre-existing anxiety disorder who do not respond well to other treatments. In some cases of alcohol dependence with high anxiety that are in effect self-medicating with alcohol, then maintenance benzodiazepines may be a safer option in terms of physical organ damage. Particularly in a person with pre-existing benzodiazepine or other substance dependence, regulated dispensing (at a minimum, weekly) is advisable.

Depression: If there is significant depression, this may lead to relapse to benzodiazepine use. It is advisable to stabilize on an antidepressant before attempting to stop the benzodiazepine.

Prevention of benzodiazepine abuse and dependence

Unless there is good reason, benzodiazepines should be prescribed only for short-term treatment (not more than 2–4 weeks), e.g. for patients with insomnia, anxiety, or for its anticonvulsant or muscle relaxant effects. In patients with incapacitating anxiety, weigh risks against benefits of benzodiazepines and tailor treatment according to the individual patient's needs.

The risks associated with prescribing benzodiazepines in-patients with a history of alcohol and other substance misuse include:

- Dose escalation/benzodiazepine dependence/benzodiazepine withdrawals
- Diversion to the black market
- Doctor-shopping
- Drug-affected presentations at the clinic
- Significant risk of interactions with other CNS depressants such as alcohol, opioids, cannabis
- Negative impact on mental acuity; impaired psychomotor performance
- Neuropsychiatric and subtle changes in mood including depressive symptoms.
  Minimize prescribing of benzodiazepines.

Benzodiazepines should be avoided in-patients with a history of alcohol and substance misuse unless:

- A compelling indication exists to use them (e.g. short-term management of acute alcohol withdrawal)
- There is no good alternative (e.g. treatment has failed with CBT and other medication options).

'Z' drugs

Zolpidem is an imidazopyridine hypnotic agent and zopiclone is a cyclopyrrolone hypnotic agent. Both have hypnotic properties similar to those of the benzodiazepines, but better (shorter) kinetics, so less likely to cause hangover. It was initially believed they would have low addictive potential, but since, a significant number of cases of abuse or dependence have emerged. Zaleplon is an even shorter $t_{1/2}$ hypnotic that can be used for middle-of-the-night insomnia to get people back to sleep with little risk of hangover. Es-zopiclone is the active enantiomer of zopiclone that is licensed in the USA and has controlled trial evidence of efficacy for 6 months.

Side effects of zolpidem are increasingly reported even at standard doses and especially at supratherapeutic doses. They include confusion, bizarre behaviour, somnambulance, sleep driving, bingeing on food, disinhibited sexual behaviour.

Zopiclone often leads to a metallic taste in the mouth, and may cause blurred vision and palpitations.

If withdrawal symptoms occur on cessation of chronic use, patients may be treated as for diazepam dependence (see above). In commencing a tapering diazepam regime one tablet of zolpidem (10 mg) or zopiclone (7.5 mg) is approximately equivalent to 5 mg diazepam.

Barbiturates

Barbiturates include amylobarbital, barbital, butabarbital, phenobarbital, pentabarbital, and secobarbital. Barbiturates bind to the GABAA receptor and enhance GABAergic transmission. They have a propensity to be fatal in overdose because at high concentrations they can directly open the chloride channels. Since the advent of the relatively safer benzodiazepines in the 1960s, they are no longer widely used.

Barbiturate overdose

The great disadvantage of barbiturates is that they have a low therapeutic ratio: the lethal dose may be only 4–5 times the therapeutic dose and the risk of mortality is accentuated if the person has taken alcohol or another CNS depressant.

Signs and symptoms of barbiturate overdose
* Lethargy
* Drowsiness
* Coma and death.

> Barbiturate induced coma can resemble a vegetative brain dead state. It is crucial to exclude barbiturate overdose prior to cessation of life support.

Treatment of barbiturate overdose
* General supportive measures: airways, breathing, circulation
* Intravenous fluids
* Alkanization of urine—with phenobarbital and barbital.

Barbiturate dependence

Typically seen in people who take barbiturates in doses of more than 500 mg a day on a daily basis for at least 1 month. Abrupt discontinuation in a dependent individual may lead to the barbiturate withdrawal syndrome.

Barbiturate withdrawal syndrome

Barbiturate withdrawal symptoms include tremulousness, sweating, anxiety, agitation, tachycardia, and hypertension in the early stages. If symptoms progress, seizures and delirum become life threatening.

Treatment of barbiturate withdrawal syndrome

General supportive measures, regularly monitor pulse rate, blood pressure and temperature. Observe for signs of agitation and barbiturate withdrawal.

The preferable approach is to manage the withdrawal syndrome by repeat doses of phenobarbital until the patient is sedated and mildly dysarthric. However, experience of using phenobarbital in this situation is rare these days. Accordingly, many authorities recommend the use of a benzodiazepine and the following regime is used instead:
* Oral diazepam 10–20 mg 4 times a day
* Reduce gradually by 10 mg every 2–3 days.

In severe cases, intravenous diazepam 10 mg may be required and repeat doses every 30 min if necessary. In such cases, nurse in a High Dependency Unit. Alternatively, midazolam or a barbiturate anaesthetic may be given.

If there are hallucinations, give haloperidol 5 mg every 4–6 h.

Further reading

Ashton H. The diagnosis and management of benzodiazepine dependence. *Current Opinion in Psychiatry* 2005; **18:** 249–255.

Baldwin DS, Anderson IM, Nutt DJ, Bandelow B, Bond A, Davidson J, Den Boer JA, Fineberg NA, Knapp M, Scott J, Wittchen H-U. Evidence-based guidelines for the pharmacological treatment of anxiety disorders: recommendations from the British Association for Psychopharmacology. *Journal of Psychopharmacology* 2005; **19:** 567–596.

Lingford-Hughes AR, Welch S, Nutt DJ, *et al.* Evidence-based guidelines for the pharmacological management of substance misuse, addiction and co-morbidity. *Journal of Psychopharmacology* 2004; **18:** 293–335.

NSW Drug and alcohol withdrawal clinical practice guidelines. Mental Health and Drug and Alcohol Office, NSW Department of Health 2007. http://www.health.nsw.gov.au

Nutt DJ, Malizia AL. New insights into the role of the GABA(A)-benzodiazepine receptor in psychiatric disorder. *British Journal of Psychiatry* 2001; **179:** 390–396.

Royal College of Psychiatrists. Benzodiazepines: risks, benefits or dependence. A re-evaluation. London: RCP, report 59, 1997.

Cannabis

Epidemiology

Cannabis is the most commonly used illicit drug in the world with estimates that it is used by an estimated 162 million adults (4% of the population) worldwide. Half of Australian men and 40% of women aged 20–40 years report having used cannabis at least once and 20% report use during the past month. Similarly in the UK over 20% of people aged 16–24 years report cannabis use in the past year. Cannabis use is particularly common among young people, and there are concerns that this is a time when the brain is still developing and may be particularly vulnerable to potential deleterious effects. Many people experiment with cannabis, or use it casually, while a proportion (perhaps up to 10% regular users in UK) become heavy or dependent users.

Pharmacology

Cannabis is derived from the Indian hemp plant, cannabis sativa. The active ingredient is delta 9-tetrahydrocannabinol (THC) which produces the desired psychological effects of cannabis smoking or eating through a stimulation of brain cannabis CB1 receptors. However, there are other components of the cannabis plant that have psychotropic properties and especially in resin, cannabidiol is present in some quantities. Cannabidiol may have effects opposite to THC and one of the explanations for new preparations of cannabis (e.g. skunk) possibly having more deleterious mental effects than seemed to occur in the past is that they contain little, if any cannabidiol so the actions of THC are not attenuated. Different preparations of the cannabis plant vary in strength, and new variants (cultivars) of cannabis grown in new ways (e.g. hydroponically) have magnified these differences.

Marijuana comes from the dried leaves and flowers. It is usually smoked in hand rolled cigarettes ('joints') or in pipes usually with tobacco or in water pipes ('bongs'). Joints typically contain 5–20 mg THC. Sometimes cannabis may be mixed in food and eaten e.g. 'hash cookies'.

It has been claimed that the development of high potency 'sinsemilla' cannabis using unfertilized female flowering heads or 'buds' and use of greenhouse technology for its growth has increased the risks associated with use of cannabis. Sinsemilla cannabis has been reported to have a THC potency of 10–18%. Hashish is made from the plant's resin. It is sold in solid pieces, and usually mixed with tobacco and smoked. Hashish oil is the most concentrated. It is often spread on tobacco and smoked.

Cannabis contains a number of psychoactive chemicals especially delta-9THC and cannabidiol. These bind to receptors specialized to respond to endogenous cannabinoids, such as anandamide. These substances are synthesized in the brain from membrane phospholipids usually as a result of neuronal depolarization. The endogenous cannabinoids act to stimulate cannabis receptors that are found in both presynaptic and post-synaptic locations where they influence second messenger processes involved in learning and memory. There are two sorts of cannabis receptors, the CB1 and CB2, which have quite different functions and locations. The main cannabis receptor is the CB1 type, which are located in areas in the brain involved with mood and memory. The psychological effects of THC are

Table 7.1 THC content of different preparations of cannabis

	Approximate THC content (depends on the plant, soil, sunlight, humidity)
Marijuana plant	0.5–18%
— Leaves and stem	0.5–5%
— Buds and heads	7–15%
— Sinsemilla (female flowering heads or buds)	10.5–18%
Hashish (resin from top of plant)	2–20%
Hash oil (concentrated hashish extract)	15–50 %

mediated through these CB1 receptors since they are lost in mice where these receptors have been deleted (knock-outs) and the effects of THC are blocked by selective CB1 receptor antagonists such as rimonabant. Other effects of smoked cannabis preparations (especially those of cannabidiol) may be mediated through the less prevalent CB2 receptors. The relative amount of THC compared with cannabidiol present in a preparation of cannabis has a major impact on the psychological and other effects.

Cannabis is fat soluble and rapidly absorbed from the alveolar membrane in the lung. Peak plasma levels are reached in 20–30 min. They show a biphasic elimination profile: the first [redistribution phase] lasts about half an hour, and reflects the distribution of THC into fatty organs such as the brain and fat. The second elimination phase last 20–80 h or more and reflects the clearance of cannabis and its metabolites via the liver and kidneys. THC is metabolized mainly in the liver to 11-nor-THC-9-carboxylic acid. Metabolites may be detected in the urine weeks after a single joint or up to 8 weeks after repeated daily use because of the residual amounts of drug and metabolites leaching out of fat stores. This very enduring presence of inactive cannabis metabolites is very easy to detect in urine screens so individuals may be found 'drug positive' weeks after the effects of cannabis have worn off (these generally disappear within a day). In practice this makes cannabis an easy target for drug testing which in some situations e.g. prisons, has the perverse effect of encouraging use of shorter acting, but more dangerous drugs, such as heroin, ketamine, or GHB.

Pharmacological effects vary with the setting, but typically include:

- Euphoria, relaxation, sleep (in some cases anxiety or restlessness)
- Floating sensations, lightness of limbs, depersonalization
- Altered perception of time, temporal disintegration
- Rapid flow of ideas, talkativeness
- Loosening of association, fragmented thinking
- Disturbed memory
- Conjunctival injection (red eyes)
- Tachycardia
- Elevations in blood pressure
- Increased appetite (the 'munchies')
- Dry mouth
- Fall in intra-ocular pressure
- Anti-emetic effect.

Current and potential therapeutic uses of cannabis

- Anti-emetic (during chemotherapy or radiotherapy-licensed as nabilone)
- Appetite stimulant (HIV/AIDS patients)
- Glaucoma
- Certain neurological disorders, such as multiple sclerosis, spinal cord injuries, movement disorders.

PET studies show that cannabis increases blood flow to parts of the brain that mediate mood and decreases blood flow to areas associated with attention and cognition.

After smoking cannabis peak levels are reached within 30 min and the effect lasts 2–4 h or more, depending on the dose. When taken orally, the effects are delayed but may last longer, for up to 12–24 h.

Core clinical syndromes

Acute cannabis intoxication

Seen with high dose of cannabis:

- **Anxiety and panic attacks:** the most common adverse emotional reactions with acute intoxication. Most often reported in naïve users and more common in those with a pre-existing anxiety disorder
- **Cannabis-induced panic attacks** lasts no more than 5–8 h, but the user may feel as if they are losing control or going mad during that time. Intoxication may also be associated with mild levels of suspiciousness and paranoid ideation, which can heighten the feeling of fear and loss of control
- **Paranoia:** may be associated with suspiciousness and some loss of insight in healthy individuals with no past or family history of psychotic disorders. While such symptoms resemble some aspects of a psychotic illness, they are transient in nature and fully resolve as intoxication clears
- **Dysphoria:** there may be a period of anxiety or lowered mood, which is usually mild, brief and self-limiting
- **Cognitive impairment:** cannabis intoxication commonly results in impaired or at least altered attention, concentration, learning, and memory
- **Perceptual distortions:** unusual somatic of visual sensations may be experienced. Occasionally, these may be reported up to a week after an episode of cannabis use, and have previously been described as flashbacks. However, because cannabis has a long half life, the experience is not strictly speaking occurring in abstinence, so cannot be called a flashback
- **Visual and auditory misperceptions or illusions** (may contribute to paranoid experiences)
- **Confusion, delirium:** delirium is more common with large doses of high potency cannabis. The disorder is short-lived, relatively benign, and recovery is usually complete within a week of stopping cannabis. Clinical features include confusion, persecutory delusions, hallucinations (auditory and visual), emotional lability, panic, and there may be depersonalization and derealization.

Death from overdose of smoked cannabis is not possible, which means it is often considered by the public to be a relatively harmless drug. However, there is an increased risk of motor vehicle accidents because of altered concentration and attention and impaired psychomotor performance. Unlike alcohol, cannabis tends to produce inhibited, rather than disinhibited driving behaviour.

Non-dependent (hazardous/harmful) use of cannabis: Cannabis may be used on a single occasion experimentally in teen-age years, or periodically at parties or other social occasions. In hazardous use no overt harms have been experienced. In harmful use, there may be complications such as respiratory infections.

Cannabis dependence

Chronic regular daily use may extend up to 14–16 h of continual smoking per day. The patient may be stoned for several hours. A proportion of regular chronic users will exhibit features of dependence with tolerance, poor control over use, unsuccessful attempts to stop or cut down, cannabis taking a higher priority over other aspects of life, continued despite clear evidence of harm (e.g. respiratory infections or psychotic episodes) and in some cases (though not all), withdrawal symptoms on cessation of use. It is associated with changes in cannabis receptor function. While in many cases cannabis may be used without any apparent adverse effects, in vulnerable individuals it may be associated with cannabis dependence, the withdrawal syndrome and other medical, neuropsychiatric, and social complications.

Cannabis withdrawal syndrome The withdrawal syndrome occurs in some cannabis dependent individuals when they cease cannabis use. The exact prevalence is not clear, but may be as high as 20% of regular heavy users. Symptoms of acute withdrawal start approximately 4 h after cessation of cannabis, peak at 4–7 days and lasts 1–2 weeks. Protracted milder withdrawals symptoms may last for up to 1 month. It has now been shown that cannabis withdrawal is to a significant extent a physical reaction since it can be precipitated by the CB1 antagonist rimonabant.

Clinical features of the cannabis withdrawal syndrome

- Lethargy
- Irritability
- Restlessness, anxiety
- Insomnia
- Mood changes
- Reduced appetite
- Muscle spasm
- Headache.

Complications

Medical complications of cannabis use:
- Increased risk of accidents, including motor vehicle accidents, especially if taken with alcohol
- Impaired pulmonary function, recurrent bronchitis, worsening of asthma, cancer of the lungs (from carcinogens in cannabis and tobacco smoke)
- Gonadal function, with heavy use inhibition of spermatogenesis and ovulation.

Neuropsychiatric complications of cannabis use:
- **Cognitive impairment:** cannabis intoxication commonly results in impaired and at least altered attention, concentration, learning and memory. Regular cannabis use can also lead to subtle cognitive impairments in memory, attention, organization and integration of complex information. It is unclear whether these effects resolve with abstinence
- **Anxiety and panic attacks:** most common adverse effect (see p. 191)
- **'Amotivational syndrome':** anecdotal reports have described an 'amotivational syndrome' in chronic regular cannabis users, which can mimic depression. This is comprised of impaired memory and concentration, apathy and lack of motivation, social withdrawal, and lethargy. It appears to be uncommon, and may be related to the effects of chronic intoxication. It may improve or resolve with abstinence, unless it reflects other factors, such as personality dysfunction and alcohol or other substance use
- **Depression:** following the euphoria usually experienced with cannabis intoxication, there may be a period of anxiety and lowered mood, which is usually brief and self-limiting. Depressive symptoms attributed to cannabis use are usually mild and transient. However, a number of recent studies have established that the rates of depression are elevated in those who use cannabis frequently or who are cannabis dependent. The cause of this is not fully clear
- **Paranoia:** cannabis intoxication may be associated with mild levels of suspiciousness, paranoia and some loss of insight in healthy individuals with no past or family history of psychotic disorders. While such symptoms resemble some aspects of a psychotic illness, they are transient in nature and fully resolve as intoxication clears
- **Delirium:** more common with large doses of high potency cannabis. Clinical features include confusion, persecutory delusions, hallucinations (visual and auditory), emotional lability, panic, and there may be depersonalization and derealization. The disorder is short-lived and relatively benign and recovery is usually complete within a week of stopping cannabis
- **Acute functional psychosis ('cannabis psychosis'):** while there is ongoing controversy around the existence of this syndrome, a number of authors have described acute psychotic episodes occurring in clear consciousness following cannabis use. These episodes are characterized by rapid onset, with a relatively benign course, usually recovering

completely within a week of abstinence even without antipsychotic agents. There is no evidence of confusion or delirium and the psychotic symptoms may be predominantly affective-like symptoms (of a manic or hypomanic type) or symptoms of a schizophreniform psychosis (with auditory or visual hallucinations; delusions of persecution; sometimes incoherent speech). Such illness is usually described in long-term or heavy users of cannabis

• **Chronic psychosis:** there is considerable debate about whether cannabis can induce chronic psychotic states, such as schizophrenia. The current consensus is as follows:
  • In patients with schizophrenia, cannabis use may trigger a relapse of the disorder and may exacerbate existing symptoms even when the patient is otherwise stable on medication
  • It is possible that regular heavy users of cannabis may suffer repeated, short episodes of psychosis and effectively 'maintain' themselves in a chronic, psychotic state. However, the psychotic symptoms will abate once cannabis use is ceased
  • Cannabis use may precipitate psychotic symptoms in an individual who is predisposed to developing schizophrenia; a genetic basis may be relevant with polymorphisms of the catechol-O-methyltransferase (COMT) gene implicated
  • Studies suggest that cannabis users have a two-fold increase in the relative risk for later developing schizophrenia, and eliminating cannabis use in those at risk would reduce the incidence of schizophrenia by around 8%. While cannabis alone does not cause schizophrenia, in some vulnerable individuals it is an important component of a complex constellation of risk factors for the disorder, particularly among adolescents.

Social complications

• Cannabis use, particularly by adolescents, is associated with impaired performance at school, absenteeism, reduced academic achievement, earlier school leaving, delinquency (It may be difficult to distinguish the behavioural changes and moodiness of adolescence from the effects of chronic marijuana use; see Adolescents, pp. 320–326)
• Impaired job performance, unemployment
• Financial problems
• Relationship problems, family problems
• Criminal activity
• Financial problems
• Legal problems.

Natural history

Information is scant on the natural history of various levels of cannabis use. Of those who have cannabis dependence, about 50% are still smoking regularly at 5 years and cannabis smoking of 30–40 years is well recognized. Studies conducted in the United States suggest that cannabis use typically begins in the mid- to late teens, and is most prevalent in early adulthood. Most cannabis use is irregular, with very few users engaging in long-term daily use. In the US and Australia, it is thought that about 10% of those who ever use cannabis become daily users, and another 20–30% use weekly. Transitions in life roles such as entry into full-time employment, getting married, or having children, are associated with reductions in or cessation of use for many people. The largest decreases are seen in cannabis use among males and females after marriage, and especially during pregnancy and after childbirth in women.

Assessment

History

Take a comprehensive history of cannabis, alcohol and other substance use. (See Chapter 2, pp. 37–41). Ask which preparation is being smoked? How is it smoked? (as joints, bongs, or pipes?) How much? How often, daily or episodic? For how long? When was the last smoke? Another important question to ask is 'for how many hours in a day are you stoned?'—being stoned for more than 4–6 h on a chronic daily basis suggests dependence on cannabis.

A past history of respiratory illnesses and a past, or family history, of psychiatric illness is also important.

Examination

Clinical examination is usually normal or the patient may have:
- Red eyes
- Tachycardia, raised blood pressure
- Signs of chronic bronchitis or obstructive airways disease.

Mental state examination may reveal anxiety, panic, depression or, in heavy users, features of psychosis (see pp. 44–47).

Opportunistic brief intervention

Cannabis users who are non-dependent, but smoking cannabis on an intermittent hazardous, or harmful basis can be offered brief intervention based on the FLAGS acronym.

Feedback: Any medical, neuropsychiatric or social harms experienced because of the individual's cannabis use.

Listen: to the patient's response—does the patient want to quit smoking?

Advice: Convey clear medical advice, e.g. the potential medical, neuro-psychiatric, and social complications of cannabis use and the benefits of not smoking cannabis. This is important particularly for young people.

Goals: Set goals tailored according to the individual patient's response.

Strategies: Set out strategies to achieve the goals. Offer follow-up to determine progress and offer support.

Management of cannabis withdrawal

Cannabis withdrawal scales are available, but they are not yet fully validated. There is also a limited evidence base to guide prescribing.

Many persons who are dependent on cannabis do not require medications to relieve withdrawal symptoms.

Advice and education about possible medical, neuropsychiatric and social complications of cannabis use, withdrawal symptoms and their time course in association with counselling and psychological interventions are often useful.

However, in those who have been unable to stop cannabis because of withdrawal symptoms, symptomatic medication is often necessary.

The following medications have been used in some centres:
- Benzodiazepines (e.g. diazepam 5–10 mg prn every 6 h for 7–10 days, then reducing to zero by 14 days). This will relieve insomnia, irritability and restlessness
- If these symptoms continue, a low dose of quetiapine may be prescribed; 25–100 mg in divided doses per day is appropriate. The patient should be warned that the first dose might cause significant sedation and to contact the prescriber if that occurs.
- Antidepressants to relieve dysphoria. Medications that have been used have included mirtazapine 15–30 mg nocte as it helps with insomnia (interestingly unlike with nicotine withdrawal bupropion worsened withdrawal symptoms).

Management of cannabis dependence

There is as yet no established pharmacological treatment specifically for cannabis dependence.

As per dependence on other psychoactive substances, the treatment involves the following 10 steps:

Steps in the management of cannabis dependence

- Provision of information and education. This may include motivational interviewing to increase chance of stopping cannabis use
- Let the patient digest the information and advice provided. The patient must then reach a point of acceptance of the need to stop and develop commitment to cease use
- Detoxification/management of cannabis withdrawal (see, p. 196)
- Pharmacotherapy: currently there is no established pharmacological treatment for treatment of cannabis dependence

Rimonabant—shows some promise but further studies are required to establish its efficacy. Note that cannabis withdrawal may also be precipitated by administration of rimonabant

- Psychological treatments: are the primary treatments currently available for cannabis dependence. This includes cognitive behavioural therapy, motivational enhancement therapy and a range of other behavioural therapies and approaches
- Treatment of co-morbidity: parallel treatment of medical and neuropsychiatric complications/underlying mental illnesses as required-referral to a psychiatrist may be necessary
- Treatment of the patient within the family or social context: Advice, education and support to help parents and family cope with the user as well as to help and support the user
- Self-help/mutual help organizations: Self-help groups such as Quit marijuana groups are available in some areas
- Follow up /after care
- Life style and environmental changes: Changes to life style, home and environment. Avoiding cannabis or other substance using friends, adopt a healthy life style, eat regular meals, exercise, re-engage with normal living activities or hobbies.

Management of complications of cannabis use

Management of acute anxiety related to cannabis use: Management involves ruling out other physical causes for symptoms and reassuring the patient the problem will resolve in the next 5–8 h. If medication is required, short term use of benzodiazepines can be tried. Because of the persistence of marijuana in the body, the patient should be warned that they may experience some minor feelings of drug intoxication over the next 2–4 days.

In managing depression, psychosis, or physical complications of cannabis use, a crucial aspect is achieving abstinence from cannabis. Standard treatment for the physical or neuropsychiatric complications may also be applied.

Prevention

Although cannabis is considered a 'soft' drug, people (particularly young people), with a past history, or family history, of schizophrenia, psychosis, anxiety or depression should be warned about the potential neuropsychiatric complications of cannabis use.

People using cannabis should be advised about the risks of driving while under the influence of cannabis, particularly if it is used in combination with alcohol.

Further reading

Budney A, Hughes A. The cannabis withdrawal syndrome. *Current Opinion in Psychiatry* 2006; **19**: 33–238.

Cannabis; Classification and Public Health. Advisory Council on the misuse of drugs. UK Home Office, 2008.

Caspi A, Moffitt TE, Cannon M, McClay J, Murray R, Harrington H-L, Taylor I, Arseneault L, Williams B, Braithwaite A, Poulton R, Craig IW. Moderation of the effect of adolescent-onset cannabis use on adult psychosis by a functional polymorphism in the catechol-O-methyltransferase gene: longitudinal evidence of a gene X environment interaction. *Biological Psychiatry* 2005; **57**: 1117–1127.

Moore THM, Zammit S, Lingford-Hughes A, Barnes TRE, Jones PB, Burke M, Lewis G. Cannabis use and risk of psychotic or affective mental health outcomes: a systematic review. *Lancet* 2007; **370**(9584): 319–328.

Nutt DJ, Nash J. *Cannabis—an update*. London: Home Office Publications, 2002. Available at: http://www.drugs.gov.uk/ReportsandPublications/Communities/1034165905/Cannabis_update_1999to2002.pdf

Rawlins M et al. (2008). Cannabis classification and Public Health. Home Office Publication. See http://drug.homeoffice.gov.uk

Opioids

Epidemiology

Illicit opioids such as heroin comprise the third most common form of illicit drug use worldwide. However, in most high income countries, less than 1% of the population have used illicit opioids in the past year. This ranges from 0.1% in Japan and Sweden, 0.5% in countries such as Australia, New Zealand, through to 0.9% in the UK. Illicit opioid use attracts much public concern, because those who die from overdose or other complications are typically young. However, illicit opioids contribute far less to the global burden of disease than do licit substances, such as alcohol and tobacco (0.8% as compared with 4% for alcohol and 4% for tobacco).

Nonetheless, dependence on illicit opioids causes considerable suffering to the drug dependent individual and to those around them, and sizeable challenges to the broader community in terms of health and social problems, especially due to hepatitis C and HIV spread.

Some illicit opioid users take only heroin, others use street methadone (orally or injected) and prescribed opioids (orally or parenteral), or if opioids are not available, many use alcohol or benzodiazepines to control their withdrawal symptoms.

Natural history of opioid dependence

One in four persons who use illicit opioids may become dependent on them. The development of dependence can be relatively rapid, after 6–8 weeks of regular use, or may follow years of intermittent use. Once dependent, users may struggle to control their use for significant proportions of their lives. There is a high morbidity and mortality associated with dependence. Some of the complications of use of illicit opioids are due to the drug itself (death from overdose, dependence); however, its illegal nature and resulting high cost further greatly contribute to the harms of illicit opioid use. As injecting of illicit opioids in most cases is not medically supervised, and is often hurried to avoid detection, a large number of medical complications may ensue, and blood borne virus infection occurs (in particular hepatitis C) in the majority of dependent heroin injectors.

Pharmacology of opioids

Opioids all act on opioid receptors in the central nervous system to produce analgesia and varying amounts of euphoria and sedation. This group includes morphine, an alkaloid of opium obtained from the poppy plant *Papaver somniferum*, and related synthetic chemicals [diacetyl morphine (heroin), methadone, dextropropoxyphene, fentanyl, pentazocine, oxycodone, pethidine, codeine and buprenorphine, etc.].

Opioids act on different opioid receptors to produce the following effects:

- **Mu receptors:** euphoria, sedation, analgesia, miosis, reduced gastrointestinal motility, respiratory depression and physical dependence
- **Kappa receptors** (principally within the spinal cord, basal ganglia, temporal lobes): drowsiness, dysphoria
- **Delta receptors:** analgesia, cardiovascular effects (hypotension, bradycardia).

Stimulation of mu (and possibly delta) opioid receptors is involved in 'reward' systems (see neurobiology of dependence, pp. 20–23). In mice that have the mu receptor 'knocked out' the rewarding effects of opioids are abolished, but the analgesic effect of delta receptor agonists may be retained.

Heroin (diamorphine) is highly lipid soluble, and crosses the blood–brain barrier more rapidly than morphine or other opioids. Within a minute or two after intravenous heroin there is a characteristic 'rush' associated with warm flushing of the skin. Heroin is metabolized in the brain and in the liver to active metabolites 6-monoacetyl morphine and then to morphine, which is then conjugated with glucuronic acid—hence, heroin is a pro-drug of morphine.

Codeine is also a prodrug of morphine—being converted to it by CYP2D6—it is misused for this reason. Persons with low functioning 2D6, e.g. as a result of blockade with drugs such as paroxetine, will get less effect from codeine. Conversely, rapid metabolizers will get greater

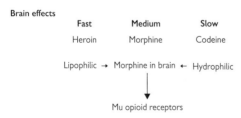

Brain effects

	Fast	Medium	Slow
	Heroin	Morphine	Codeine

Lipophilic → Morphine in brain ← Hydrophilic

↓

Mu opioid receptors

Fig. 8.1 Heroin and codeine are 'prodrugs' of morphine.

effects perhaps with dangerous consequences. A case report has been described where a lactating woman was taking codeine for pain and, because she was a rapid metabolizer, her baby died of morphine toxicity.

With repeated administration, tolerance develops to most opioid effects, except miosis and constipation, and withdrawal may occur on cessation of use. Cross-tolerance is the norm among the opioids as they share a common target receptor.

Oral morphine has a high first pass effect and for a therapeutic effect, the oral dose is higher than the parenteral dose. Morphine is metabolized by conjugation in the liver, but one of the major metabolites, morphine-6-glucuronide, is also a mu receptor agonist and is used as an analgesic.

Methadone and buprenorphine are long acting opioids primarily used in substitution treatment for opioid dependence. However, they are sometimes misused or diverted to the black market.

Methadone A synthetic opioid mu receptor agonist with properties similar to morphine and other opioids. It was first developed in Germany during World War II as an analgesic. It is available as a syrup or in the form of tablets. Methadone tablets are used for the relief of pain, while methadone syrup is indicated for the treatment of opioid dependence, as it is easier to supervise.

On single dose, effect of 30 mg of methadone is equivalent to 15 mg of morphine.

Methadone has a much longer plasma half-life than morphine (mean 22 h, range 15–32, versus 2 h for morphine). This long half-life enables once daily administration.

Methadone is well absorbed after oral administration, and reaches a peak at about 4 h, and readily crosses the blood–brain barrier. 90% is bound to plasma proteins. It is extensively metabolized by *n*-demethylation and cyclization in the liver, and excreted in the urine and bile. Some of the details of methadone's neuropharmacology and metabolism remain poorly defined.

Rifampicin and phenytoin accelerate the metabolism of methadone by inducing cytochrome P450 enzymes and may precipitate withdrawal symptoms. In contrast, fluvoxamine decreases the metabolism of methadone and may result in symptoms of opioid intoxication.

Buprenorphine is a partial agonist with a high affinity for both the mu and kappa receptors.

Buprenorphine competes with and displaces heroin or methadone from the mu receptor sites and is sometimes referred to as a mixed agonist-antagonist. Because of its low intrinsic activity and 'ceiling effects', it has lower risk of respiratory toxicity and, thus, is relatively safer than either heroin or methadone.

Buprenorphine is more potent than either heroin or methadone. The smallest sublingual dose of buprenorphine (0.4 mg) is equivalent to 10 mg morphine (intramuscular injection), and 2 mg of sublingual buprenorphine is equivalent to 30 mg oral methadone.

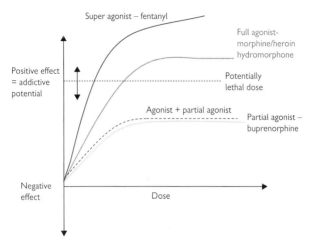

Fig. 8.2 Mu partial agonists—safety and antagonist action.

Buprenorphine is highly lipophilic and slowly released from fat stores. It undergoes extensive first pass metabolism and, hence, needs to be given sublingually (though depot preparations and patches are under development). Onset of action occurs within 30–60 min. Peak plasma levels are reached in 1–2 h and the half-life is approximately 20–70 h (average 35 h), Steady state levels are achieved in 3–7 days. Duration of action is dose-dependent and ranges from 4 to 12 h for low doses to 48–72 h for high doses.

Buprenorphine undergoes enterohepatic circulation. Metabolism is by hepatic microsomal enzyme systems, CYP3A4 and by conjugation with glucoronic acid. Most (70%) is excreted in the faeces and the rest in the urine.

Characteristics of buprenorphine

- More potent than morphine or methadone per mg (up to 30×)
- Good sub-lingual absorption (60%+) in most patients
- Poor gastric absorption and high first pass metabolism (only 10% of dose enters systemic circulation)
- Partial agonist at the mu opioid receptor
- High affinity means it blocks access of other opioids to the mu receptor so reduces 'on-top' use.
- Half-life (inc. active metabolite) from one to several days as dose increases
- If there has been recent use of other opioids, buprenorphine can displace these off opioid receptors, precipitating a withdrawal reaction in dependent users (because of its high affinity and lower activity at the opioid receptor).

Table 8.1 Comparison of the pharmacology of three opioids

	Heroin	Methadone	Buprenorphine
Receptor	mu agonist	mu agonist	Partial mu agonist Kappa antagonist
Administration	IV	Oral usually. May be given in reduced dose, IM or subcutaneously when a person is nil by mouth	Sub-lingual
Peak plasma levels	1–2 min	2–4 h	1–2 h
Plasma half-life	2 h	22 h	Approx 36 h (20–72 h, increases with dose)
Onset of effect	Minutes	30–60 min	30–60 min
Peak effect	1–2 min	3–6 h	1–4 h
Duration of effect	4–5 h	16–30 h dose dependent	12 h, low dose 72 h, high dose
Liver metabolism	Hydrolysis	MEOS CYP3A4	MEOS CYP3A4 Conjugation
High first pass metabolism	Yes	No	Yes
Drug interactions	MAOIs Sedatives	MAOIs Sedatives Protease inhibitors	MAOIs Sedatives Protease inhibitors
		CYP3A4 inducers: Phenytoin Rifampicin Carbamazepine Methadone has complex effects on 3A4, induces and blocks	Antimycotics Ca channel blockers Macrolide antibiotics
		CYP3A4 inhibitors Fluvoxamine	

Pathophysiology

In contrast to the widespread toxic effects of alcohol, the pathological effects of opioids are discrete. These effects reflect the pharmacological effects of the parent drugs and some of the metabolites. There is not the same extensive breakdown to toxic metabolites as seen with alcohol.

The acute complications of opioid toxicity are directly related to the pharmacological effects, of sedation, and in severe cases, respiratory depression.

Release of histamine may occur through degranulation of mast cells. Leakage in endothelial cell vessel lining may lead to pulmonary oedema.

Contraction of smooth muscles occurs with acute opioid use. With chronic use, the opposite of the acute effect tends to occur with smooth muscle becoming hypotonic, leading to risk of gastroparesis.

Opioids decrease bowel motility and both illicit and prescribed opioid misuse can cause chronic and sometimes severe constipation.

The dry mouth resulting from opioid use chronically results in dental decay. This is because saliva has antibacterial properties. In addition heroin dependent individuals rarely prioritize dental care, because of the preoccupation with drug use.

Norpethidine is an opioid metabolite which causes adverse effects. Morphine is metabolized to several glucuronides which are excreted by the kidneys.

Many of the medical complications of illicit heron use are complications of unsafe injecting practices, e.g. viral or bacterial infections (pp. 207–209; 367–74).

Core clinical diagnoses

A person may use illicit opioids, but not meet criteria for an ICD or DSM diagnosis. These individuals are described as either using or misusing the illicit opioid(s). Alternatively an individual may meet the criteria for a diagnosable drug use disorder, either in the past 12 months (current) or in the past.

Non-dependent opioid use

A person meets the criteria for harmful opioid use (ICD-10) if they have experienced complications of use, e.g. overdose or hepatitis C infection or injuries from violence associated with purchasing the drug, but are not dependent on opioids.

If the individual experiences recurrent social problems as a result of their repeated illicit opioid use, but are not dependent on opioids, their diagnosis is heroin (or other illicit opioid) abuse (DSM IV-TR).

Opioid dependence

An individual has heroin or other illicit opioid dependence if they use opioids repeatedly and meet 3 or more of the following criteria:

- **Impaired control over use**
- **Craving/compulsion to use:** this may manifest as unsuccessful attempts to cut down
- **Preoccupation** with heroin use to the neglect of other responsibilities
- **Tolerance:** a heroin user first may have only inhaled the drug; after some time they find they need higher doses, and then may revert to injecting to get the desired effect. Injectors may increase their use from a 'half a quarter' a day up to 1 g (street gram) per day or, in financial terms, from \$25 per day to hundreds of dollars per day
- **Withdrawal or use of opioids to prevent or relieve withdrawal:** the dependent user typically describes withdrawal symptoms ('hanging out') when they are overdue for their next hit of heroin, with low energy, runny nose, aches and pains (see below)
- **Persistent use despite clear evidence of physical or psychological adverse consequences**.

In practice, if a person experiences clear physical withdrawal, sufficient criteria to diagnose dependence will always be present.

The opioid withdrawal syndrome

Simple opioid withdrawal resembles a flu-like illness and simple withdrawal is not life-threatening. Symptoms include low energy, aches and pains, rhinorrhoea, nausea and vomiting. Insomnia and craving for opioids are prominent (see p. 214 for assessment and management of opioid withdrawal).

Complications of opioid use

Acute complications

Complications may be experienced by those who use opioids by oral, intravenous or inhaled routes

Opioid overdose Relatively common among heroin and other opioid users and a cause of death from respiratory depression; even controlled use of heroin is associated with marked drops in oxygen saturation. (See p. 212 for assessment and management of overdose.)

QTc prolongation and ventricular arrhythmias has been reported with methadone, particularly in high doses, but in practice is very rare. Concomitant use of other medications, which prolong QT interval may increase the risk.

Medical complications of injecting opioid use (Also see pp. 367–374 for complications of injecting drug use in general)

Heroin is typically used by the intravenous route. Other common routes of self administration of opioids include oral use and inhalation of heroin vapours—'chasing the dragon').

Complications of illicit drug use may arise from:
- The pharmacological effects of the drug itself (e.g. overdose)
- The adulterants and contaminants in the drug (unknown potency, purity and sterility)
- Unsafe injecting practices including needle sharing
- Social complications related to the illegal nature and high cost of drugs.

Complications related to contaminants and adulterants

Illicit heroin is typically non sterile and the potency is unknown. It may be contaminated or 'cut' with a variety of substances, usually added to reduce the cost to the dealer of pure heroin, and so increase their profit. The user may experience unexpected pharmacological or toxic effects. Particulate matter may result in emboli.

Acute heroin reaction (rare): An acute reaction or allergic reaction to pyrogenic material or contaminants in the illicit drug preparation. It is more common with heroin than with other illicit drugs. The acute heroin reaction is typically associated with sudden onset severe occipital headache, fever, tremor/shaking (occasionally with rigors), tachypnoea, leucocytosis, non-cardiogenic pulmonary oedema, cyanosis, coma, and death from respiratory depression.

Complications relating to unsafe injecting practices

Infections: Injecting illicit drugs and sharing of injecting equipment places individuals at risk of infections with a variety of agents including blood borne viruses (hepatitis C, B, and HIV), as well as bacteria and fungi.

Bacterial infections are common. These may become systemic and life-threatening. In cases of high unexplained fever, or chronic fever, in an injecting drug user always consider endocarditis or another hidden focus of serious infection.

Do blood cultures in all febrile injecting drug users

Bacterial infections are most commonly caused by *Staphylococcus aureus*. They also may be caused by *Streptococcus viridans*, *Clostridium*, or other organisms. Presentations may be local, distant or systemic and include:

- Local infections:
  - Abscess, cellulitis
  - Septic thrombophlebitis
  - Necrotizing fasciitis (mainly with clostridium following subcutaneous injection), necrotizing ulcers
- Embolic or distant infection:
  - Metastatic abscesses
  - Bacterial endocarditis—mainly *Staphylococcus aureus*. Also *Streptococcus viridans*, *Pseudomonas aeruginosa*. May affect the tricuspid valve or mitral or aortic valves.
  - Osteomyelitis, septic arthritis
- Septicaemia and disseminated infections (mainly streptococci).

Viral infections: Injecting drug users are at risk of one or more blood borne virus infections, and in particular hepatitis C, B, and HIV.

Hepatitis C: Injecting drug use is responsible for 90% of cases of hepatitis C in the developed world. Hepatitis C is associated with acute hepatitis and with a significant burden of chronic liver disease, including cirrhosis and hepatocellular carcinoma. In most countries, the majority of chronic regular IV drug users will be infected with hepatitis C (e.g. 65–70% in Australia and higher in countries without ready access to sterile injecting equipment). Hepatitis C has high infectivity. It is spread not only by sharing of needles and syringes, but also by sharing of other injecting equipment (e.g. spoons used for dissolving the drug, swabs, tourniquets). In addition, putting injecting equipment down on a bench or other surface which may have been contaminated by another users' blood, can potentially lead to infection.

Hepatitis B is a less common complication than hepatitis C, and may be acquired through unsafe injecting practices or unprotected sex.

HIV: In some countries (e.g. in many parts of Asia) HIV infection in injecting drug users is a relatively common complication, with consequent risk of spread to other segments of the community. In other countries, such as Australia, with active harm reduction measures such as needle syringe services and availability of opioid maintenance treatment, the prevalence of HIV in injecting drug users has remained low (<5%).

Fungal and other infections: Particularly Candida albicans:

- Distant or systemic infection including endocarditis, fungal ophthalmitis
- Illicit injection of diverted sublingual buprenorphine tablets increases the risk of blood borne or mouth organisms, including *Candida*.

Vascular complications

- Vasculitis, vascular damage
- Vascular spasm due to local trauma of injecting
- Inadvertent or deliberate injecting into arteries, can be associated with distal ischaemia

- Embolism, strokes
- Aneurysms:
  - Arteriovenous aneurysm
  - Mycotic aneurysms
  - Pulsatile pseudoaneurysms (caused by vascular injuries, *Staph. aureus* is the main pathogen).

Other acute medical complications: May also be due to the property of the opioid, the injecting practices and/or the associated lifestyle:
- Pulmonary complications:
  - Infections: including tuberculosis, pneumonias—due to poor living conditions, nutrition, and self-care, associated smoking of tobacco, cannabis and of crack cocaine
  - Lung complications may follow inhalation of opioids
  - Atelectasis
  - Pulmonary emboli, pulmonary infarction (from septic thrombophlebitis or coincident cocaine use)
  - Non—cardiogenic pulmonary oedema (heroin)
  - Pulmonary granulomas (from insoluble additives).

Sexually transmitted infections: Chlamydia, syphilis, gonorrhoea, etc., may be acquired through unprotected sex, either as part of sex work to raise money for drugs, or when under the influence of drugs (e.g. sedated with heroin, alcohol and/or benzodiazepines; or increased libido with stimulant use).

Rhabdomyolysis: May result from pressure following prolonged unconsciousness with heroin (and/or benzodiazepines, alcohol); also reported with cocaine or amphetamine use. May lead to acute renal failure if not diagnosed and appropriately treated.

Chronic complications

Several of the above complications may have acute or chronic manifestations.

Medical complications

Chronic infection with either hepatitis C or B poses a risk of cirrhosis, and also the risk of infection to others beyond the drug user.

HIV infection: HIV carrier status poses the risk of transmission to others. Should immunodeficiency develop the individual can present with a range of unusual and/or severe infections.

Dental complications: As opioids (illicit or prescribed) dry the mouth, bacteria can reproduce more readily that cause dental decay. Combined with sometimes poor dental hygiene, dental decay is common. This can result in acute or chronic pain, and dental infections (pp. 375–378).

Constipation: For heroin dependent individuals and for patients on opioid maintenance programmes, constipation may be a troublesome complication. Occasionally reduced bowel motility becomes a medically serious complication with gastroparesis or intestinal pseudo-obstruction.

Renal disease: Glomerulonephritis or interstitial nephritis may occur with injecting drug use (an uncommon though severe complication).

Psychiatric complications
Depression and anxiety
Individuals who are opioid dependent are five times more likely than the general population to have a depressive disorder. As for the general population, these rates are higher in women than men. The rates of anxiety disorders are about 3 times higher than the general population. Because opioid users are more likely than the general population to be exposed to traumatic events (particularly physical assault), they may also have an increased risk of post-traumatic stress disorder.

Protracted abstinence syndrome. After acutely withdrawing from heroin or other opioids, opioid dependent individuals often continue to feel uncomfortable for up to 6 months. This protracted withdrawal syndrome varies from a vague sense of feeling abnormal to symptoms of low level lethargy, insominia irritability, depression, anxiety, reduced self-esteem, and hypersensitivity to stress. This may be accompanied by mild physiological changes in blood pressure, respiration and temperature. These symptoms leave the ex-user vulnerable to drug cravings and relapse.

Social complications
The social complications of heroin dependence are typically considerable:
- While acutely intoxicated the user is vulnerable and may become the victim or violence, sexual abuse, or theft
- Chronically, because heroin is illegal and high cost, many users are drawn into crime (drug dealing, theft, etc.) or sex work to make money
- Many users become victims of violence through association with the illicit drug and criminal scene
- A history of imprisonment is common (e.g. either for possession or sale of drugs, or for crimes committed to obtain money for drugs). Long periods of imprisonment may disrupt personal relationships and a criminal record may make finding a job very difficult, even when abstinent from illicit drugs
- Family problems and/or child neglect may occur
- Considerable marginalization often accompanies illicit drug use and heroin dependence in particular.

Further reading
Cherubin CE, Sapira JD. The medical complications of drug addiction and the medical assessment of the intravenous drug user 25 years later. *Annals of Internal Medicine* 1993; **119**: 1017–1028.

Dore GJ, Thomas DL. Management and treatment of injecting drug users with hepatitis C virus (HCV) infection and HCV/Human Immunodeficiency Virus co-infection. *Seminars in Liver Disease* 2005; **25**:

Gordon RJ, Lowy FD. Bacterial infections in drug users. *New England Journal of Medicine* 2005; **353**: 1945–1954.

Identification of illicit opioid use and opportunistic intervention

A significant proportion of the heroin users (or persons with other opioid misuse) within the community are not yet seeking treatment. They may be occasional and non-dependent users (e.g. episodically smoking or injecting heroin), or may be dependent users, but not wishing to stop.

   While the effectiveness of opportunistic and brief intervention has not been examined, the general principles of brief intervention can be considered when offering assistance.

Feedback: Most heroin users are well aware of the harms they have experienced through their heroin use, so any feedback is most often given in the form of empathy rather than new information: e.g. 'I can see that your heroin use has been making your life very difficult'. If no harms have been experienced, the clinician can check if the client is aware of the risks associated with use (e.g. dependence, blood borne viruses in injectors).

Listen: To the patient's response—is there any ambivalence about opioid use, that can be capitalized on in a motivational interviewing style approach? Is the individual adamant that he or she wishes to continue using? Has the individual tried to stop many times and is very ready for assistance?

Advice: Convey your medical advice empathically and non-judgementally. This may include, for example, the reflection that if the individual is prepared to go onto opioid maintenance treatment, their life would be simpler—they would not have to constantly seek the funds for heroin and their prospects of remaining/becoming healthy would be greatly improved. Were they aware that methadone or buprenorphine is currently the best proven way to cease illicit opioids?

Goals: While the clinician's goal will generally be abstinence from illicit opioids (typically achieved through opioid maintenance treatment), the patient may be unwilling or unable to accept this goal at this point. In that case, the patient and clinician may be able to discuss an interim goal, e.g. for an intermittent user, trying to ensure that heroin use dose not exceed once weekly; or for the dependent user who is not willing to cease, safer injecting practices or attending to hepatitis monitoring or treatment of a co-morbid psychiatric condition.

Strategies: If the patient is prepared to accept referral to a specialist addiction treatment centre or other opioid maintenance treatment prescriber, suggest that they attend to discuss treatment options. If the patient does not want treatment for their dependence, he or she may still be prepared to discuss harm reduction strategies, or approaches for managing co-morbid or complicating physical or psychiatric conditions. It is always important to offer further assistance if or when the patient wishes to change their opioid use.

Assessment and management of opioid overdose

Opioid overdose is a life-threatening condition. Take a good medical and drug history if patient is able to communicate:

• Obtain collateral information if available
• Look for needle track marks
• Look for signs of opioid overdose—typical signs include pin point pupils and slowed respiration.

Clinical features of opioid overdose

Symptoms
• Nausea, vomiting
• Drowsiness.

Physical signs
• Stuporose
• Cool moist skin
• Slow deep respiration (2–7/min)
• Hypothermia
• Bradycardia
• Hypotension
• Pin-point pupils (may be dilated if there is brain damage)
• Coma
• Risk of death from respiratory depression.

NOTE: Generalized seizures may occur in pethidine overdose.

Morphine overdose may be associated with a confusional state, with agitation and, in some cases, psychosis.

Resuscitation

General supportive and symptomatic measures:

• **ABC:** maintain:
  • Airway (O$_2$/monitor and maintain oxygen saturation, artificial respiration if necessary)
  • Blood pressure
  • Circulation

• **Antidote:** naloxone 0.4–2 mg intravenously.

  i) *For heroin overdose:* initial dose 0.4 mg As naloxone has a short half-life the patient may lapse back into a coma. Constant observation is essential and it may be necessary to repeat the dose after 15–20 minutes, and then every 30–60 minutes until the level of consciousness is stable. Naloxone is sometimes given outside the hospital* for observation as opioid withdrawal symptoms may occur.

  If high doses of naloxone are administered quickly to reverse overdose in an opioid dependent person, a withdrawal reaction may be precipitated, and result in angry and difficult behaviour.

---

* In some centres 'take-home' naloxone ampoules are made available to opioid dependent patients so that in the event of an accidental overdose, family or friends can administer the antidote before the emergency services are called.

ii) *For methadone overdose*: methadone has a long half-life (approximately 20 h). Thus, in cases of methadone overdose, repeated doses of IV naloxone 0.4–2 mg or a 24-h infusion may be required and the patient should be monitored for up to 72 hours.

iii) *For buprenorphine overdose*: while overdose of buprenorphine by itself is uncommon, there is a possibility of overdose if patients use heroin concurrently in larger than usual doses after ceasing buprenorphine and/or use benzodiazepine or other sedative drugs in association with buprenorphine

Buprenorphine has a long half-life and, in rare instances of overdose, the patients should be monitored for more than 72 h. Vasopressor agents may be required. Naloxone is of limited usefulness in the treatment of buprenorphine overdose as buprenorphine is not easily displaced by naloxone because of its high affinity for the mu receptor. The dose of naloxone may have to be increased to 15–20 times and assisted ventilation may be required.

Other measures in the management of opioid overdose
- Give intravenous fluids
- In rare cases of non-cardiogenic pulmonary oedema, treat as for pulmonary oedema.
- If the patient does not respond to naloxone, and a combination of opioids and benzodiazepine overdose is suspected, consider careful addition of the benzodiazepine antagonist flumazenil (0.5–2 mg by slow IV infusion; p. 178).

Warning: flumazenil may precipitate a withdrawal syndrome in benzodiazepine dependent patients
- Exclude medical complications of injecting drug use (see p. 367), and treat complicating or concurrent medical conditions
- Exclude polysubstance overdose: many opioid overdoses also involve alcohol and/or benzodiazepines
- Exclude other causes of coma: e.g. head injury, metabolic diseases, electrolyte abnormalities
- Urine drug screen should be dispatched: although results will typically only be available once the overdose is resolved, they indicate the extent and range of substance use at the time of overdose, which may inform future management.

Further assessment

If the patient is able to provide any history, or if collateral information is available (e.g. ambulance officers, general practitioner, family or friends) try to assess recency and type/range of drug use (including alcohol), and typical pattern of drug use. Once overdose has resolved and consciousness is fully restored, a full history can be taken, including substance use (recent and usual), medical and psychiatric history (pp. 39–41). A psychiatric assessment is important where there is suspicion of a suicidal intent.

Education and advice

Once overdose has resolved and consciousness is fully restored:

Provide education and advice: About the complications of opioid use, particularly in combination with alcohol, benzodiazepines and other CNS depressants. Offer referral to a specialist Drug and Alcohol Unit for on-going treatment, support and encouragement and/or discuss NA, and other agencies and self-help groups.

Management of the opioid withdrawal syndrome

The intensity of withdrawal symptoms varies with the severity, duration of use and level of health of the individual. Typical and uncomplicated opioid withdrawal is not life threatening.

Withdrawal symptoms occur within hours of cessation of heroin.

The symptoms of opioid withdrawal resemble a flu-like illness with aches and pains, rhinorrhoea, nausea and vomiting. Insomnia and strong cravings for opioids may be distressing.

Table 8.2 Onset and duration of opioid withdrawal symptoms

Drug	Onset	Peak effect	Duration
Heroin	4–6 h	18–72 h	5–10 days
Methadone	24–48 h	3–4 days	2 to several weeks
Buprenorphine	2–3 days	5 days	Several weeks

Features of opioid withdrawal

Physical symptoms
- Rhinorrhoea
- Lacrimation
- Sweating
- Hot and cold flushes
- Piloerection ('cold turkey')
- Abdominal cramps
- Nausea, vomiting, diarrhoea
- Bone and muscle aches and cramps

Neuropsychiatric symptoms
- Insomnia
- Restlessness, anxiety, irritability, agitation
- Depression
- Intense 'craving' ± drug seeking behaviour

Physical signs
- Yawning, rhinorrhoea, lacrimation
- Fever (low grade)
- Skin:
  - Needle track marks
  - Sweating
  - Piloerection ('cold turkey')
- CVS
  - Tachycardia, hypertension (mild)
- CNS—Restlessness, anxiety, agitation
  - Dilated pupils

Management of opioid withdrawal

Opioid withdrawal is not usually an indication for hospital admission, unless there is intercurrent illness, severe vomiting or pregnancy, or concurrent benzodiazepine or alcohol dependence, or withdrawal from these substances.

It is not necessary for an opioid user to complete withdrawal from opioids before commencing opioid maintenance treatment (see below). However, if an individual does not wish to go onto maintenance treatment, or such treatment is not appropriate or locally available, three options are set out below for withdrawal management ('detoxification').

In most cases, tapering dose buprenorphine treatment provides the simplest and most effective management of withdrawal symptoms. It provides greater rates of completion of detoxification than does symptomatic treatment alone or going 'cold turkey' (i.e. just putting up with the symptoms without treatment). Buprenorphine provides swifter and safer relief of withdrawal symptoms than methadone, because the dose can be increased relatively swiftly, and weaning off buprenorphine also tends to be quicker and easier.

However, in some cases buprenorphine may not be a feasible option (e.g. in Australia general practitioners have to be accredited to prescribe opioids for addiction, and there may be no local prescriber available). In other cases, methadone may be more appropriate (e.g. coincident acute severe pain where methadone may facilitate control of pain; or recent history of long acting opioid use, where buprenorphine may precipitate a withdrawal reaction).

In some countries, rapid or ultrarapid detoxification using naltrexone is keenly sought by members of the public, often through private treatment providers.

Whichever option for management of opioid withdrawal symptoms is chosen, general supportive measures, such as reassurance, rest, hydration, and good nutrition are useful adjuncts.

Monitor regularly with an opioid withdrawal scale. (See Appendix pp. 438–439).

Option 1: Tapering opioid replacement therapy

Short-term detoxification or withdrawal therapy with either buprenorphine or methadone.

Short-term detoxification or withdrawal therapy by substitution with small to moderate doses of either methadone or buprenorphine may be used. Buprenorphine typically provides more rapid relief of withdrawal symptoms as doses can be increased more rapidly. However, there is a risk of precipitated opioid withdrawals if buprenorphine is administered too early after use of opioids (see below).

Buprenorphine: 4–8 mg sublingually on day 1, increase by 2–4 mg daily to 10–12 mg/day (tablets should be dissolved under the tongue, taking 4–7 min). Then reduce by 2 mg/day to zero. Reductions may be slower if desired, and once the dose has reached 2 mg reductions may be by 0.4 mg steps.

Before initiation of buprenorphine treatment, it is important to wait until at least 8 h after the last dose of heroin or 24 h after low dose methadone (up to 30 mg methadone per day) until opioid withdrawal symptoms are present in order to avoid precipitating withdrawal. While recently buprenorphine has been commenced 24 h after higher doses of methadone (30–60 mg), precipitated withdrawal symptoms are more likely following higher doses.

OR

Methadone: 30 mg methadone syrup/solution orally on the first day, then reduce by 5 mg every day to 0. Reduction may be slower if desired.

NB: Short-term detoxification does not confer the benefits obtained from longer term opioid maintenance treatment for relapse prevention, and there is a high risk of relapse after detoxification with increased risks of death from overdose. However, exposure to these medications and to treatment staff in an out-patient or in-patient detoxification setting may encourage later engagement with maintenance therapy.

Option 2: Symptomatic treatment
Simple opioid withdrawal symptoms may require no treatment. However, if symptoms are distressing, the following regime may be instituted:
- **Diazepam:** 5–10 mg orally nocte (or in some cases every 6 h) for 3–4 days and then taper off over 2–3 days (for insomnia, anxiety, restlessness). Daily dispensing is recommended to reduce the risk of misuse
- **Hyoscine butylbromide:** 20 mg orally 6-hourly (for abdominal cramps)
- **Loperamide:** 2 tablets initially, then 1 tablet after each unformed stool (maximum 4 tablets/day) or atropine sulphate: diphenoxylate (Lomotil) 2 tablets 3–4 times a day (if diarrhoea is a problem)
- **Clonidine:** 150–300 mcg orally (or in some countries lofexidine is used instead as it causes less hypotension) 3–4 times a day reduces opioid withdrawal symptoms. Clonidine and lofexidine decrease central sympathetic outflow by stimulating central presynaptic inhibitory alpha-2-receptors on the noradrenaline neurons. As they can lower blood pressure regular monitoring is necessary. If diastolic pressure is <60 mmHg before any dose, omit that dose. Reduce clonidine/lofexidine in a stepwise fashion over a period of 1 week. (A small test dose of 50 mcg with monitoring of blood pressure is advisable prior to administering the full dose of clonidine.)
- Hydroxyzine or other sedating antihistamines may be used to help with insomnia.

NB: Quinine bisulphate is no longer recommended for the treatment of muscle cramps because of the risk of thrombocytopaenia.

Option 3: Accelerated 'Rapid Detoxification' or 'Ultra Rapid Opioid Detoxification (UROD)' induced by naltrexone
Naltrexone, a specific mu opioid antagonist, which acts by competitively blocking opioid receptors, may precipitate opioid withdrawal if administered soon after use of heroin or other opioids. To shorten the period of detoxification, strategies whereby naltrexone is administered to induce opioid withdrawal either under general anaesthesia (Ultra Rapid Opioid Detoxification) or light sedation (rapid detoxification) have been trialled. The resulting severe opioid withdrawal symptoms are treated symptomatically with clonidine, anti-emetics, and sedatives. Detoxification is then typically followed by 6–12 months maintenance treatment with naltrexone

to prevent relapse. While abstinence rates of more than 60% have been claimed, there is currently insufficient evidence of efficacy or safety to endorse this form of treatment as routine for opioid dependence.

Naltrexone induced withdrawal may be severe with vomiting, confusion, agitation, delirium, and depression. The risks of prolonged anaesthesia or sedation are significant of themselves. As it is associated with greater risks than conventionally treated (or, indeed, untreated heroin withdrawal), Ultra Rapid Opioid Detoxification or Rapid Detoxification is employed only as part of formal ethics approved studies or in selected private clinics. It is not standard practice in most mainstream drug and alcohol treatment units.

Sometimes patients and families place unrealistic expectations that rapid (or, indeed, any form of acute) detoxification may 'cure' their opioid dependence in one step. As with all substance dependence, management of the withdrawal syndrome is just an early step in achieving the desired outcome of long-term abstinence. Relapse prevention remains the main challenge.

Management of opioid withdrawal (opioid detoxification)

Detoxification may be defined as a process of helping patients to cease heroin and other drug use, by treating their withdrawals so that they are comfortable when they stop using.

Monitor with an opioid withdrawal scale.

1. Opioid substitution therapy with either

- Buprenorphine (Subutex 2 mg; 8 mg sublingual tablets) 4–8 mg sublingually on Day 1, increase by 2–4 mg/day to 10–12 mg/day. Then reduce by 0.4–2 mg/day to zero (Unless the patient wishes to undergo long term buprenorphine maintenance therapy—see relapse prevention section below).

NOTE: Before initiation of buprenorphine treatment, it is important to wait until opioid withdrawal signs and symptoms become evident— least 8 h after the last dose of heroin or 24 h after the last dose of low dose methadone, to avoid precipitation of opioid withdrawals.

OR

- Methadone 30 mg/6 mL orally on Day 1, reduce by 5 mg/day over the next 5 days to zero (unless patient wishes to undergo long-term maintenance therapy; p. 223).

2. Symptomatic treatment (if required):

- **Diazepam (Valium):** 5–10 mg orally nocte or qid orally for anxiety, agitation, insomnia
- **Metoclopramide (Maxolon):** 10 mg tds orally or intramuscularly for nausea and vomiting
- **Hyoscine butylbromide (Buscopan):** 20 mg qid orally or intramuscularly for abdominal cramps
- **Loperamide (Imodium):** 2 mg tablets orally, 2 tablets initially followed by one tablet after each unformed stool 9 max. 8 tablets/day) for diarrhoea.
- **Clonidine (Catapres):** 150 mcg tablets, 150–300 mcg orally tds (initial test dose of 75 mcg, monitor BP closely) or lofexidine
- **Hydroxyzine** or other sedating antihistamines may be used to help with insomnia.

NB: Naltrexone-induced Accelerated Rapid Detoxification or Ultra Rapid Opioid Detoxification is not recommended in a standard clinical setting.

Comprehensive assessment of opioid users

As described in the Chapter 2 (p. 37) comprehensive assessment should include:

History
Opioid use history
Amount, frequency, route, recency and duration of opioid use.
- Quantity of heroin is often described in street grams, quarters (approx 0.25 g) or points (approximately 0.1 g). As the purity of heroin varies these weights are only very approximate guides to the amounts used
- Money spent on heroin provides not only an indication of amount being used, but also the likely social impact of use
- Frequency of use—number of 'hits' per day, number of days per week
- Route: injected or inhaled?
- Recency: when was the last hit? Are you 'hanging out' (withdrawing) now?
- **Duration of use:** age of first use, age when use became daily. Since that time, how many years have you used and how many have you been 'clean' (abstinent from heroin).

Presence of dependence: In particular, does the individual experience withdrawals between doses of heroin or if heroin runs out?

Types of treatment tried
- What was the longest period of abstinence? How did you achieve this?
- What treatments have you tried? Why did you relapse?

Complications of heroin use
- In particular, viral hepatitis status (Hepatitis B,C): when were you last tested? Have you been vaccinated against Hepatitis B? What are your LFT's usually like?

Other drug use history
Including illicit and prescribed; in particular ask about benzodiazepines. Also, alcohol and tobacco use/dependence.

Other medical and psychiatric history
- Past hospitalizations
- Screening questions for mental health disorders? E.g. 'are you bothered much by anxiety or depression? Have you ever had treatment for a mental health disorder?

Family history/brief social history: including does partner or close friends use heroin?
Medications

Physical examination: As described on p. 42.
In particular, look for signs of intoxication or withdrawal, and consistency of physical signs with the history of recent drug use.

Check for signs of complications of opioid injecting, such as vein damage, stigmata of liver disease, cardiac murmurs.

Laboratory tests
- FBC
- EUC
- LFTs (isolated elevation of ALT suggests chronic hepatitis C infection; levels may fluctuate)
- Serological investigation for blood borne viruses (see below)
- Tests for sexually transmitted infections
- Urine drug screen—is useful both at initial assessment and as part of monitoring, as an objective measure of heroin or other drug use
- Other tests as indicated:
  - TFTs
  - CPK
  - BSL

Other investigations as indicated
- Chest X-ray (e.g. if fever)
- CT head/MRI (e.g. potential intra cerebral infection).

Assessment of viral infections
Assessment of viral infections should be undertaken at the Drug & Alcohol clinic or general practice as these patients will often not attend another specialty service whilst still having problems with injecting drug use.

> Offer serological testing for hepatitis C and B, and HIV on all patients with a history of injecting drug use, and where appropriate, tests for sexually transmitted infections.

- Serology for blood borne viruses:
  - Hepatitis C: Anti-HCV
  - If hepatitis C Ab positive, can periodically test HCV RNA (PCR) to assess if viral replication is occurring
  - If HCV RNA positive, further tests to define genotype and viral load if treatment is considered
  - Hepatitis B: HBsAg, HBsAb, HBcAb (see below)
  - HIV: Anti-HIV

Pre- and post-test counselling is important, not only to avoid stress, but as an opportunity for raising awareness of the risks of blood borne virus infection associated with injecting drug use, the need for testing for the presence of infection for up to 6 months after the last episode of injecting and for ongoing monitoring should viral hepatitis be present.

Interpretation of hepatitis C serology

- Hep C Ab positive—current or past infection (60–70% of injecting drug users are Anti-HVC positive)
- HCV RNA (PCR) positive—active replication of virus, infectivity
- Hepatitis C genotype (if treatment is being considered)—treatment efficacy varies by genotype (pp. 233, 373).

All HCV RNA positive patients should be informed of the availability and efficacy of treatment and offered referral.

Interpretation of hepatitis B serology

- Hep BsAg positive—acute or chronic infection with hepatitis B:
  - If Hep B eAg is also positive there is a high level of viral replication, higher level of infectivity, higher risk of progression of HBV liver disease
- Hep B core Ab—exposure to the virus:
  - Where HBsAg is negative, core antibody (IgG) represents past exposure to hepatitis B
- Hep BsAb positive—reflects immune state secondary to either vaccination or past infection.

Injecting drug users who are not immune to hepatitis B should be offered vaccination.

Hepatitis B antigen positive patients should be referred for possible treatment and their contacts followed up and tested.

In some cases, liver ultrasound and CT scan may be indicated to assess the severity of viral hepatitis, or the presence of a complication, such as hepatic carcinoma.

Serology for HIV

Anti-HIV positive—probable HIV infection, confirm with HIV RNA PCR or western blot.

If positive, refer to an appropriate specialist for monitoring and consideration for treatment.

Management of opioid dependence

After detoxification alone there is a high rate of relapse to opioid dependence. Tolerance to opioids reduces after periods of abstinence and so relapse is associated with an increased risk of death from overdose.

Therefore, it is most important to consider the long-term management of opioid dependence.

As with management of dependence on any psychoactive drug, treatment can be described by 10 steps:

1. Provision of information and education

Advice and education are provided. This may employ the principles of motivational interviewing.

2. Patient acceptance and commitment

Let the patient digest the information and advice provided, and consider their current status and available options. For treatment to be successful the patient must then reach a point of acceptance of the need to change their opioid use and to develop commitment.

3. Detoxification

Opioid detoxification is rarely indicated in injecting drug users. It has a place prior to entering a residential programme or therapeuatic community. Otherwise it should be employed cautiously given the evidence for increased morbidity and mortality following detoxification. There is no need to complete withdrawal before commencing methadone or buprenorphine.

4. Pharmacotherapy

Opioid maintenance therapy

Explain treatment options, including that opioid substitution treatment (with methadone, buprenorphine or Suboxone®) is currently the most effective way to help them achieve a goal of abstinence from heroin, resume daily work or other important activities, and avoid or minimize harm associated with injecting drug use.

The long-acting opioid provides relief from craving and withdrawal symptoms, and allows the patient to escape the domination of illicit opioids over the rest of life. The large amounts of time previously spent getting money to buy heroin, being intoxicated, or withdrawing is now freed up by the use of a single daily dose of a supervised, pure and long-acting opioid.

Once stability has been achieved and sustained, the opioid maintenance treatment can be slowly reduced and, in stable cases, weaned off altogether.

Maintenance opioid treatment of heroin dependence results in 70% reduction in heroin use and improved treatment retention compared with non pharmacological treatments, with 40–50% of patients remaining in treatment at six months. It avoids the multiple complications of injecting drug use (pp. 207, 367), substantially reduces criminal activity and enables re-engagement in routine life.

Legal and administrative requirements in prescribing methadone and buprenorphine

The legal restrictions on prescribing opioid maintenance treatment vary considerably between countries.

In Australia, for example, in order to prescribe methadone or buprenorphine to heroin-dependent patients, medical practitioners must be accredited by the State or Territory health department after completing a training course. In addition, each patient who is to commence methadone or buprenorphine for treatment of opioid dependence must be approved by the state authority. This is to prevent the same patient presenting for opioids at more than one service. There are clearly defined guidelines on the need for supervision of methadone dosing (by a clinic or pharmacy). In the early stages of maintenance, all doses are supervised at a clinic. Once a person is stable they generally have the option of transferring to pharmacy dosing, and gradually increasing the number of unsupervised ('takeaway') doses per week, to a maximum of 4 takeaways of methadone per week. For Suboxone® the number of takeaways can be progressively increased so that a very stable patient collects their medication from a pharmacy only once a month. In Australia if a patient is under the age of 18 years a second opinion from an approved prescriber is necessary in some regions. In some regions patients under the age of 16 years cannot be prescribed methadone unless court approval is obtained.

In UK there are less restrictions on prescribing, which can be by trained psychiatrists or GPs. Consumption of the opioid dose is usually monitored at community pharmacies or in specialized clinical drug treatment settings, though stable patients may graduate to take supplies home on a weekly basis.

Methadone maintenance treatment

Induction to methadone maintenance

Informed consent should always be obtained from the patient before entry into an opioid maintenance programme. In particular, persons entering into methadone maintenance should understand that reduction off methadone is a slow process which may take months.

Commence treatment with 20–30 mg methadone orally daily. Maximum starting dose is 40 mg to avoid risk of overdose. If the patient has been abstinent from heroin for a period of time, starting dose should be low (e.g. 20 mg). Do not administer methadone if patient is drowsy or intoxicated. Steady state levels are reached by 5–7 days. During the induction phase, patients should be reviewed daily (e.g. by a nurse or doctor).

Increase the dose of methadone by increments of 5 mg every three or four days until the patient is stable. An adequate dose should provide the patient with 24 h relief of cravings and withdrawal symptoms.

A maintenance dose of 60–90 mg/day is sufficient for many patients to relieve withdrawal symptoms and then to facilitate their ceasing heroin use. However, some patients may require considerably higher doses.

If there is ongoing regular heroin use (especially greater than weekly), the patient is offered an increased dose of methadone, so that any slip up to heroin use is less likely to produce significant euphoria. If the heroin use is only intermittent (e.g. fortnightly on payday), in some cases it may be more appropriate to try to address this via behavioural means (e.g. ensuring they have an activity with a non-using friend organized for pay day.)

A second specialist opinion should be obtained for doses >150 mg (this is required in Australia).

• Occasional individuals are rapid metabolizers of methadone and average doses do not relieve withdrawal symptoms (or achieve a therapeutic plasma concentration). If clinically a patient seems to require a dose greater than 200 mg, first measure trough methadone levels (i.e. before the day's methadone dose is due), to document that plasma levels are low despite adequate attendance at dosing. Perform an ECG to check for QTc prolongation. Some rapid metabolizers of methadone may need to switch drugs, use higher doses, or split the methadone dose twice daily, rather than daily)

• The patient should be maintained at an adequate dose for at least 6 months.

• If the patient wishes to cease methadone maintenance treatment, reduce the dose by 2.5–5 mg every 1–2 weeks, or slower if necessary, to zero. If there is no need for haste, reducing by 2.5 mg fortnightly often ensures a smooth and relatively symptom-free reduction in dose. At this rate it is often only when methadone doses fall below 40mg that withdrawal symptoms are felt. If withdrawal symptoms have become problematic by the time the methadone dose has fallen to ≤30 mg daily, the patient may transfer to buprenorphine maintenance at least 24 h after the last dose of low dose methadone (see below).

Further reading

Henry-Edwards S, Gowing L, White J, Ali R, Bell J, Brough R, *et al. Clinical guidelines and procedures for the use of methadone in the maintenance treatment of opioid dependence.* Canberra: Australian Government Department of Health and Ageing, 2003. Available at: http://www.health.gov.au/internet/wcms/publishing.nsf/Content/health-pubhlth-publicat-drugpubs.htm/$FILE/methadone_cguide.pdf

Buprenorphine maintenance treatment

Buprenorphine is a partial agonist with high receptor affinity but low activity, so to avoid precipitating withdrawals, wait at least 8 h after the last dose of heroin. Longer periods of time are needed following longer acting opioids.

Induction to buprenorphine maintenance: Depending on the severity of heroin dependence, commence with 4–8 mg buprenorphine on day 1. In a person who has had a longer period of abstinence from heroin, a lower starting dose may be needed, e.g. 2 mg.

Increase buprenorphine by 2–4 mg daily until the patient is comfortable up to a maximum daily dose of 12–24 mg/day. Follow-up the patient every week with further increments 2–4 mg every 4 days until stabilization has been achieved. The maximum daily dose is 32 mg. A second specialist opinion is required for doses >32 mg.

Some centres use a more rapid induction regime but this is still being evaluated.

The patient should be advised against using heroin, street methadone or other opioids during the period of dose stabilization. If they do, difficulties in dose stabilization and opioid withdrawal symptoms (in the case of buprenorphine) may develop and require symptomatic treatment. Overdose is a risk particularly with the combination of heroin and methadone.

Side effects of buprenorphine are often few. Many people report feeling very normal on buprenorphine. Headache and nausea may occur, and may suggest the need for a lower dose. A 'racing' or 'speed-like' effect has been reported with buprenorphine. This tends to resolve with a lower dose.

If the patient wishes to cease buprenorphine treatment, reduce the dose by 2 mg weekly to zero. To avoid insomnia after cessation of buprenorphine, the final stages of reduction (e.g. once the patient has reached 2 mg daily) can be slowed down to 0.4 mg weekly.

For most patients, weaning off buprenorphine is relatively symptom-free when conducted at this pace.

Advantages of buprenorphine

- Long duration of action:
  - Alternate day dosing is typically possible, using double the dose, up to a maximum of 32 mg
  - In some patients higher doses (triple dose to a maximum of 32 mg) can used to provide 3 day weekend cover
- Less euphoria
- Less sedation than methadone—'feel more normal' (though not all want to)
- Less severe withdrawals on dose reduction and cessation
- Relatively safe in overdose because of 'ceiling effect', e.g. if accidentally taken by children.

Disadvantages of buprenorphine

- Need for sublingual administration (takes 4–7 min to dissolve)
- Easy diversion if not properly supervised
- May precipitate withdrawals in opioid dependent patients
- Naloxone is only partially effective in overdose; dose of naloxone may have to be increased to 15–20 times, and assisted ventilation may be required.

Precautions with buprenorphine

Drug interactions
- **MAOIs**
- **CNS depressants:** alcohol, benzodiazepines, antihistamines, tricyclic antidepressants, major tranquillizers (additive depressant effect). *Deaths have been reported following the combined use of buprenorphine with benzodiazepines and/or alcohol*

- **Hepatic CYP3A4 enzyme inhibitors**: slow the metabolism of buprenorphine: Protease inhibitors, antimycotics, calcium channel blockers; macrolide antibiotics, fluoxetine and fluvoxamine (particularly the latter)
- **Hepatic CYP3A4 enzyme inducers**: metabolism is enhanced by phenobarbital, rifampicin, phenytoin, carbamazepine, and cortisol.

Concomitant medical conditions
- As for all opioids: use with caution where there is recent head injury, acute abdomen or chronic airways limitation
- Significant liver disease.

Concomitant psychiatric conditions
- **Psychosis**
- **Pregnancy:** is listed as a contraindication to buprenorphine by the manufacturers in Australia, but not in UK and many European countries. There is a growing body of evidence to the safety of buprenorphine if the patient wants to use it.

Contraindications
- Acute intoxication with alcohol or other CNS depressants
- Severe hepatic or renal insufficiency
- Suboxone® is contraindicated in pregnancy.

Principles of methadone maintenance and buprenorphine maintenance treatment
- Initial doses must be modest (no more than 40 mg with methadone and 8 mg with buprenorphine)
- Approximately 4 half-lives are needed to achieve steady state trough levels, i.e. about 4–6 days for methadone and may be 5–10 or more days for buprenorphine
- Drug interactions: methadone and buprenorphine both are metabolized by some common pathways such as cytochrome P450. Fluoxetine and fluvoxamine both inhibit the breakdown of agonist treatments, most substantially with the latter . Metabolism is enhanced by rifampicin, phenytoin and cortisol. Anti-retroviral zidovudine metabolism is slowed by methadone but not by buprenorphine
- Optimal doses of methadone are typically 60–90 mg. Usually dose is titrated according to clinical response
- Optimal doses of buprenorphine are typically in the 12–24 mg range. Maximum dose is 32 mg for daily or second daily dosing.

Further reading

Lintzeris N, Clark N, Winstock A, Dunlop A, Muhleisen P, Gowing L, *et al. National clinical guidelines and procedures for the use of buprenorphine in the treatment of opioid dependence.* Canberra: Australian Government Department of Health and Ageing 2006. Available at: http://www.nationaldrugstrategy.gov.au/internet/drugstrategy/publishing.nsf/Content/buprenorphine-guide

Suboxone®

Suboxone® is a combination tablet containing buprenorphine and naloxone in the ratio 4:1. It is taken sublingually in a dose of buprenorphine the same as that of buprenorphine alone. Naloxone, a mu opioid receptor blocker, has no effect when taken sublingually/orally. It is added to buprenorphine in order to prevent diversion and illicit intravenous use for naloxone is active when administered intravenously. This means that if the buprenorphine: naloxone combination is injected intravenously, naloxone will to some extent block the effect of buprenorphine, but more importantly it will precipitate withdrawals in opioid dependent persons. In this way diversion to replace street heroin use is reduced. The combination has the advantage of increasing the possibility of unsupervised takeaways. The buprenorphine–naloxone combination is contraindicated in pregnancy and the need for contraception is required if considering it.

Choosing between methadone and buprenorphine/Suboxone®

Patients will often have a strong preference as to which form of opioid maintenance treatment they prefer.

There is not yet a firm evidence base to guide choice, but clinical practice suggests that:

- Methadone may offer advantages to patients:
  - With co-morbid psychiatric conditions, where the sedating side effects of methadone may be beneficial
  - Where craving is not adequately relieved with appropriate doses of buprenorphine
  - Where engagement has been (or is predicted to be) difficult with buprenorphine, e.g. challenging behaviour, severe opioid dependence. The fact that withdrawal is experienced earlier after a missed dose of methadone, encourages more regular attendance.
- Buprenorphine may offer particular advantages to patients:
  - Who have a shorter duration of opioid dependence, or less severe dependence
  - Who prefer to avoid any sedating side effects
  - Who need the flexibility of future takeaway (unsupervised) doses, e.g. for work. Because of the relative safety of the Suboxone® formulation, in some regions, in a very stable patient, tablets can eventually be dispensed monthly
  - Who are known to be fast metabolizers of methadone or are on medications that will interact with methadone, more than with buprenorphine.

Prescribing methadone or buprenorphine for in-patients

If a patient is documented to be already on a methadone maintenance programme, methadone is continued in hospital unless specific contraindications like head injury or unconsciousness are present. It is important to check the date and amount of the last dose given with the dispensing point.

If the patient is nil by mouth, a reduced dose (e.g. two thirds the oral dose is often given intramuscularly—as divided twice daily doses).

Patients on methadone who experience *acute pain* (e.g. broken bones) and who require opiate analgesia will typically need the analgesia *in addition to* their usual dose of methadone. Forms of analgesia which are not compromised by opioid tolerance, such as tramadol (which has serotonergic, as well as opioid actions), or strong non-steroidal anti inflammatory drugs (e.g. ketorolac) may provide relief for some patients.

If a patient has heroin dependence and is not yet on methadone or buprenorphine, they can be offered the option of commencing maintenance treatment while in hospital, provided that a prescriber and dosing point will be available when they leave hospital. Informed consent should be obtained, as per standard induction onto treatment.

Follow-up and monitoring for out-patients on opioid maintenance treatment

A nurse, pharmacist or doctor assesses whether the patient is overdosed or withdrawing at the time of each supervised dose.

The prescribing doctor reviews the patient on the methadone or buprenorphine programmes regularly with urine drug screens as required, initially at weekly intervals. Once stable, the patient is reviewed at monthly to three monthly intervals. At review, recent drug use is assessed and the patient is examined for fresh needle track marks and signs of opioid intoxication or withdrawal.

In drug and alcohol treatment services a case worker is typically allocated who:
- Monitors progress
- Provides support, advice and counselling
- Assesses and monitors any concerns in relation to any children under the care of the patient
- Assists with (or refers for assistance with) accommodation, employment, and other needs
- Provides harm minimization interventions where indicated.

Missed doses of opioid maintenance treatment

As tolerance to opioids can reduce with a period of opioid abstinence, if a patient misses 3 or more doses of maintenance treatment the dose should be reduced.

Methadone
- Patients who miss 3–5 consecutive doses need assessment for the extent of intervening heroin use and presence of intoxication or withdrawal. Then the previous dose is usually halved, as tolerance may have reduced, then gradually increased back to the original dose over the ensuing days.
- If the patient has missed more than 5 doses, they recommence methadone via the induction regimen above.

Buprenorphine
- Patients who miss 1 or 2 doses of buprenorphine may receive the usual dose subsequently (this dose should always be at least 8–12 h after any heroin use)
- Patients who miss 3–5 days consecutive daily dosing (or of alternative day dosing):

- If there is no likelihood of precipitated opioid withdrawals (no heroin in the past 8–12 h, no long acting opioids in the past 24 h), the next dose of buprenorphine is administered in a dose of half to two thirds of the usual dose, up to a maximum of 24 mg. The dose is increased gradually back to the usual dose
- The patient who has used heroin in the past 8–12 h should be asked to re-present after >4 h to assess for intoxication or withdrawals

- Patients who miss more than 5 consecutive doses require re-induction onto buprenorphine as per the initial induction regime.

Switching over maintenance agents

From methadone to buprenorphine: Slowly taper the dose of methadone to preferably less than 30 mg/day (wherever possible not more than 40 mg/day). Maintain on this dose for at least 1 week. To avoid precipitating opioid withdrawals, wait at least 24 h after the last dose of methadone before commencing buprenorphine. Ideally, the patient should be starting to experience opioid withdrawal symptoms before buprenorphine is started.

Starting dose: 2–4 mg buprenorphine on Day 1; increase by 2–4 mg/day according to response to maximum of 12–24 mg/day. Subsequently, monitor the patient every week, with further increments of 2–8 mg/week according to response, until stabilization has been achieved (maximum daily dose 32 mg).

In some centres there have been recent trials of transferring patients from higher doses of methadone to buprenorphine, but in these situations, precipitated withdrawal is likely. Transfers from higher dose of methadone should generally be undertaken by a specialist unit and, in some cases, as an in-patient.

From buprenorphine to methadone: Taper dose of buprenorphine to at least 16 mg/day for several days before transfer. Wait at least 24 h before commencing methadone 20–30 mg/day (maximum daily dose 40 mg). Increase by 5 mg methadone every 3–4 days until stabilization is achieved.

Pregnancy

In the latter half of pregnancy, methadone requirements may increase gradually. Then, typically after the baby is born, the dose may need to be reduced somewhat. In each case, dosage is titrated against clinical symptoms.

Buprenorphine is not currently recommended by the manufacturers for use in pregnancy, but early studies suggest it may be as safe or safer than methadone.

Concurrent benzodiazepine use

Up to 35% of patients in an opioid treatment programme are known to use benzodiazepines. This may emerge via the history or via routine urine drug screen (which should always test for benzodiazepines). The concurrent use of benzodiazepines carries the additional risk of overdose, especially if either drug is used IV.

Where dependent on benzodiazepines, a supervised benzodiazepine reduction regime may be required once opioid treatment is stabilized (p. 179).

How long should maintenance treatment be continued?
Patients should be on opioid maintenance treatment for as long as is necessary to achieve stability (typically at least 6 months, in some cases many years). Not all patients feel safe to stop opioid maintenance treatment and their self-assessment of risk of relapse is important.

If the patient has been free from illicit heroin use (preferably for at least 6 months), their life is relatively stable and they would like to commence reduction of maintenance treatment, a gradual reduction of dose can be planned with the patient. In many centres, a flexible script can be written, so that the patient has the option to reduce their dose (by a defined amount) when they feel comfortable to do so.

Weaning off maintenance treatment

Weaning off methadone
- Slowly reducing the dose to zero may take weeks to several months
- For methadone maintenance—reduce by 2.5–5 mg every 1–2 weeks or slower if necessary to zero
- Ideally, 2.5 mg reduction no more than fortnightly, to minimize withdrawal
- If withdrawal is troublesome despite a slow rate of dose reduction, the patient can switch to buprenorphine
- The switch to buprenorphine is easier if methadone dose as been 30 mg or lower for at least a week.

Weaning off buprenorphine
- For buprenorphine maintenance—reduce the dose by 2 mg weekly down to a dose of 2 mg. The rate of reduction may then be slowed to 0.4 mg weekly.

There are typically fewer withdrawal symptoms when weaning off buprenorphine than off methadone.

Heroin maintenance: Trials of heroin maintenance treatment are under way in some centres in the UK. In some countries like the UK, heroin prescription has been a niche treatment for a small number of heroin dependent individuals. There has been some resurgence of interest in heroin prescription in recent years with findings from controlled trials in Switzerland, the Netherlands, and now the UK.

Dealing with other challenging situations: More detailed guidelines are available to assist with situations such as missed doses, accidental overdosing, vomited doses, etc., for example from:
- **Australia:** NSW Health. *New South Wales Opioid Treatment Programme. Clinical guidelines for methadone and buprenorphine treatment of opioid dependence.* Sydney: Mental Health and Drug and Alcohol Office, New South Wales Health, 2006. Available at: http://www.health.nsw.gov.au/policies/gl/2006/pdf/GL2006_019.pdf
- **UK:** *Drug Misuse and Dependence—Guidelines on Clinical Management.* London: Stationery Office, 2007. Available at: http://www.nta.nhs.uk/publications/documents/clinical_guidelines_2007.pdf

Maintenance treatment with an opioid antagonist: naltrexone

Pharmacology

Naltrexone, a specific mu antagonist, acts by competitively blocking opioid receptors. It possesses no intrinsic opioid-like effects and there is no risk of dependence. Peak plasma levels are reached in 1 h. It is metabolized in the liver to 6-beta naltrexol and excreted primarily in the urine. The half-life of naltrexone is about 4 h and that of 6-beta naltrexol is 12 h. Unlike naloxone, naltrexone is effective orally and the longer duration of action enables once a day dosage. Depot preparations with much longer durations of action are currently under investigation.

Naltrexone is an alternative to methadone or buprenorphine for relapse prevention in opioid dependent patients who wish to remain drug free. It is indicated as part of a comprehensive treatment and rehabilitation programme with extensive psychosocial support, individual and family counselling and follow-up to enhance compliance. It works best in individuals for whom compliance can be made mandatory, e.g. doctors and pharmacists.

As naltrexone may precipitate severe opioid withdrawal signs and symptoms if taken soon after dependent patients have recently used opioids, treatment should not be initiated until the patient has remained heroin free for at least 7–10 days. This is best achieved by a period of detoxification either in a detoxification unit or at home under professional supervision.

An opioid-free state is verified by urine drug screens and a naloxone challenge test. If signs and symptoms of opioid withdrawal are observed after the challenge, a waiting period of 24 h is recommended before repeating the challenge. Because of the long half-life of methadone (approximately 20 h) or buprenorphine (up to 72 h depending on the dose), a drug-free period for 2–3 weeks is recommended prior to initiating treatment with naltrexone.

Patient acceptability of naltrexone is poor, and lack of compliance and high drop out rates, particularly in the first month of treatment, are commonly encountered.

Whilst on naltrexone, attempts to self administer heroin or other opioids will have no effect.

Precautions with naltrexone

- Patients with chronic pain on opioid analgesics.
- Discontinue for at least 72 h prior to elective surgery. In emergencies, blockade may be overcome by greater than normal doses of opioids, but this carries the risk of respiratory depression and histamine release.

Further reading

Bell J, Kimber J, Lintzeris N, White J, Monheit B, Henry-Edwards S, et al. Clinical guidelines and procedures for the use of naltrexone in the treatment of opioid dependence. Canberra: Australian Government Department of Health and Ageing 2003. Available at: http://www.health.gov.au/internet/wcms/publishing.nsf/Content/health-pubhlth-publicat-drugpubs.htm/$FILE/naltrexone_cguide.pdf

Naltrexone maintenance treatment in opioid dependence

- An alternative to methadone or buprenorphine
- Patient compliance is a major limitation—needs high patient commitment
  - Treatment retention may be as low as 5%
- May precipitate withdrawals in opioid dependent patients. (Ensure that there is an interval of at least one week between the last dose of heroin and the first dose of naltrexone)
- 50 mg naltrexone blocks the effects of 25 mg heroin for up to 24 h
- Reduces tolerance to opioids—after ceasing naltrexone self-administration of opioids at doses previously safely used, may now lead to coma or even death
- Requires a comprehensive treatment and rehabilitation programme with counselling, psychosocial support and follow up to enhance compliance.

Side effects

- >10% patients may complain of non specific side effects, mainly gastrointestinal symptoms
- Depression
- Anxiety, nervousness
- Low energy
- Headache, joint, and muscular pain
- Dose-related hepatocellular injury
- Sedation
- Confusion
- Rarely visual hallucinations.

5. Psychological treatments

These can be provided to some extent by the treating doctor, but in many cases, also referring the patient to a psychologist or counsellor has significant advantages. As well as supportive counselling, a number of specific approaches are commonly employed:

- **Motivational enhancement therapy:** can be used both to help enhance engagement with treatment (initially and on an ongoing basis), and to address illicit opioid use.
- **Cognitive behavioural therapy:** e.g. may include increasing understanding and methods for dealing with the triggers to drug use; training to enhance skills in problem solving, assertiveness, communication, behavioural self management, relaxation, stress or anger management, or alcohol and drug refusal)
- A range of other approaches are employed in some centres, such as behaviour modification programmes (e.g. community reinforcement approach; contingency management).

6. Treatment of complications and co-morbidity

Parallel treatment of underlying medical, neuropsychiatric co-morbidity or complications, e.g. treatment of hepatitis C, depression.

Monitoring and management of blood borne virus infection

Patients often believe that, if they feel well, there is no need for monitoring or treatment for blood borne viruses. The patient should be well educated about the value of monitoring as an early warning system should harms or disease progression occur.

Hepatitis C

Patients with chronic hepatitis C infection are generally asymptomatic. If symptoms occur, the main symptom is tiredness or lethargy.

Any patient who is hepatitis C antibody positive needs regular monitoring of LFTs (usually twice yearly) and periodic monitoring of HCV RNA (PCR), unless he or she has cleared the virus [HCV RNA (PCR), negative]. Viral clearance without treatment occurs in about 20% of cases.

Effective treatment with pegylated interferon and ribavirin is now available and all HCV RNA positive patients should be informed of its availability and efficacy. If HCV RNA remains positive it indicates active replication of the virus as well as infectivity. Such patients should be encouraged to undergo treatment to prevent progression of the disease and further spread of hepatitis C viral infection, if their lifestyle is sufficiently stable. If treatment is being considered, test for viral load and genotype and refer to a liver specialist.

Where there is persistent LFT elevation or evidence of reducing liver function (e.g. falling platelets or rising INR, even in the presence of normal LFTs), referral to a liver specialist should be particularly prompt.

Assessment for treatment will usually include liver ultrasound and or CT scan. Some centres perform liver biopsy prior to treatment, though, in an attempt to remove barriers to treatment, this is becoming less routine in other countries (e.g. Australia).

Treatment with pegylated interferon and ribavirin is effective, and can optimally produce sustained viral response in 40–50% of genotype 1 and 4 infections, and up to 80% of genotype 2 and 3 infections.

All patients with hepatitis C should be advised not to drink alcohol to excess as this aggravates viral hepatitis. There is not clear evidence as to what level of drinking is safe in this condition. Some clinicians advise limiting consumption to half the recommended limit for a healthy person, and ensuring the consumption is not daily.

Patients should be educated on avoiding spread of hepatitis C (e.g. taking care with blood spills, avoid sharing toothbrush, comb or razor where their may be microscopic blood transfer).

Hepatitis B

Injecting drug users who are not immune to Hepatitis B should be offered vaccination.

Hepatitis B antigen positive patients should be referred for possible treatment, and their contacts followed-up and tested. Advice on preventing spread should be provided (e.g. vaccination of key contacts, protected sex with non immune partners).

In persons with established cirrhosis, regular monitoring will include AFP, to screen for hepatic carcinoma. Wherever possible, treatment and monitoring will be conducted in association with a liver specialist.

HIV

Patients who are HIV Ab positive should be referred to the appropriate HIV specialist (e.g. immunology or infectious diseases specialist) to assess the need for treatment and for monitoring.

Treatment of co-morbid psychiatric symptoms

Depression and anxiety

For some individuals, opioids may be used to self-medicate a pre-existing depression. However, for a significant number, depressive symptoms remit once the individual's opioid problem is treated. This suggests the symptoms may be caused by the stresses and chaotic lifestyle associated with the disorder, as well as the pharmacological instability related to altering states of intoxication and withdrawal.

As a general guideline, consider starting an antidepressant medication if the depression persists for more than 4 weeks after initiating treatment, or there is a clear history of depression during previous periods of abstinence for 4 weeks or more.

Depressed patients with hepatitis C require treatment of depression prior to commencing treatment with interferon as depression is a contra-indication to treatment.

Protracted abstinence syndrome: There is no effective treatment for symptoms such as insomnia, lethargy, irritability, depression, anxiety, reduced self-esteem and an abnormal response to stressful experience, but the patient should be reassured that the symptoms are normal, and will improve and abate over time (for insomnia see p. 354). Cognitive behavioural strategies may be useful to help the individual gain some control over the symptoms. Some patients with pre-existing anxiety or depressive disorders will find these re-emerge once they withdraw from opioids and medication should be instituted in such cases.

7. Support for and of family and friends

Families of users require support, assistance, and advice on how to cope with living/interacting with the user. Families also need information and advice on how to best support and help the user.

8. Self-help (mutual-help) organizations

Narcotics Anonymous (NA): As with AA for alcohol dependence, NA can be offered to opioid dependent patients who are seeking to maintain abstinence, particularly those who are not taking opioid maintenance treatment. As NA groups have traditionally discouraged opioid maintenance treatment, patients on opioid maintenance treatment are not generally referred to NA.

Nar-Anon and Nalteen are associated organizations developed to provide education and support for partners and teenage children of drug-dependent patients.

9. Continual care/follow-up

Regular monitoring and support, and the maintenance of a therapeutic and relationship is highly important. At follow-up the clinician can regularly reassess the situation (gathering new information, revising diagnoses and treatment plans accordingly).

Residential in-patient treatment/rehabilitation programmes

While the cost effectiveness of residential in-patient treatment and rehabilitation programmes are subject to debate, residential in-patient treatment programmes are appropriate for some patients who have failed to respond to out-patient treatment, who are polysubstance users (e.g. alcohol and/or benzodiazepines, or chaotic stimulant use), have no social support, and who have co morbid psychiatric or medical illnesses. Such programmes have demonstrated efficacy.

In addition to providing food and shelter and some 'time out' in safer environment, residential treatment programmes provide a structured daily routine and staff directed programmes, and daily activities. Ideally, the programmes should be tailored according to the needs of individual patients.

Patients with severe co-existing psychiatric or medical problems who are unable to look after themselves may require longer term care either in residential facilities or in a nursing home.

10. Changes to lifestyle, home, and environment

Many heroin dependent individuals find they are only able to cease illicit opioid use by reducing or cutting off contact with heroin using friends.

Re-engaging with activities of normal living (e.g. training, employment or recreation), helps reduce boredom, improve self esteem, and reduces the risk of drug use. Simple measures like increasing level of exercise, can improve mood and self esteem, and reduce the risk of relapse. Where the individual has unstable or unsuitable housing, assisting them to address this can have an important impact on drug use.

Further reading

Godfrey C, Stewart D, Gossop M. Economic analysis of costs and consequences of the treatment of drug misuse: 2-year outcome data from the National Treatment Outcome Research Study (NTORS). *Addiction* 2004; **99**: 697–707.

Teesson M, Mills K, Ross J, Darke S, Williamson A, Havard. A. The impact of treatment on 3 years' outcome for heroin dependence: findings from the Australian Treatment Outcome Study (ATOS). *Addiction* 2008; **103**: 80–88.

Harm reduction/palliation

It is common for some injecting drug use to continue in the induction phase of opioid maintenance treatment, until adequate doses are reached. Other individuals have great difficulty totally eliminating injecting drug use, and sporadic use continues while on treatment. Even while efforts proceed to help the individual cease heroin use, it is important to provide realistic harm reduction advice.

Patients on methadone maintenance treatment in particular should be warned of the risk of overdose if they use heroin on top of methadone. This risk is further increased by use together with other sedatives such as benzodiazepines and alcohol.

For those individuals who continue to inject (whether or not they have accepted treatment for their dependence), check if they are using clean needles, and are aware of the risk of transmission of Hepatitis C from other injecting equipment.

Any patient who is not yet immune to Hepatitis B (or currently infected) should be offered Hepatitis B vaccination. In pregnant women, defer vaccination till after birth of the baby. Patients with chronic hepatitis C infection, particularly those who are HCV-RNA positive should be considered for treatment.

Prevention

Control supply has been the measure most widely used to prevent illicit opioid use.

There is evidence that when supply of heroin is reduced (whether by international factors or local controls) that rates of heroin overdose decrease. However some users will switch to use of other illicit or licit substances when heroin is less available.

Community education methods are used to attempt to reduce demand for heroin, but evidence for the effectiveness of these is limited.

There has not been a great deal of research specifically into prevention of illicit opioid use, however general measures to reduce the risk factors for illicit drug use are likely to be beneficial: e.g. early intervention for children in troubled families, addressing disadvantage in communities, increasing opportunities for individuals at risk to feel connected to and valued by society and quality treatment of mental health disorders.

Summary

Illicit opioid use often causes deaths and sickness among young people, and chronic opioid dependence typically runs a course of relapse and remission. Accordingly, opioid users may regularly come into contact with the health care system. Any contact may provide the opportunity for engagement of the individual with treatment and/or harm reduction services. Treatment has well documented efficacy. Currently opioid maintenance treatment is the most effective treatment available. While the person is engaged in treatment, their concurrent or complicating medical conditions (in particular, hepatitis C) and psychiatric conditions can be treated.

Further reading

Law F Daglish MRC, Myles JS, Nutt DJ. The clinical use of buprenorphine in opiate addiction: evidence and practice. *Acta Neuropsychiatrica* 2004; **16**: 246–274.

Lingford-Hughes AR, Welch S, Nutt DJ, *et al.* Evidence-based guidelines for the pharmacological management of substance misuse, addiction and co-morbidity: recommendations from the British Association for Psychopharmacology. *Journal of Psychopharmacology* 2004; **18**: 293–335.

NSW Health. *New South Wales Opioid Treatment Programme. Clinical guidelines for methadone and buprenorphine treatment of opioid dependence.* Sydney: Mental Health and Drug and Alcohol Office, New South Wales Health 2006. Available at: www.health.nsw.gov.au, via: http://www.health.nsw.gov.au/policies/gl/2006/pdf/GL2006_019.pdf

Psychostimulants

The psychostimulants are a group of drugs that increase central nervous system arousal and are typically sympathomimetics, acting like noradrenaline to increase cardiovascular tone and activity. The term psychostimulants is reserved for those drugs whose primary actions are central nervous stimulation.

Naturally occurring psychostimulants have been used by human beings for thousands of years. These include cocaine (found in coca leaves), betel (areca nut; p. 291) and khat (p. 289). In addition, there are numerous synthetically manufactured psychostimulants, such as amphetamines and their derivatives.

Amphetamines were used by armed forces in the 20th century for the prevention of fatigue and sleep ('wakies'). They were commonly used in South East Asian countries such as Japan in the 1950s and 1960s. The last decade, has seen a marked increase in the illicit production of amphetamine-type stimulants, and they are now the second most common illicit drug used after cannabis in both high income and low income countries. Considerable public concern has been expressed about incidents of violence, and dependence relating to potent and long acting preparations such as methamphetamine ('ice').

Prescribed amphetamine type stimulants (ATS) such as dexamphetamine and methylphenidate are used for the treatment of narcolepsy and attention deficit hyperactivity disorder (ADHD). Diethylpropion hydrochloride and phentermine were previously prescribed as appetite suppressants, but because of concerns about dependence and other cardiovascular side effects are now rarely used.

Amphetamine-type stimulants are available in illicit preparations, and less often as prescribed drugs which are diverted into recreational use.

Illicit psychostimulants

Illicit psychostimulants are commonly manufactured in backyard laboratories. The exact potency, content, and purity is uncertain.

Table 9.1 Commonly used illicit stimulants

Chemical name	Vernacular 'street' names
1. Amphetamine type stimulants (ATS)	
Amphetamine sulphate	Speed, goey, whiz
Crystalline methamphetamine (purity of 70–85%)	Ice, crystal, shabu, glass, hot, meth
Methamphetamine base (purity of 40–50%)	Paste
3,4-Methylenedioxymethamphetamine (MDMA)	Ecstasy, E, eckies, love drug
Paramethoxyamphetamine (PMA)	PMA
2. Cocaine	Coke, charlie, snow, blow, nose candy, toot
3. Benzylpiperazine (BZP)	Herbal party pill, legal X

Epidemiology

Methamphetamine and amphetamine are the major amphetamine type stimulants used worldwide, followed by 3,4 methylenedioxymethamphetamine (MDMA or 'ecstasy' as it is commonly known).

Use of amphetamine-type stimulants is relatively common. Between 3.5 to 4% of Australian and New Zealand adults report having used amphetamines in the past year, as do 1.5–2% of UK and US adults. MDMA use varies between countries, with 1% of US adults, 2% of NZ and UK adults, and up to 4% of adult Australians using it in the past year. Amphetamines are most likely to be the first illicit drug to be injected. There are currently 73,000 methamphetamine dependent users in Australia (compared with 19,000 who are heroin dependent) in Australia. The use of methamphetamine varies greatly between countries, and in the UK there is little abuse because the preferred ATS is amphetamine sulphate. In the USA there is much methamphetamine use especially in the gay scene and driven by both imports from South and Central America and local laboratories often run by 'biker' gangs. Reasons for such large national variations are not well understood but include historical allegiances to drugs and availability of precursors such as pseudoephedrine.

Increases in the prevalence of stimulant use over the past decade, and the growing availability of more potent forms such as methamphetamine have been associated with increased presentations to the Emergency Departments. Individuals typically present with agitated, aggressive and chaotic behaviour and psychosis which has led to increased rates of admissions to psychiatric hospitals.

Overall cocaine is used less widely, although the prevalence varies greatly with availability from country to country. Use is concentrated in North America, Latin America and some European countries. In the US use of cocaine (2.8%) is more common than use of amphetamine-type stimulants. In the UK cocaine and crack cocaine are more prevalent and commonly used than either amphetamine or methamphetamine. In contrast, cocaine is more expensive in Australia where its use is less prevalent than that of amphetamines. Although complications associated with use of cocaine are not dissimilar to those observed with amphetamine use, the incidence and severity of such complications are often greater, though the acute effects are shorter-lived on account of its shorter half-life than amphetamines.

Up to two-thirds of users become dependent on cocaine, particularly those who inject or smoke it. In the UK, cocaine (and MDMA) are classified as Class A drugs (most harmful), while amphetamines are in the Class B category (intermediate category). Methamphetamine has recently been reclassified to A in the UK scheme in an attempt to prevent its use escalating.

Pharmacology

All stimulants cause CNS arousal, excitation and have sympathomimetic effects similar to noradrenaline.

Amphetamines and amphetamine type stimulants

The primary action of amphetamines is to activate the release of the monoamines dopamine, noradrenaline, and serotonin from central storage sites in presynaptic nerve terminals, and to a lesser extent to inhibit their reuptake. Amphetamines act as substrates for transporters of these biogenic amines and increase central synaptic concentrations of dopamine, noradrenaline and serotonin. Noradrenaline release contributes to the sympathomimetic effects, dopamine to central stimulant and rewarding effects and serotonin to psychotomimetic effects.

Pharmacological effects of amphetamine type stimulants (ATS)

Central stimulant effects:
- Euphoria
- Increased energy and mental alertness
- Insomnia
- Nervousness or anxiety
- Reduced appetite and weight loss
- Enhanced self-confidence
- Increased libido
- Increased body temperature.
- May precipitate psychosis (p. 266)

Sympathomimetic effects:
- Tachycardia
- Raised blood pressure
- Sweating
- Dilated pupils, blurred vision
- Tremor.

Methamphetamine has similar effects to amphetamines, but higher brain levels are reached for the same dose and smoking of crystal methamphetamine (ice) produces a very rapid brain entry, and so a greater euphoria.

Amphetamines and amphetamine-type stimulants (ATS) can be smoked, snorted, injected, or taken orally, including rubbing on gums. Occasionally, they are taken anally ('shelving'). In Australia most amphetamine is injected, but the opposite applies in most European countries. Onset of effect is rapid and depends on the mode of administration, occurring within minutes after intranasal administration and even faster after inhalation or intravenous administration (see Table 9.2, p. 245). Most amphetamine users take the drug for the 'rush' or 'high' associated with use, but some use amphetamines to stay awake longer (students and truck drivers), to give more energy (e.g. at dance parties), to lose weight (young women), or for increased sexual desire or performance.

Metabolism: Amphetamines are metabolized in the liver by isoenzymes of cytochrome P450 to active metabolites. Methamphetamine is partly converted to amphetamine and amphetamine to 4-hydroxyamphetamine. Depending on the pH of the urine, a significant proportion is excreted unchanged by the kidneys. As renal excretion is increased in acidic urine, overdose can be treated by acidifying the urine. Urine drug screen remains positive for 2–4 days.

3,4-Methylenedioxymethamphetamine (MDMA, Ecstasy)

MDMA, a synthetic derivative of amphetamines and related drugs, possesses both central nervous system stimulant and empathetic (entactogenic) effects. It is popular at dance parties and 'raves', and is generally taken for its euphoric and stimulant effects, and for generating feelings of closeness with others (sometimes called a 'hug drug'). MDMA was previously used as an appetite suppressant or to induce a state of improved empathy and consciousness during psychotherapeutic sessions.

Like the amphetamines, MDMA releases central monoamines such as dopamine, noradrenaline and serotonin by reversing the action of their transporters, particularly the serotonin transporter. MDMA also inhibits tryptophan hydroxylase, the rate limiting enzyme in serotonin synthesis, which is followed by acute depletion of central serotonin levels. The acute release of central serotonin is profound and may lead to permanent serotonin depletion with chronic use.

MDMA is usually taken orally but can be injected or inserted anally. Typically, it is taken as 1–2 tablets at weekly to monthly intervals, but occasionally a number of tablets are taken consecutively ('stacking'), and uncommonly dependence may occur. Onset of effect occurs within 30–60 min and peaks at 90 min. Duration of effect is approximately 8 h.

MDMA is metabolized in the liver to an active metabolite MDA.

Pharmacological effects of MDMA

CNS stimulation:
- Euphoria
- Increased alertness and energy
- Diminished appetite
- Heightened empathy and feelings of closeness (entactogenic)
- Psychedelic/hallucinogenic effects (high doses)

Sympathomimetic effects:
- Tachycardia
- Hypertension.

Cocaine

Pharmacology of cocaine

Cocaine is an alkaloid present in the leaves of erythroxylum coca. Cocaine hydrochloride is a crystalline white water soluble compound which is readily absorbed following either intranasal administration ('snorting', 'sniffing') and intravenous administration. The cocaine free base (crack), formed when cocaine is heated in an alkaline solution, is usually smoked or inhaled. It is more rapidly absorbed and, thus, has greater addictive potential.

A mixture of heroin and cocaine is known as 'speed balling'.

Cocaine is similar in structure to amphetamine sulphate, but is significantly more potent and effective. Cocaine inhibits the reuptake of dopamine, noradrenaline, and serotonin from the central synaptic cleft by blocking the transporters of these biogenic amines. Cocaine is thought to produce its rewarding effect primarily by increasing dopamine concentrations in the nucleus accumbens. The block of the noradrenaline transporter produces the sympathomimetic effects.

Cocaine's vasoconstrictor and local anaesthetic actions have led to its use as a topical anaesthetic when a blood free field is necessary.

Onset of effect of euphoric effect of cocaine is rapid, occurring within minutes, and within seconds when inhaled as free base. Duration of effect is short, approximately 30–90 min depending on the mode of administration. Because of its short duration of intense euphoria, cocaine is at times used repeatedly, in a binge pattern over several hours, which places the user at increased risk of toxicity and transmission of sexually transmitted infections and HIV/AIDS.

Pharmacological effects of cocaine

Central nervous system stimulation:
- Intense euphoria
- Increased energy, hyperactivity, excitability
- Enhanced confidence and libido
- Increased performance of repetitive tasks
- Insomnia
- Increased risk of aggressive, violent, erratic and high risk behaviours and drug induced psychosis (p. 250)

Sympathomimetic and vasoconstrictor effects:
- Tachycardia
- Hypertension
- Vasoconstriction

Local anaesthetic effects (via stereo-isomer procaine—present in equal amounts in cocaine).

Metabolism of cocaine

Cocaine is metabolized, mainly in the liver, by choline esterase to an inactive demethylated metabolite benzoylecgonine and ecgonine methyl ester. A small proportion (1–2%) is excreted unchanged in the urine. Metabolites can be detected in blood or urine 36 h and in the hair for weeks to months after use.

When cocaine is used with alcohol a longer-acting metabolite co-caethylene is formed that can have more prolonged stimulant and cardiotoxic actions.

Many of the acute complications of cocaine tend to result from over stimulation of the CNS sympathomimetic effects and/or vasospasm.

The differential diagnosis of stimulant toxicity includes thyrotoxicosis, the serotonergic syndrome, other drug overdose and the neuroleptic malignant syndrome.

Table 9.2 Half life and approximate time course of pharmacological action of various stimulants

Psychostimulant	Approximate $t_{1/2}$	Onset of action	Duration of effect
Amphetamines (ATS)	7–12 h (up to 36 h)	Rapid after IV use through to 20 min after oral use	8–36 h
Methamphetamine	7–12 h	Within minutes after smoking	As for amphetamines
MDMA	7–9 h	30–60 min	8–9 h
Cocaine	Variable and dose-dependent: 18 min	5–10 s (inhalation)	Up to 20 min
		½–2 min (IV)	Up to 90 min
		1–3 min (intranasal)	Up to 90 min (metabolite benzoylecogonine can be detected in urine 48 h later)

Note that the time course differs with the route of administration.

The stimulant 'crash'

Individuals typically may experience 'coming down' or a 'crash' after a brief period of stimulant use (e.g. binge use for 1–2 days), even when they are not dependent on the drug being used. The 'crash' often occurs a few days after weekend stimulant use.

The 'crash' commences as the effect of the stimulant wears off, approximately 8–36 h after use ('suicide Tuesday'). The crash and subsequent comedown may last several days. Acute cocaine intoxication may be followed by a shorter 'crash' phase, which lasts from hours to days with depression and fatigue.

This crash is characterized by fatigue, hypersomnia, hyperphagia and low mood due to acute monoamine depletion. Extreme lethargy, irritability, and argumentativeness and/or depression can also be experienced.

Symptoms of the stimulant 'crash' or come down

- Lethargy, fatigue
- Malaise, dysphoria
- Depression, with increased risk of suicide
- Headache
- Anxiety
- Irritability, which may result in argumentativeness or aggression.

These 'come down' effects are not universal, however, and some individuals continue to feel positive and energized even when binge use of the drug ceases. Some MDMA users in particular continue to experience positive effects on mood and a sense of well being for several days after use. Others notice a 'come down', which is milder than that experienced with amphetamines and cocaine. The crash is briefer and less intense than the more prolonged withdrawal which can occur with stimulant dependence.

Pathophysiology of psychostimulants

Acute side effects and complications of psychostimulant use may be due to sympathomimetic effects. The additional vasoconstriction with cocaine use is responsible for a number of complications, such as peripheral ischaemia, myocardial infarction, cerebral haemorrhage, ischaemic stroke, bowel ischaemia. In pregnancy, vasoconstriction may threaten placental blood supply.

Inhibition of ADH caused by MDMA in some people: In response to hyperthermia, sweating, and dehydration, both from the drug and from increased physical activity (e.g. dancing), large amounts of water may be consumed. The resulting hyponatraemia may be exacerbated by ADH inhibition. Water intoxication and hyponatraemia may lead to cerebral oedema and, in rare cases, death.

Acute neurotransmitter depletion: The 'crash' phase following acute intoxication is attributed to acute depletion of neurotransmitter stores, as well as exhaustion from excessive activity.

There is growing evidence that chronic use of psychostimulants may have a long-term effect on neurotransmission. Recent positron emission tomography (PET) studies in chronic methamphetamine users demonstrated a reduction in dopamine transporter concentration suggesting a loss of dopamine projections. This reduction was significantly associated with the duration of methamphetamine use and the severity of persistent psychiatric symptoms. (See neuropsychiatric complications, pp. 249–251).

There is limited evidence that MDMA may have permanent neurotoxic effects on serotonergic nerve terminals which are involved in memory and regulation of mood. Chronic serotonin depletion may result in premature cognitive impairment, as well as sleep disorders, anxiety states, depressed mood, impulsiveness and hostility. There is conflicting evidence on whether this damage to serotonergic neurons is permanent, but MDMA users need to be warned of these potential risks.

Core clinical syndromes

Non-dependent stimulant use disorders
- Psychostimulants are typically used intermittently, rather than on a daily basis. Recreational users are those who use irregularly, often in a social setting, but some use large amounts intermittently in a binge pattern.
- Among those with non dependent use (with diagnoses of harmful use or abuse), which represent the majority of users of these drugs, complications are still common. These include local and systemic effects of snorting or injecting use, aggression and violence, psychotic symptoms, and the ever-present risk of progression to dependence.

Psychostimulant dependence
Dependence on psychostimulants occurs in 30–40% of people who use amphetamines repeatedly after an average period of use of 3–4 years, with much variation. It is more common among heavy male users, in those who smoke or inject the drug and in those with a history of drug and mental health problems. Dependence is more likely to occur following use of methamphetamines, amphetamines and cocaine than for MDMA. Cocaine dependence develops in approximately 55% of repeated users in western societies.

Dependent users typically consume a large amount of the drug over several days, going without sleep (a binge) before ceasing use through physical exhaustion or running out of money. Daily use to avoid withdrawal symptoms is a less frequent pattern of use in this group.

A diagnosis of stimulant dependence is made if three or more of the following criteria have occurred repeatedly over the past 12 months:
- **Loss of control:** awareness of an impaired ability to control use
- **Craving or compulsion to use:** a significant amount of time is usually spent in drug use and associated activities, to the detriment of other aspects of their lives
- **Tolerance:** requiring high doses of the drug (often several grams) to achieve the desired affect
- **Withdrawal:** some individuals experience a withdrawal syndrome on cessation or reduction of use
- **Relief or prevention of withdrawal by further use:** daily use to avoid withdrawal symptoms is a less frequent pattern of use in stimulant users.
- **Continued and persistent use despite clear evidence of harm**.

Psychostimulant withdrawal
In many ways the withdrawal is an exaggeration of the 'crash'. It occurs in stimulant dependent individuals following cessation of or reduction in stimulant use. The period of withdrawal may follow the 'crash' phase (see p. 245).

Time course of stimulant withdrawal
- Amphetamine withdrawal typically starts 2–4 days after last use, peaks at 7–10 days, then subsides over 2–4 weeks.
- Cocaine has a shorter half-life, and accordingly withdrawal symptoms typically commence and resolve earlier, starting at 1–2 days, peaking at 4–7 days, and subsiding over 1–2 weeks.

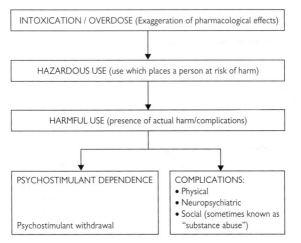

The 'coming down' or 'crash' occurs after a brief period of psychostimulant use, even when the patient is not dependent on the psychostimulant being used; withdrawal occurs only in those who are psychostimulant dependent .

Fig. 9.1 Psychostimulant use disorders.

The withdrawal period is characterized by craving, low mood, anergia, irritability, sleep disturbance, and appetite disturbance. It usually diminishes gradually over 2–4 weeks although dysphoric symptoms may persist for up to 10 weeks. Depressive symptoms and anxiety are common features of the withdrawal syndrome in stimulant dependent patients. These symptoms can include intense feelings of depression, anhedonia, anxiety, agitation, and fatigue, in combination with over-eating and over-sleeping. They often fluctuate in intensity. Similar neurobiological mechanisms involving decreased function and activity of the monoamine transmitters are responsible for the overlap between the symptoms of depression and those of withdrawal.

Extinction phase: After the withdrawal symptoms have subsided, there is often then a prolonged 'extinction' phase (analogous to protracted withdrawal symptoms in alcohol dependence) which may last from weeks to months as the mood gradually normalizes. Fluctuations in mood and energy levels are common during this phase, with evidence of fatigue, low mood, anxiety, irritability and disturbed sleep.

Cravings for stimulants may occur during all phases of withdrawal and contribute to relapse. Mood will gradually normalize if relapse can be avoided.

Complications of psychostimulant use

Complications of psychostimulant use

1. From expected pharmacological effects
- Restlessness, hyperactivity
- Insomnia, sleep disorders
  - Users may take 'downers'—CNS depressants such as benzodiazepines, cannabis, alcohol or opioids to overcome the effects of CNS stimulation. Polydrug use is common in stimulant users.

2. Stimulant 'crash'

3. Psychostimulant dependence and withdrawal

4. Psychostimulant intoxication/medical complications (pp. 257, 258, 259)
Complications include:
- Enhanced libido and engaging in risky sexual behaviours carries an increased risk of sexually transmitted infections, including HIV/AIDS
- Blood borne viral infections (hepatitis C, B, and HIV) can also be transmitted through sharing of snorting or injecting implements
- Other complications of injecting drug use: In addition to complications specific to stimulants, injecting users are prone to the array of medical complications of injecting drug use (p. 367).

5. Neuropsychiatric complications
- Anxiety, panic attacks
- Depression and increased risk of suicidality (related to stimulant withdrawal)
- Agitation, aggression, violent, erratic and sometimes criminal behaviour
- Stimulant induced psychosis—a transient drug induced psychotic state following use of psychostimulants (see p. 250)
- Hypomania, mania
- Perceptual disturbances, depersonalization
- Confusion, delirium.

6. Social complications
See (p. 251).

Neuropsychiatric complications
Psychostimulant use, particularly of amphetamines and cocaine, mimics a variety of psychiatric disorders. Severe psychiatric disturbances appear to be generally less common with MDMA than with cocaine and amphetamines.

Stimulant induced psychosis: A transient drug-induced psychotic state following use of psychostimulants. Usually occurs after chronic use of high doses, but can be seen with one or several large doses.

Risk factors for stimulant-induced psychosis
- Young males
- Injector or smoker of stimulants (rather than oral use)
- Binge users
- Stimulant dependence
- Previous episodes of psychosis
- Polysubstance use (particularly alcohol, benzodiazepines, cannabis)
- Prolonged insomnia.

The clinical picture of stimulant-induced psychosis resembles paranoid schizophrenia and sometimes mimics mania, but is differentiated by the rapid improvement when drug use stops. Also, abnormal physical findings may be apparent if the patient first presents while intoxicated.

The acute episode is typically characterized by suspiciousness, unusual thought content or hallucinations (with more visual and somatic content than is usual in schizophrenic psychosis). Once stimulant use ceases, the psychosis usually clears within days. It may last for a week, sometimes up to a month, especially with metamphetamine.

Features of stimulant induced psychosis
- Mood is fearful, agitated and often labile
- Repetitive, compulsive, meaningless behaviour (foraging for rubbish, cleaning for hours, dismantling objects)
- High level of suspiciousness with paranoid delusions in a state of clear consciousness. Patient has no insight and may be very frightened, which can lead to panicky or aggressive behaviour and sometimes result in unprovoked violence or homicide
- Hallucinations—auditory, tactile (e.g. formication—perception that bugs are crawling under the skin), visual ('snow lights'), gustatory or olfactory.

See p. 266 for management of stimulant induced psychosis.

Chronic or recurrent psychotic states: There is no evidence that stimulants cause a chronic psychotic state. However, stimulants may precipitate psychosis in an individual with an underlying vulnerability to psychosis (such as schizophrenia). Stimulants may also trigger and exacerbate psychotic symptoms in those with pre-existing disorders. This can occur even when patients are stable on antipsychotic medication.

Depression: The combination of stimulant abuse or dependence and depression places the individual at increased risk for suicide. Suicide risk assessment should be undertaken regularly if indicated.

Depressive symptoms are common in the crash phase, and in withdrawal, however the persistence of depressive symptoms beyond 2–4 weeks after stopping amphetamine use may suggest that there is an underlying depressive illness and should be treated, since left unmanaged its presence represents a high risk of relapse. It is useful to delay commencing antidepressants until after the individual has stopped using for 2–4 weeks to reassess the depressive symptoms. The advantages of waiting are improved diagnostic accuracy, avoidance of potentially unnecessary medication, and probably an improvement in compliance and efficacy.

Anxiety: Even with lower doses of stimulants (20–50 mg), individuals can experience anxiety, nervousness, tachycardia, palpitations, and hyperventilation. Chest pain may also develop in association with these symptoms and the individual may believe they are having a heart attack. Stimulant effects can also result in a feeling of panic that the user is losing control or going mad. High dose stimulants can produce an obsessive-compulsive state (for example, a compulsive desire to pull objects apart and reassemble them; compulsive foraging for things).

Hypomania or mania: With increased use of high dose cocaine or amphetamines, the user experiences symptoms of euphoria, increased energy levels, disinhibition, grandiosity, impulsiveness, decreased need for sleep, increased feelings of sexuality, decreased appetite, impaired judgement, hypervigilance, compulsively repeated actions, and marked psychomotor agitation. Up to 80% of regular cocaine users experience these effects which may result in illegal activities, uncharacteristic sexual behaviour or accidents. Physical symptoms of sympathetic nervous system over activity is clinically similar to hypomania or mania, but subsides rapidly depending on the duration of action of the drug taken (e.g. within 30 min of cocaine use though can be for much longer with methylamphetamine).

Delirium: Stimulant-induced delirium can occur with confusion, disorientation, persecutory delusions, hallucinations and thought disorder. Signs such as bruxism and repetitive compulsive behaviours may alert the clinician to the cause, as does the high prevalence of visual hallucinations.

Social complications

The social complications of stimulant use can be considerable, and may put a burden not only on the individual and their family and friends, but also on hospital emergency departments, corrective services and social work departments. The social impacts of stimulant use can occur after a single episode of use. However, repeated use and, in particular, dependent use, usually leads to a chaotic lifestyle with major social impacts.

Social problems associated with repeated stimulant use

- **Work difficulties:** poor performance, absenteeism, job loss
- **Interpersonal/relationship problems:**
  - Domestic violence
  - Separation, divorce
  - Neglect of care of children may be a major problem in the chaos surrounding repeated and regular stimulant use
- **Financial problems:**
  - Poverty
  - Risky behaviour to obtain money: gambling, break enter and steal, prostitution
- **High risk behaviour:**
  - Violence (perpetrator or victim) including assault
  - Rape
  - Other antisocial and criminal behaviour
- Forensic problems due to chaotic, dangerous lifestyle.

Natural history

Little information is available on the natural history of stimulant use. Methamphetamines and cocaine are known to be highly addictive, with ecstasy and amphetamines, having lesser addictive potential.

The course of amphetamine dependence is typically a chronic one with periods of non-use and episodes of relapse. Approximately 60% will be dependent after 3 years, but the long-term natural history (over 10–20 years) has still to be determined. At 3 years, mortality is 5% with most of the deaths occurring from accidents, suicide, and homicide, and a smaller proportion as a result of blood borne infections.

Identification and opportunistic intervention

The routine questioning of patients about illicit drug use assists in the early detection of amphetamine use. This can facilitate earlier intervention, including assistance to stop drug use in those wishing to change, or provision of harm reduction advice for those not yet willing or able to change their stimulant use.

Brief intervention is typically most useful for the non-dependent patient with harmful psychostimulant use.

As for all substance use disorders, the clinician can adopt the model used for alcohol use disorders, which is described by the FLAGS acronym (p. 56) to provide an opportunistic intervention for stimulant-use disorders.

Feedback: Personalized feedback on experience of medical, neuropsychiatric or social harms, or major risks that are being faced, e.g. sexual risk taking, risk of the non-sterile and unknown content of illicitly prepared stimulants, risk of strokes. In giving the feedback, be aware that the individual is likely to know many stimulant users who have 'got away with it' and had no adverse effects.

Listening: To the patient's response, readiness to change, and past attempts to change.

Advice: Providing clear advice on substance use and its complications. Provide clear advice and raise the patient's awareness of the medical, neuropsychiatric and social complications associated with psychostimulant us. Advise patients with a history of mental health problems (anxiety, depression, psychosis) that they should avoid use of stimulants because of the increased risk of precipitating, prolonging, or exacerbating their psychiatric problems. Advice may also include elements of harm reduction.

Goals: The clinician's goal is abstinence from psychostimulants; however the patient may not yet be ready to accept this goal so using motivational interviewing techniques, an interim goal can be negotiated (e.g. decreasing frequency of use, or reducing the harm from each episode of use).

Strategies to achieve the goal: Practical steps to try to reduce or cease stimulant use might include minimizing alcohol use, if stimulant use tends to occur as a result of alcohol intoxication; limiting time or contact with stimulant using friends; taking less money when going out to a party; looking for less hazardous ways to get a 'high', e.g. through sport or exercise. In the case of a person unwilling to change their stimulant use, motivational interviewing techniques can be employed and harm reduction strategies can be discussed (see p. 269).

Follow up: Offer follow-up and support. Psychostimulant dependent patients and polysubstance users are best referred to a Specialist Drug & Alcohol Treatment Service. Substitute ATS prescribing, e.g. oral amphetamine sulphate is used in some centres, although the evidence of efficacy is not yet proven.

Assessment and management of psychostimulant use/intoxication

(Also see Chapters 2 and 3)

Principles

- Be alert to the possibility of stimulant use, e.g. suspect stimulant use in a young person with an unusual medical presentation
- Polysubstance use is common among psychostimulant users
- Be aware that co-morbid psychiatric disorders are commonly present in psychostimulant users
- In particular, inquire about sleep disturbances and the use of benzodiazepines
- Is stimulant dependence present? Or stimulant abuse/harmful use?
- Is the patient intoxicated, or in withdrawal?
- What are the physical, psychiatric and social complications of substance use?

History

Take a thorough *drug and alcohol history* (pp. 37–41).

Drug use history

- Which substance or substances are being used? In particular, check for concurrent use of alcohol, benzodiazepines, cannabis and opioids.
- For each drug, record:
  - Quantity, frequency and pattern of use (whether daily, intermittently or in a binge pattern)
  - Duration of use
  - Time of last use
  - Route(s) of administration
  - Is the patient dependent on any substances?

What is the diagnosis with regard to stimulant use?

- Does the individual use stimulants, without evidence of current harms?
- What are the physical, psychiatric and social complications of psychostimulant (and/or alcohol and other substance) use?
- Is their use harmful? (psychological or physical harms have occurred, but use of amphetamines is voluntary rather than compulsive, and criteria for dependence are not met)
- Is there evidence of social harms? Abuse is diagnosed where there are recurrent social harms from stimulant use but the patient is not dependent on stimulants
- Is the patient dependent on the stimulant?
  - e.g. check for degree of control over use—are you able to stop when you want to, or avoid using when you want to?
  - Is the patient aware of harms they have experienced from stimulant use, but continues to use?
  - Has the amount of stimulant they require to get an effect (or the money they spend on stimulants) gone up? etc.

Medical history: Including screening for common complications, including overdose, and complications of injecting (pp. 367–374) where relevant.

Psychiatric history: Including past suicide attempts, complications and co-morbidities (such as anxiety, depression, psychosis). A past history of ADD/ADHD can lead to the use of ATS as a form of self medication (the patient may say that in contrast to his peers ATS makes him/her calmer and less active).

Family history: Of alcohol and other substance use and psychiatric illness is also important.

Clinical examination Look for features of **psychostimulant use and complications** [See pp. 257–259 for specific features of amphetamine (ATS), MDMA and cocaine intoxication.]

Investigations for psychostimulant intoxication
- Routine investigations:
  - FBC
  - EUC
  - LFTs
  - TFTs
  - BSL
  - Serological tests for hepatitis C, B and HIV
  - Screen for STIs.
- Other investigations:
  - Urine drug screen (for cocaine request plasma benzoylecgonia, the demethylated metabolite of cocaine, as cocaine itself has a variable and short half-life)
  - ECGs: to exclude arrhythmias in toxicity
  - Cardiac enzymes, troponin levels—where ischaemic heart disease is suspected (cocaine)
  - CPK to exclude rhabdomyolysis
  - Chest X ray where indicated
  - CT or MRI head: if indicated e.g. to exclude cerebrovascular accidents.

Clinical features of psychostimulant use disorders and their complications

General appearance
- Weight loss, poor self-care
- Clenched jaw, bruxism
- Fractures or other trauma
- Sweating, (or dehydration)
- Fever, hyperthermia (either dehydration or water intoxication due to drinking excess water)
- Repetitive movements
- Dilated pupils

Dental
- Loss of teeth, caries, broken teeth, periodontal disease (jaw clenching, tooth grinding, ischaemia).

Nose (with cocaine)
- White powder in nostrils
- Rhinorrhoea, sinusitis, epistaxis
- Nasal septal necrosis

Skin changes
- Needle track marks
- Thrombophlebitis, cellulitis, skin abscess
- Excoriations, sores on face arms or legs (formication).

CVS
Tachycardia, tachyarrhythmias, hypertension, myocardial infarction (cocaine), heart murmurs/infective endocarditis (from injecting drug use)

Respiratory
Dyspnoea, tachypnoea, infections

Pulmonary oedema
GIT
Jaundice, hepatomegaly, and/or stigmata of chronic liver disease (hepatitis C from injecting)

Renal
Acute renal failure (secondary to rhabdomyolysis)

CNS
Seizures, cerebral haemorrhage, stroke

Neuropsychiatric
Restlessness, disinhibition, erratic behaviour, rapid speech, anxiety, agitation, hypervigilance, aggression, violence, paranoia, psychosis. May also be depressed or suicidal in the crash/withdrawal phase (p. 245).

Infections
Sexually transmitted infections, HIV/AIDs.
(Also see complications of injecting drug use—p. 367).

Features of stimulant intoxication

Features of intoxication with amphetamines and ATS

- Nausea, vomiting
- Jaw clenching/grinding (bruxism)
- Stereotypic movements/formication (scratching, excoriations)
- Hyperthermia.

Sympathomimetic effects
- Tachypnoea
- Sweating
- Dilated pupils, blurred vision
- Tachycardia
- Hypertension
- Cardiac arrhythmias
- Cardiovascular collapse.

CNS stimulation
- Restlessness, hyperactivity
- Agitation
- Anxiety, panic attacks
- Insomnia, sleep disorders
- Twitching
- Seizures
- Cerebral haemorrhage, stroke
- Delirium.

Psychiatric complications
- Amphetamine induced psychosis (resembles paranoid schizophrenia; p. 250)
- Depression during the 'crash phase': watch out for suicidality.

Other complications
- Hypersexuality (increased risk of HIV/AIDS and sexually transmitted infections)
- Rhabdomyolysis.

If not treated appropriately, amphetamine toxicity may lead to coma and death.

Features of MDMA intoxication

Unpredictable

General
- Fatigue
- Nausea
- Dry mouth
- Restlessness
- Insomnia
- Jaw clenching (bruxism)
- Hyperthermia.

Cardiovascular system (sympathomimetic effects)
- Hypertension
- Tachyarrhythmias
- Asystole
- Arteritis, vasculitis
- Cardiovascular collapse.

Gastrointestinal system
- Hepatotoxicity.

Musculoskeletal
- Muscle cramps
- Rhabdomyolysis.

Fluid and electrolytes
- Dehydration (sweating)
- Water intoxication and hyponatraemia (drinking excess water to overcome dehydration; exacerbated by inappropriate ADH secretion).

Renal
- Acute renal failure (secondary to rhabdomyolysis).

Central nervous system
- Restlessness in the legs
- Transient gait disturbance
- Increased tactile sensitivity
- Impaired memory and learning
- Cerebral haemorrhage (or cerebral oedema due to water intoxication and hyponatraemia).

Neuropsychiatric complications (pp. 249–251)
- Agitation
- Hallucinations/psychosis.

Hyponatraemia in combination with hypoglycaemia and/or hypokalaemia suggests PMA toxicity.

Deaths in MDMA users: While most MDMA users experience few acute adverse effects, sporadic deaths occur, sometimes in persons who have used relatively small doses. These are believed to reflect, at least in part, individual sensitivity. Deaths are typically due to:
- Hyperthermia
- Hyponatraemia, cerebral oedema

- Disseminated intravascular coagulation (probably due to hyperthermia)
- Hepatic failure (idiosyncratic reaction)
- Acute renal failure
- Cardiovascular collapse.

Features of cocaine intoxication

- Tremor
- Sweating
- Hyperthermia
- Epistaxis

Cardiovascular system
- Tachycardia
- Hypertension
- Tachyarrhythmias
- Myocardial infarction
- Peripheral ischaemia, gangrene.

Respiratory system
- Dyspnoea, tachypnoea (non-cardiogenic pulmonary oedema, pulmonary infarction)
- Haemoptysis: pulmonary infarction and or haemorrhage (due to vasoconstriction).

Gastrointestinal tract
- Abdominal pain, bloody stools, bowel ischaemia, bowel infarction (due to vasoconstrictor effect)
- Hepatic ischaemia, hepatic necrosis (due to vasoconstrictor effect).

Muscular: Rhabdomyolysis
Renal: Acute renal failure (secondary to rhabdomyolysis)
Central Nervous System
- Tics and other stereotyped muscle activity
- Seizures
- Intracranial haemorrhage
- Ischaemic stroke
- Cerebral vasculitis.

Neuropsychiatric symptoms (see below pp. 249–251)
- Paranoia, paranoid psychosis
- Violent and erratic behaviour
- Hypomania, mania
- Perceptual disturbances, depersonalization
- Confusion
- Delirium.

Enhanced libido and risky sexual activity
- Sexually transmitted infections, hepatitis C, HIV/AIDs.
(Also see other complications of injecting drug use—p. 367).

Suspect cocaine intoxication in a young person with an unusual medical presentation.

Management of stimulant intoxication

- There is no specific antidote for psychostimulant toxicity
- General symptomatic and supportive measures—nurse in a calm, quiet and soothing environment; allow patient to sleep.
- Monitor closely: 2–4 hourly observations of temperature, blood pressure, pulse rate, respiratory rate. Place on ECG monitor if tachyarrhythmias are present or if the patient complains of chest pain.
- Ensure clear airways, breathing and circulation
- If hyperthermic, promote cooling
- Rehydrate and correct fluid and electrolyte disturbances.
- Acidification of urine, e.g. with ammonium chloride may help speed the excretion of amphetamines and ATS
- If the patient is acutely agitated, sedate with benzodiazepines (e.g. diazepam 10–20 mg orally and repeat after 2 h until the patient is calm and mildly sedated; typical dose required 60–80 mg in the first 24 h)
- If the patient is extremely agitated or violent, it will be necessary to give intravenous diazepam (10 mg slowly), titrating dose according to response. This may be repeated after 30 min if necessary. Then aim to switch to oral diazepam as above
- As an alternative intravenous midazolam 2.5–10 mg (intravenously or intramuscularly) may be given, repeated as necessary after 10 min, and with further doses given according to response up to a maximum of 20 mg
- Note that patients requiring parenteral benzodiazepines should always be nursed in a high dependency or intensive care unit because of the risk of respiratory depression, aspiration, airways obstruction or hypotension requiring assisted respiration
- A sedating antipsychotic agent (e.g. olanzapine or quetiapine) may be needed in addition to a benzodiazepine (do not give phenothiazines which lower seizure threshold; also see p. 266 for management of stimulant induced psychosis)
- Dialysis may be required for rhabdomyolysis, which does not resolve with good hydration
- When the acute phase is over, monitor closely for depression and suicidality
- Protect from risk of self-injury.

Additional steps in management of MDMA (or PMA) intoxication
In addition to measures described above:
- Emesis or gastric lavage is indicated if the patient has MDMA toxicity from oral intake, is alert and has taken MDMA less than 4 h previously
- Rehydrate and correct fluid and electrolyte imbalance, particularly hyponatraemia.

Additional steps in the management of cocaine intoxication
Any person with chest pain after cocaine use should be admitted for observation (see management of suspected myocardial infarction, p. 261).

Hypertension may be treated with an alpha blocker (phentolamine) or a combined alpha and beta adrenergic blocker (e.g. labetalol). Labetalol reverses cocaine-induced increase in blood pressure but has no effect on cocaine-induced coronary vasoconstriction. Alternatively nitroprusside may be used.

Beta blockers (e.g. propranolol) should be avoided as they exacerbate cocaine induced vasoconstriction of coronary arteries. Calcium channel blockers should also be avoided because seizures have been reported.

Management of complications of stimulant intoxication

- In severe intoxication acute rhabdomyolysis may occur. This needs to be diagnosed urgently as there is a risk of renal failure (for which dialysis may be required)
- Cocaine-induced myocardial infarction is due to increased myocardial oxygen demand, tachycardia, increased blood pressure, and vasoconstriction of the coronary arteries. Admit all patients who present with chest pain after cocaine use. Risk is highest in the first hour after use. Monitor with serial ECGs, cardiac enzyme and troponin levels for at least 12 h. Administer sublingual glyceryl trinitrate for chest pain and treat as for myocardial infarction but note that cocaine has local anaesthetic effects. Avoid beta blockers; also avoid aspirin if cerebral haemorrhage is suspected.

Management when intoxication resolves

- Monitor closely for depression and suicidality
- Protect from risk of self-injury
- Provide brief intervention if this was an isolated incident of use or use is low level
- Offer ongoing treatment or referral for harmful stimulant use, abuse or dependence
- Be alert to the likely onset of the 'crash'. Adopt suicide precautions where necessary. Keep away from verandas, high windows that can be opened, knives.

Management of psychostimulant withdrawal: detoxification

A dependent patient may go into psychostimulant withdrawal when admitted to hospital, for example for a psychotic episode. Alternatively cessation of psychostimulant use may be a planned (elective) process, known as detoxification, so that withdrawal symptoms can be appropriately managed under supervision.

Patients are educated about withdrawal symptoms and their time course, and reassured that, if necessary, medication will be provided for any withdrawal symptoms; that these symptoms will gradually resolve if they remain abstinent from stimulant use.

Setting for elective detoxification

Home detoxification: Simple and uncomplicated stimulant withdrawals may be managed in a supportive home environment, where there is a live-in carer and a nurse and/or general practitioner able to visit daily. An alternative is ambulatory detoxification where, the patient visits the hospital/treatment centre or general practitioner on a daily basis.

However, severely dependent patients with medical or psychiatric complications, or without a supportive home environment, are best managed in a detoxification unit or hospital setting. The clinical features of stimulant withdrawal may be complicated by withdrawal from co-existing alcohol or other substance dependence because many psychostimulant users are polysubstance users (particularly alcohol; benzodiazepines or opioids). Psychiatric co-morbidity further adds to the complexity of the withdrawal features.

A supportive safe, quiet and non threatening environment is essential for rest and sleep.

Other aspects of management

- Adequate diet: because a significant component of the withdrawal syndrome is probably related to neurotransmitter depletion, recovery may be delayed because of anorexia associated with amphetamine use. It may be useful to provide some nutritional supplements or a well balanced diet rich in monoamine precursors phenylalanine, tyrosine or l-tryptophan, e.g. pumpkin seeds, chocolate, marmite or vegemite, bananas.
- Short-term benzodiazepines may be prescribed for insomnia and agitation, e.g. diazepam 5–10 mg 3–4 times daily
- If patient is psychotic: olanzapine 10–20 mg daily
- The 3 Ds technique may be helpful in managing cravings. This involves:
  - Delay the decision to use or not for 1 h
  - Distract yourself with some activity during this hour
  - Decide whether it is worth using after the hour is up
- It is important to treat co-morbid psychiatric disorders. Recognize that the combination of stimulant use and depression places the person at increased risk of suicide. Suicide risk assessment should be undertaken regularly if indicated.

- **The role of antidepressants:** the benefits of antidepressants in managing stimulant withdrawal symptoms are clearer where there is pre-existing depression and when administered 4–6 weeks following abstinence (see below). Tricyclic antidepressants and SSRIs appear to have limited efficacy in reducing symptoms of depression in stimulant dependence unless there is co-morbid depression
  - Tricyclic antidepressants may place the patient at risk of toxicity overdose if the patient is suicidal. Tricyclic antidepressants may cause CNS depression if combined with other antidepressants
  - SSRIs may cause the serotonin syndrome if combined with stimulants.

In the management of psychostimulant dependence, detoxification, and management of withdrawals is the first important step to ongoing pharmacological, psychological, and social interventions in association with self-help programmes, life style changes, and residential care, if required.

Management of stimulant dependence

Steps in the management of stimulant dependence

- **Provision of information and education** regarding stimulant use and its complications. This may include brief intervention and motivational interviewing
- **Let the patient digest the information provided** and consider where they are at. The patient must then reach a point of acceptance of the need to stop and develop a commitment to stop stimulant use
- **Detoxification** is a necessary first step for cessation of stimulant use and other drug use in polydrug users (see above for management of stimulant withdrawal)
- **Pharmacotherapy:** to date, there are no widely accepted and evidence-based pharmacotherapy regimens for the treatment of stimulant dependence. There are several promising pharmacotherapies, which are described below. In addition, consider use of antidepressants for chronic co-morbid depression
- **Psychological treatment:** This very important component of treatment includes brief advice, Motivational interviewing, cognitive behavioural therapy (CBT), psychological counselling and behavioural treatments to deal with impaired cognition. They help to attract and retain users who present to treatment facilities. Cognitive behavioural therapy involving skills training and practice to deal with craving and high risk situations associated with relapse, and contingency management is effective in preventing relapses. It may involve 1:1 individual counselling by skilled counsellors using standardized manuals or group drug counselling
- **Treatment of co-morbidity:** parallel treatment of underlying physical, neuropsychiatric co-morbidity or complications. Consult a psychiatrist.
- **Treatment of patient within the family and social context.** Families of users require support, assistance and advice on how to deal with the user and how to access community services, mental health services and correctional services. Families also need information and advice on how to support and help the user
- **Self Help Groups or mutual support groups** based on 12-step fellowship (AA, NA) with abstinence as a goal. Weekly 12-step programmes are effective and patients who participate in both formal drug treatment and weekly 12-step programmes have higher rates of abstinence
- **Continual care:** treatment is not just a brief one-off; follow-up and if necessary, residential care is important
- **Life style change:** Changes at work, home and environment.

Pharmacological treatments under study

A variety of medication regimes are currently under study.

Long acting psychostimulant replacement therapy: Including dexamphetamine, methylphenidate, and phentermine. Small scale studies have shown that agonist substitution engages people in treatment and there are some early indications of benefit in terms of reduction of psychosocial harm and drug offences. Prescribing of psychostimulants as substitution agents is not possible in most countries, and in those where it can be undertaken special authorization is necessary.

Disulfiram has been reported to reduce cocaine use. It acts as a central inhibitor of dopamine beta hydroxylase, causing an increase of dopamine and decreased synthesis of noradrenaline. As a result it may attenuate the cocaine 'high' causing a decreasing desire to use more cocaine.

Modafinil is a non-stimulating alerting agent used in narcolepsy and other disorders of daytime excessive sleepiness. It is being tried as a substitute for ATS dependence as it has low abuse potential.

Bupropion is an antidepressant that has a dopaminergic mode of action but has low abuse potential. As well as lifting depression, it also helps people stop smoking nicotine. It may help reduce cravings and provide some restoration of energy and drive in ATS withdrawal states.

Management of neuropsychiatric complications of stimulant use

Stimulant-induced psychosis

- General supportive measures, a low stimulus environment, reassurance and support, while waiting for the symptoms to remit spontaneously with abstinence
- If the symptoms are severe and the patient becomes a danger to him/herself or to others, the patient should be placed under the Mental Health Act, medicated and hospitalized
- Exclude other causes of an organic brain syndrome
- **Benzodiazepines** are prescribed as the first line treatment for stimulant induced psychosis:
  - Diazepam—10–20 mg orally; repeat 2-hourly if necessary, until the patient is calm and mildly sedated; monitor vital signs every hour, maximum dose 120 mg in 24 h (see p. 115). If more diazepam is required, seek specialist advice
  - In severe cases, it may be necessary to give diazepam 10 mg slowly IV, repeated after 10 min if necessary. Alternatively midazolam 5 mg IM or IV may be administered, then repeat after 10–30 min if required.

Precautions

- Patients requiring intravenous benzodiazepines should always be nursed in a high dependency unit or intensive care unit
- Patients with chronic airflow limitation may require lower doses of benzodiazepines. Do oximeter readings before and after each dose, may require transfer to a high dependency or intensive care unit
- Patients with hepatic decompensation: give a shorter acting benzodiazepine such as oral oxazepam.

Antipsychotic agents: Antipsychotics are used to supplement benzodiazepines particularly when there is a sub-optimal response.

- Haloperidol 2.5–5 mg intramuscularly three times daily or olanzapine: 5–10 mg orally, intramuscularly or as a wafer; OR
- Quetiapine 25–100 mg every 6 h, titrated according to response
- Review antipsychotic medication after a few days. Refer to a psychiatrist
- A diagnosis of a possible underlying or persistent psychotic disorder must be deferred until a reassessment can be made in a drug free state. Those with florid psychoses usually remit within a few days and the user returns to normal functioning although some retain a vulnerability to such episodes. Only a minority (1–15%) persist beyond one month and many of these will have underlying psychiatric disorders.

Chronic or recurrent psychotic states

- Stimulants may precipitate psychosis in an individual with an underlying vulnerability to psychosis (such as schizophrenia) or trigger and exacerbate psychotic symptoms in those with pre-existing disorders
- A diagnosis of a possible underlying or persistent psychotic disorder must be deferred until a reassessment can be made in a drug free state.

Many of those whose psychotic symptoms persist for more than a month after abstinence from stimulants will have underlying psychiatric disorders

- The prognosis is variable and those who have experienced an acute psychotic episode are more vulnerable to future episodes (possibly through sensitization) on exposure to the drug, often at lower levels
- The underlying psychotic disorder must be appropriately treated and cessation of stimulant use is important as there appears to be some recovery of dopamine system function with abstinence.

Management of depression in persons with stimulant abuse/dependence

Severely depressed and suicidal patients need to be managed in an inpatient setting, and the Mental Health Act may need to be used.

The efficacy of antidepressants in reducing stimulant drug use is confined to those who are depressed. It is useful to delay commencing antidepressants until after the individual has stopped using for 2–4 weeks to reassess the depressive symptoms. The advantages of waiting are improved diagnostic accuracy, avoidance of potentially unnecessary medication and probably an improvement in compliance and efficacy. Doxepin or fluoxetine may be helpful.

In patients with a well-documented history of a pre-existing mood disorder occurring during periods of abstinence, or with a strong family history of a mood disorder, medication should be started early during the withdrawal phase.

The combination of psychostimulants and antidepressants (SSRIs, MAOIs), may place the person at risk of the serotonin syndrome. SSRIs should not be prescribed if the patient continues to use a psychostimulant. Patients prescribed SSRIs must be warned of the risk of developing the serotonin syndrome if they relapse to stimulant use. Tricyclic antidepressant drugs should be used with caution because of their potential lethality in suicidal patients.

Other drugs that may be prescribed for intercurrent conditions, such as tramadol or fentanyl for pain, and St John's Wort may also be associated with serotonergic syndrome and must be prescribed with caution (see below for assessment and management of serotonin syndrome).

The serotonin syndrome: A potentially fatal syndrome due to excess central serotonergic activity. May be precipitated when psychostimulant use is combined with use of SSRI's or other medications, which increase serotonin levels.

Clinical features
- Hyperthermia
- Tremulousness, agitation
- Dilated pupils
- CVS: hypertension
- GIT: hyperactive bowels, diarrhoea
- CNS: hyperreflexia, hypertonia, clonus, coma.

Investigations: see p. 255.

Management
- General supportive measures airways, breathing, circulation
- Intravenous fluids: ensure adequate amounts and adequate urine output (for rhabdomyolysis, dehydration, hypotension)
- External cooling
- Sedation with benzodiazepines
- Consider a serotonin receptor antagonist such as cyproheptadine or an atypical neuroleptic, e.g. olanzapine or quetiapine, (after ensuring that an anticholinergic agent has not been taken concurrently)
- The patient may require intubation and mechanical ventilation.

Anxiety Provided underlying medical illness and a pre-existing anxiety disorder have been ruled out, treatment involves reassuring the patient the reaction is due to the drug and will resolve completely as the drug is metabolized. If medication is required, short-term use of a benzodiazepine (e.g. diazepam) is appropriate.

Harm reduction/palliation for psychostimulant users

Individuals with a history of mental health problems (anxiety, depression, psychosis) should be warned not to use stimulants because of the potential to exacerbate these psychiatric problems.

Given the relatively high prevalence of psychostimulant use, harm reduction measures are important. In the health care setting, individual stimulant users who are not willing or able to change their stimulant use can be engaged in motivational interviewing and interventions about reducing the risks of their use.

Sometimes harm reduction measures are targeted to high risk settings such as dance clubs, to avoid the effects of hyperthermia and to seek urgent medical help should problems occur.

Examples of advice to reduce harm from stimulant use

- Advise that inhaling or injecting stimulants place the individual at risk of dependence and various medical, neuropsychiatric, and social complications
- If individuals insist on injecting stimulants, check that they are aware of sources of supply of clean needles and the risk of transmission of hepatitis C and HIV/AIDS from injecting paraphernalia
- Avoid effects of hyperthermia—ensure a well ventilated dance floor. Rest and rehydrate, but be aware that drinking excess quantities of water may cause water intoxication
- If someone feels unwell, do not delay in seeking help—call an ambulance urgently
- Do not drive under the influence of stimulants because of the increased risk of accidents
- Individuals with a history of mental health problems (anxiety, depression, psychosis) should not use stimulants because of their potential to precipitate, exacerbate or prolong these psychiatric problems
- Advise patients not to use psychostimulants if they are on prescribed SSRI antidepressants (e.g. citalopram, fluoxetine, paroxetine, fluvoxamine, sertaline) because of the risk of developing the serotonin syndrome.
- Avoid combining stimulants with other drugs, (especially with alcohol, cannabis, benzodiazepines, opioids) as polydrug use increases the risk of overdose, accidents and other complications
- Do not use stimulants if you are pregnant or liable to become pregnant or if you have underlying cardiovascular or other medical problems

Prevention of uptake of stimulant use

As for illicit drug use generally, efforts have been made to reduce or prevent use through control supply (policing, importation restrictions, restrictions to purchase of precursors), and to reduce demand for the drug, through community and school education programmes.

Supply control has been difficult for amphetamine-type substances because of the ease of back-yard manufacture.

School and community education has been widely employed, although the evidence base for this is variable. In general, education, which aims to increase young people's skills in making independent choices and in drug refusal have been shown to be more effective in preventing uptake than education about the risks of substance use. As for other drugs, increasing young people's resilience may prevent uptake of substance use, e.g. through increasing sense of connectedness to family, school, sporting, cultural, or religious group or community.

Further reading

Dawe S, McKetin R. The psychiatric co-morbidity of psychostimulant use. In Baker A, Lee NK and Jenner L (Eds). *Models of intervention and care for psychostimulant users (Second Edition)*, National Drug Strategy Monograph Series number 51. Canberra, 2004

Katzung BG. *Basic and clinical pharmacology*, 10th edn. London: McGraw Hill Lange, 2007.

Latt N, White J, McLean S, Lenton S, Young R, Saunders JB. Central nervous stimulants: In: Management of alcohol and drug problems. Ed. Hulse G, White J, Cape G (Eds) Oxford: Oxford University Press, 2002: 124–140.

Management of patients with psychostimulant use problems—Guidelines for General Practitioners. Canberra: Commonwealth of Australia, 2004. Available at: http://www.dcita.gov.au/cca

Management of patients with psychostimulant Toxicity: Guidelines for Emergency Departments. Canberra: Commonwealth of Australia, 2006.

Other drugs

Hallucinogens

These include:
- Lysergic acid diethylamide (LSD)
- Psilocybin (magic mushroom).

Pharmacology

These drugs probably act through altering brain 5HT function especially in the cortical and hippocampal regions. They have high affinity for 5HT 2 receptors and probably act as agonists or partial agonists at these. Recent studies suggest that the psychedelic 5HT agonists produce different actions on intracellular second messengers or subpopulations of cortical pyramidal cells than do other non-psychedelic 5HT 2 acting drugs, which probably explains their effects.

Acute effects

- Psychedelic effects: thought, mood and sensory distortion and altered perception but can mimic psychosis
- Anxiety/panic
- Dilated pupils
- Lateral nystagmus, in some cases
- Agitation
- Tachypnoea
- Dry flushed skin.

Management of toxicity

- Supportive reassurance and reorientation. Most effects are self-limiting, lasting 4–12 hours
- If required, sedation with diazepam: 10–20 mg orally; titrate dose according to response
- Antipsychotics are not typically required, but may assist in settling acute agitation e.g. haloperidol, olanzapine
- Treat hyperthermia, hypertension, tachycardia, seizures, rhabdomyolysis as appropriate.

Chronic effects

- Dependence does not occur, though compulsive use may be seen
- Exacerbation of underlying mental health disorders
- Flashbacks
- Psychosis.

Hallucinogenic drugs and psychiatric symptoms

Hallucinogens and flashbacks

Flashbacks may occur in the form of similar perceptions and emotions experienced during drug intoxication. The most common forms are visual hallucinations including flashes and trailing of colour, geometric pseudo-hallucinations, perceptions of movement in the peripheral field of vision, after-images, halos around objects, macropsia, and micropsia. These seldom interfere with the individual's functioning, but can be distressing. Flashbacks are more common after a crisis or after using another drug, such as cannabis, stimulants, antihistamines. Flashbacks usually reduce in intensity over time and cease altogether, though up to 50% may experience the symptoms for up to 5 years. Treatment involves reassurance that the symptoms are not a feature of mental illness and will pass. Occasionally, benzodiazepines are helpful.

Hallucinogen-induced psychosis

Visual hallucinations are the most marked feature, and may be accompanied by persecutory delusions. The emotional state may vary from panic to depression to manic-like features. However, the drug user may retain insight that the symptoms are drug-induced. Symptoms usually clear within hours to days to weeks depending on the drug taken. If psychotic symptoms persist despite abstinence, it probably reflects a pre-existing psychiatric disorder.

Hallucinogens and anxiety

The stimulation and perceptual alterations with hallucinogenic drugs may create anxiety and panic in the user who may believe he is losing his mind. This is one example of a 'bad trip'. Such anxiety reactions are more common in inexperienced users of these drugs, and when the drug is used alone, or in an unfamiliar or unpleasant setting. The length of such a reaction is determined by the duration of action of the drug, e.g. 8–12 h for LSD. Treatment generally involves reassuring the individual that their mental state will return to normal once the effects of the drug wear off. If the reaction is severe, a short course of diazepam will reduce anxiety symptoms.

Amotivational syndrome: While some users have symptoms similar to the 'amotivational syndrome' reported by cannabis users, it is difficult to establish a cause and effect relationship. The features of social withdrawal and amotivation have often been present prior to the onset of drug use.

Hallucinogens and organic brain syndrome

An **acute organic brain syndrome** can develop due to toxicity or overdose, or as part of a drug-induced psychosis (another example of a 'bad trip'). Symptoms include disorientation, agitation, delusions and hallucinations. In this state, individuals sometimes assault others or harm themselves because of bizarre beliefs (e.g. that they can fly).

Chronic organic brain syndrome: Concerns have been raised that hallucinogens might cause permanent brain impairment with reduced abstract reasoning and intellectual functioning, but this has not been confirmed.

Further reading

National Institute on Drug Abuse. Hallucinogens and dissociative drugs. Rockville, MD: National Institutes of Health; 2001. Available at http://www.nida.nih.gov/ResearchReports/Hallucinogens/Hallucinogens.html

Party drugs

GHB (gammahydroxybutyrate)

Also known as Fantasy, Liquid Ecstasy, G, or Grievous Bodily Harm.

Epidemiology

First synthesized in 1964 as an anaesthetic, GHB has been increasingly common as a recreational drug used by those associated with the dance music and gay drug scene. Although it is used therapeutically and legally in some countries as a sleep agent, and in the management of alcohol and opioid withdrawal, in the UK it is classified as a Class 3 drug. At low doses stimulant effects predominate, at higher dose significant CNS and respiratory depression can occur. With a narrow therapeutic index, GHB is the dance drug most associated with overdose especially when combined with alcohol. GHB or its pro drugs (GBL, 1,4 butanediol) are typically sold as colourless, odourless liquid, which may have slightly salty taste. Typically, doses are sold as plastic ampoules holding 5–10 mL, often in small plastic fish-shaped containers similar to those used for soy sauce.

Pharmacology and pathophysiology

GHB is an endogenous short-chain fatty acid found in the CNS and elsewhere in the body and is a putative neurotransmitter. Its use leads to a transient decrease followed by increase in dopamine levels in association with an increase in endogenous opioid release.

Often prepared in crude home laboratories, there is inconsistent composition and purity that, when added to marked variation in individual tolerance, makes titration difficult. Usually added to other fluids to lessen the aversive taste, the effects come on rapidly, commencing within 15–30 min, peaking at between 30–60 min after use, with a duration of effect of 2–4 h (the effects of the pro-drugs may be slower and may be delayed further when mixed with alcohol). Intoxication may resemble alcohol intoxication with slurring of speech and sedation. GHB has a half life of 27 min and is excreted as CO_2 and H_2O. It is not routinely detected on urine drug screens.

Complications and management

Presentations to emergency departments will characteristically be that of overdose. Patients will present unconscious, with or without a history of nausea and vomiting (see Table 10.1). Coma may precede respiratory arrest. There is no specific antidote to reverse the effects, and management is supportive. Airway patency needs to be maintained with adequate oxygenation. If a patient who is seen out of hospital can tolerate a Guedel's airway, transfer to hospital is likely to be needed. Ventilation may be required. Typically patients wax and wane in their recovery but may also come round very suddenly and can be both disorientated and aggressive. Patients are often unrousable and GCS scores of <5 are not uncommon. If overdose is as a result of GHB or its pro-drugs, patients should recover within 3–5 h. Should sedation or coma persist beyond this point other causes should be explored. Attribution as to the cause of the overdose may be impaired by poor recall of substances and amounts consumed, since GHB is an amnestic drug. Patients should be advised not to return to use and advised of the risk of combining GHB with a alcohol or stimulant medication.

Dependence can occur and may be associated with a prolonged undulating withdrawal syndrome not unlike alcohol withdrawal, but with less marked autonomic disturbance. Doses of benzodiazepines far in excess of that typically used to mange alcohol withdrawal may be required.

Signs suggestive of GHB overdose

- Nausea and vomiting
- Sedation, unconsciousness and coma (usually of rapid onset)
- Weakness, slurred speech, tremors and collapse
- Hypotension, bradycardia, respiratory depression
- Ataxia and nystagmus
- Agitation, anxiety
- Delirium and hallucinations
- Amnesia, disorientation and confusion
- Evidence of alcohol or other substance use.

Further reading

Gonzalez A, Nutt DJ. Gammahydoxybutyrate abuse and dependency. *Journal of Psychopharmacology* 2005; **19**: 195–204.

Ketamine

Also known as K, Special K.

Epidemiology

Ketamine [2-(2-chlorophenyl)-2-(methylamino)-cyclohexanone] was first synthesized as an anaesthetic. Ketamine is still used in a range of clinical areas including emergency anaesthesia, paediatric analgesia, and in veterinary practice. It is described as a dissociative anaesthetic producing a 'lack of responsive awareness'. Since the 1990s ketamine has become an increasingly popular drug of abuse, most commonly associated with the dance music scene. Ketamine exerts short-lived but significant psychedelic effects, with sensory and perceptual distortion, synaesthesia, cognitive impairment and thought disorder, euphoria and out-of-body experiences. Ketamine may seem to have stimulant effects, like many other CNS depressants, because of suppression of inhibitory control. Its effects, like those of other psychedelics, are highly sensitive to set and setting. Typically sourced from diverted licit supplies of the commercially produced solution, it may be injected or more commonly dried to its crystalline form, when it is snorted (typical doses 100–400 mg). It may be taken orally (typical dose 350–500 mg) though because of extensive first pass metabolism it has relatively poor oral bioavailability (20%). However, oral consumption does result in higher levels of its primary metabolite, nor-ketamine, which is psychoactive and thus oral consumption, although associated with a slower onset and less intense effects, does result in a longer duration of action. Although marketed in its own right, ketamine occasionally may be found as part of pills sold as ecstasy. In the UK ketamine is classified as a Class C drug.

Pharmacology and pathophysiology

Ketamine, like PCP, is a non-competitive NMDA antagonist though it has a shorter half-life and is associated with less problematic emergence phenomena. It has actions at many receptor sites upon many neuro-transmitter systems, most significantly glutaminergic and monoaminergic neurotransmission, responsible for its sympathomimetic effects (see Table 10.2). The majority of the parent drug is eliminated within 24 h though extended effects due the presence of active metabolites can be seen. Ketamine has a short half-life (17 min). Following intranasal or intravenous use it has a rapid onset of action with a duration of effect of 1–2 h. Repeated dosing over the course of a using session is common, often in association with other drugs. Because ketamine, like GHB, can impair memory, it may become difficult to remember the total number of doses consumed and other drug consumption over a period of time, leading to additional complications.

Table 10.1 Adverse short-term outcomes associated with ketamine use

Physical	Psychological
Tachycardia, palpitations and chest pain	Out of body experiences/floating
Difficulty breathing	Hallucinations/sensory distortion
Nausea, vomiting	Panic/anxiety
Ataxia, temporary paralysis (may induce cataleptic state)/ inability to speak	Brief psychotic picture
Blurred vision	Derealization/depersonalization
No awareness of pain	Amnesia
Trauma, accidental injury. Rarely rhabdomyolysis	Exacerbation of pre existing disorders

Signs suggestive of ketamine intoxication

- Tachycardia
- Mydriasis
- Tachycardia, elevated BP
- Slurred speech and ataxia,
- Delirium
- Blunted affect
- Nystagmus [not always < phencyclidine (PCP)].

Although it demonstrates a wide safety margin, in clinical practice serious adverse incidents occur, particularly through accidents, trauma and risky sexual behaviours. Toxicological adverse effects are short lived (<5 h) and include frightening hallucinations/out of body experiences, thought disorder, confusion and dissociation (the K hole). These are similar to those that may be seen after LSD ingestion, though typically with ketamine they come on after a shorter period following use but recede more quickly. Other adverse effects are associated with sympathetic over-stimulation (see Table 10.1), with hospital admissions most commonly prompted by complaints of chest pain and palpitations. A brief self-limiting psychotic picture that may encompass both positive and negative symptoms may also be seen.

Most adverse effects are self limiting, requiring only supportive cardio-vascular monitoring, reassurance and reorientation, preferably in a quiet low stimulation room. Excitation and hyper-arousal may be treated with benzodiazepines which may usefully be provided in combination. For example, while midazolam negates the perceptual disorder associated with the use of ketamine, lorazepam has a more significant effect upon the associated mood disorder. Propranolol may be helpful to reduce CVS excitation. Chlorpromazine should be avoided (anticholinergic effects) and haloperidol is largely ineffective.

Dependence or compulsive use has been reported but is rare. Longer-term cognitive impairment has been reported in chronic users.

Further reading

Nutt DJ, Williams TM. Ketamine—an update. 2000–2004. Available at:
   http://www.drugs.gov.uk/ReportsandPublications
Wolff K, Winstock AR. Ketamnine: from medicine to misuse. *CNS Drugs*. 2006; **20(3)**: 199–218.

Proprietary or 'over the counter' medicines

Epidemiology

Proprietary or 'Over the counter' medicines (OTCs) are medicinal products that can be sold to the public without the need for a prescription. They are mainly sold from community pharmacies (retail pharmacies), where supervision of a qualified pharmacist is often mandatory. Some must be sold from pharmacies but do not require a pharmacist to supervise. However, many products are available for general sale from non pharmacy outlets.

In the developed world, access to OTCs is subject to regulation based on the level of risk of harm associated with their use. The availability of individual OTCs varies from country to country. Product use may be restricted within certain groups, or the use may be precluded due to medical conditions, pregnancy, and/or the use of other medicines. In addition, products which contain ingredients which are known to be liable to misuse are often more tightly regulated by law, or by professional codes of practice.

Community pharmacists are generally aware of OTC misuse, and are particularly concerned about sedating antihistamines and those containing opiates. Because many OTCs have the potential to interact with other medicines, or to be misused and cause related harms, health professionals need to be aware of the issue and to include OTC medicine use in medical history taking.

What is OTC misuse?

Before describing some of these products, their ingredients and the problems associated with their misuse, it is important to define what is meant by misuse. Misuse can be defined or construed as 'intentional' or 'unintentional'. A more sophisticated classification has been proposed—see Table 10.2 (for a fuller explanation see Wills 2005: 240–241).

Table 10.2 Types of over the counter (OTC) substance misuse

Type of OTC misuse[*]	Example
1. Inappropriate medical use	Taking the OTC for the wrong indication or at the wrong dose, usually due to lack of knowledge
2. Medication dependence	Where a person starts to take a medication for correct reasons but becomes dependent on it
3. Altered body image	Laxative abuse for weight loss
4. Intentional psychotropic abuse	Drug used for a non medical reason for its 'high'
5. Abuse support	OTCs are used to as part of OTC abuse, e.g. in the manufacture of drugs of misuse

[*] 3–5 are generally considered 'intentional' misuse.

Which substances are intentionally misused and why?

Opioids/opiates

Many pain remedies contain small amounts of codeine and, in some countries, dihydrocodeine combinations with non-opioid analgesics are also available. Furthermore in the UK, kaolin and morphine mixture is available OTC for the treatment of diarrhoea. Abuse/misuse exists among those dependent on these OTCs, and also amongst street drug users when they are unable to access drugs, such as heroin. There is significant risk from using large amounts of combination OTCs, in particular due to the paracetamol content—consuming excessive amounts of paracetamol can lead to liver failure and death. Historically, in geographically isolated countries such as New Zealand, where the supply of heroin is irregular, drug users extract codeine from codeine-containing analgesic OTCs to produce a product known locally as 'homebake'.

Dextromethorphan

Dextromethorphan was developed as a cough suppressant, and although structurally similar to opiates, has distinct properties of its own. When misused it tends to produce effects such as hallucinations, dissociation, and euphoria. There have been reports of long-term, high dose use, and ceasing after chronic use can produce withdrawal symptoms and craving. When abused, serious, rare, adverse effects can occur and include psychosis and mania. More common adverse effects include tachycardia, sleepiness, dizziness, insomnia and confusion. There tends to be a general lack of awareness amongst health professionals of misuse of this drug.

Sedating antihistamines

These are generally misused for their ability to cause euphoria and hallucinations, especially at high doses. The main drugs of concern in this group are believed to be cyclizine, diphenhydramine, and dimenhydrinate, and it is hypothesized that it is their antimuscarinic properties that may be responsible for these effects. Discontinuation after prolonged use can result in withdrawal symptoms. There have also been reports of cyclizine being injected. Adverse effects of cyclizine include confusion, agitation, drowsiness, raised heart rate, and seizures.

Sympathomimetics

Drugs in this class are generally ingredients in OTCs, which are used as decongestants, and are included in cold and flu remedies. Their active ingredients work as peripheral vasoconstrictors. Some are also centrally active and have mild stimulant properties, thus making them liable to misuse. The use of ephedrine as a performance enhancer in gyms has been reported and it is also used to combat fatigue. Use as a weight loss aid occurs, and products containing this are marketed for this purpose in some countries. Furthermore, ephedrine and pseudoephedrine are sought as precursors for the clandestine manufacture of methamphetamine. Thus, doctors and pharmacists need to be alert to requests for large or repeated quantities of the drugs on their own or in combination products.

Adverse effects associated with their use at high doses include tachycardia, hypertension, insomnia, agitation, anxiety, and gastrointestinal (GI) disturbances. Psychosis has also been reported. Long-term use in escalating doses has reported to produce dependence.

Laxatives

These drugs are misused by people who are trying to lose or control their weight, or by those who are obsessed with having a regular bowel movement. In the first case, laxatives are abused in the mistaken belief that fewer calories will be absorbed from food, and abusers of laxatives tend to be younger females. In the latter case, the group who tend to abuse laxatives are the elderly as many in the western world believe that a daily bowel evacuation is required to keep healthy. In some, tolerance to the effects of laxatives such as senna results in increasing doses.

Other products

Other products which have been reported to be misused include those containing caffeine, antimuscarinics (e.g. hyoscine), and menthol and camphor. In addition, many chemicals available OTC from pharmacies have been used in the illicit manufacture or preparation of illegal drugs.

What interventions can be helpful?

Community pharmacists use a number of strategies to avoid or deal with the issue—mainly from a supply reduction perspective, including not stocking the drug, training staff to recognize potential misuse issues, keeping potentially misused substances out of sight and sharing information with colleagues.

Once a practitioner is aware of OTC misuse or abuse, it may also be possible to intervene from a harm reduction perspective. However, much of misuse/abuse behaviour is likely to be covert and difficult to change. In the case of misuse for altered body image, unintentional misuse, and medication dependence, interventions may be more successful.

What can be done?

Health professionals and professional bodies need to be alert and vigilant. Emphasis is currently on regulation of supply and efforts by pharmacists to avoid selling to known or suspected abusers, but there is still scope to explore the potential for interventions designed to help and support those with OTC abuse problems and to provide treatment for those who want to quit, or who have co-morbidities associated with their misuse. The pharmaceutical industry needs to be aware of the potential for misuse of OTC products, not just with regard to the ingredients, but also with respect to formulation such as liquid filled capsules, the contents of which are easy to inject.

Finally, whilst not a major issue from a public health perspective, OTC misuse for some people is highly problematic, and is something which should not be ignored by health care professionals.

Further reading

Hughes G, McElnay J, Hughes C, McKenna P. Abuse/misuse of non-prescription drugs. *Pharmacy World & Science* 1999; **21**: 251–255.

MacFayden L, Eadie D, McGowan T. Over-the-counter medicine misuse in Scotland. *Journal of the Royal Society for the Promotion of Health* 2000; **121**: 185–192.

Matheson C, Bond C, Pitcairn M. Misuse of over-the-counter medicines from community pharmacies: a population survey of Scottish pharmacies. *Pharmaceutical Journal* 2002; **269**: 66–68.

Pates R, McBride A, Li S, Ramadan R. Misuse of over-the-counter medicines: A survey of community pharmacies in a South Wales health authority. *Pharmaceutical Journal* 2002; **268**: 179–182.

Wills S. *Drugs of Abuse*. London: Pharmaceutical Press, 2005.

Anabolic steroid misuse

Epidemiology

Steroid misuse is common in body-builders and professional athletes, but true prevalence figures are difficult to obtain because of the illicit nature of this misuse. Lifetime prevalence for males may approach 1%. Highest prevalence rates are seen in male adolescents (up to around 5%) and amongst gymnasium attendees (up to around 25%), and the gay male population. All prevalence figures are derived from US populations. Anabolic steroids are misused for their muscle-building properties. In gay male communities they also have a reputation for instilling a subjective sense of power and dominance. They have numerous adverse effects both physical and psychological.

Patterns of misuse

There are three methods widely used:
- **Stacking**: using oral and injectable steroids in high doses
- **Pyramiding**: increasing dose and number of preparations taken over a set period
- **Cycling**: alternating periods of high use (stacking or pyramiding) with periods of abstinence.

Many steroid misusers consume other drugs to treat steroid adverse effects. These include oestrogen antagonists (tamoxifen), analgesics, and oral hypoglycaemics.

Pharmacology

Anabolic steroids are compounds chemically related to testosterone and sharing its actions on the body. Testosterone itself is not active orally (high first pass effect) and it is usually given as 17 α-alkyl substituted molecules (orally active) or parenterally as testosterone esters.

Pathophysiology

Physical effects

Anabolic steroid misuse is associated with a wide range of important adverse effects. These include:
- Elevated lipid profiles
- Increased blood pressure
- Increased heart size
- Decreased thyroid-stimulating hormone (TSH)
- Decreased sperm count
- Carcinoma of the liver
- Hirsutism
- Insulin resistance
- Testicular atrophy (clitoral growth in woman)
- Gynaecomastia
- Prostate hypertrophy
- Prostatic carcinoma.

Psychological effects

While low doses of anabolic steroids are not normally associated with psychiatric adverse effects, the huge doses used by body-builders and athletes cause a wide range of serious psychological sequelae. These include:

- **Aggression**: often severe, provoking violent acts against other people or property, often accompanied by irritability and mood instability.
- **Depression**: usually characterized by low mood, insomnia, anxiety and, more rarely, suicidality. Suicide has been widely reported amongst current steroid misusers, and may represent the ultimate outcome of steroid-induced concurrent aggression, depression and lack of impulse control.
- **Hypomania and mania**: common symptoms include euphoria, grandiosity, over-confidence, irritability, increased libido, and poor judgement.
- **Psychosis** is less often seen than aggression or mood disorders. Symptoms may include paranoid delusions, auditory hallucinations, delusions of reference.
- **Dependence**: anabolic steroids may provoke endogenous opiate release and dependence is not uncommon. Naloxone can usually be shown to illicit an acute opiate-type withdrawal reaction in heavy misusers. On cessation of misuse, an acute hyperadrenergic state is experienced followed later by depression, fatigue, joint pain, and craving.

Treatment of psychological effects

There are no formal guidelines for the treatment of steroid-induced psychological effects. Some suggestions are given below:

- **Aggression**: haloperidol, olanzapine, lorazepam
- **Depression**: standard antidepressants
- **Mania**: standard treatments
- **Psychosis**: standard treatments
- **Withdrawal**: clonidine, lofexidine acutely; antidepressants in the medium term. NSAIDs may be required for muscle and joint pain.

Further reading

Graham S, Kennedy M. Recent developments in the toxicology of anabolic steroids. *Drug Safety* 1990; **5**: 458–476.

Pope HG Jr, Katz DL. Affective and psychotic symptoms associated with anabolic steroid use. *American Journal of Psychiatry* 1988; **145**: 487–490.

Trenton AJ, Currier GW. Behavioural manifestations of anabolic steroid use. *CNS Drugs* 2005; **19**: 571–595.

Polysubstance use

Epidemiology

Polysubstance use is defined as the hazardous or harmful use of two or more psychoactive substances. Tobacco and alcohol are most commonly implicated, and there are several diseases for which alcohol and tobacco are synergistic risk factors. The term 'polysubstance use' also embraces various combinations of illicit drugs (such as opioids, cocaine, amphetamines, MDMA and cannabis) and prescribed medications (in particular benzodiazepines and/or opioids) and also over the counter (proprietary) medications.

The true prevalence of polysubstance use is difficult to determine. The pattern of use may be intermittent, 'recreational use', e.g. at parties, or it may involve hazardous or harmful use for some drugs combined with daily use progressing to dependence for others. Individuals may thus be dependent on one or more drugs, or classes of drugs, while using another drug or drug combinations on an intermittent (non-dependent) basis. To add to the complexity of the problem, the mode of administration may vary and the drug may be used orally, intranasally, intravenously, or by a combination of different routes.

Illicit drug users, patients with mental illness, chronic pain, or insomnia, the unemployed, adolescents, and partygoers are subgroups at particular risk of multiple substance use.

Reasons for polysubstance use

Polydrug use often has functional value for the individual. People use multiple substances to:

Accentuate the effects of drugs: The effects of drug can be increased by various combinations for example heroin and cocaine ('speed balling'). Illicit drug users often use multiple substances for additive pharmacological effects. Opioid dependent individuals may use opioids (heroin, methadone, or buprenorphine) in combination with other central nervous system depressants, such as alcohol, cannabis or benzodiazepines to enhance the effects of opioids. The combined use of these drugs carries the risk of fatal overdose. The danger of multiple drug use is highlighted in a toxicological review of heroin-related deaths in New South Wales. A single drug was found in only 27% of cases, while two or more drug classes were detected in 71% of cases, alcohol being found in 45% and benzodiazepines in a quarter of cases.

Reverse or reduce the effects of drugs: Sometimes drug combinations are used because their pharmacological effects are the opposite of the drug that was recently taken (or is to be taken) Thus, central nervous system depressants, such as alcohol, benzodiazepines, or opioids may be used to reverse or reduce the agitation, paranoia, and stimulant effects caused by amphetamines, cocaine, and other psychostimulants.

Psychostimulant users may seek to terminate their hyperactive state by taking alcohol or a sedative-hypnotic. Individuals who use psychostimulants commonly use benzodiazepines to help them sleep or come off the 'high', particularly after stimulant binges lasting several days.

Relieve withdrawal symptoms: Alcohol dependent individuals as well as opioid dependent individuals take benzodiazepines for relief of withdrawal symptoms such as anxiety, insomnia, restlessness or agitation. This may progress to polysubstance dependence.

Relieve pain: Patients with chronic pain are at risk of misusing or becoming dependent on prescribed opioids. They are also at risk of drinking excess alcohol or misusing benzodiazepines prescribed for insomnia or relaxation of skeletal muscles. They may see a range of different doctors to seek opioids and other psychoactive substances, including benzodiazepines. Others may obtain these medications from the black market or Internet to alleviate pain, anxiety, sleep disorders, insomnia, withdrawal syndromes, or simply to achieve temporary alteration in mental state. (See also pp. 360–366.)

Alleviate psychiatric co-morbid symptoms: Up to 25% of patients with psychiatric disorders are reported to use multiple drugs. Alcohol use disorder and cannabis use disorder are the commonest co-existing disorders. It is unclear whether patients with psychiatric illnesses self medicate because of the underlying illness or to alleviate psychiatric symptoms or the side effects of prescribed medication or whether the polydrug use itself has led to psychiatric co-morbidity.

Smoking is very common in individuals with mental health disorders.

Increase the pleasurable effects of drugs e.g. by adolescents and party goers
- Alcohol and cocaine are commonly combined. Cocaethylene, a metabolite of alcohol and cocaine, is thought to enhance and extend the euphoria and abate the 'crash' following a cocaine binge. While sometimes the combination is planned, in other cases the use of alcohol or a similarly disinhibiting substance can lead to unplanned use of another substance such as cannabis, cocaine or methamphetamines. Alcohol is a particularly powerful cue for cocaine use.
- 'Party drugs' or 'club drugs' mainly used by young people in various combinations include tobacco, alcohol, cannabis, benzodiazepines (diazepam, temazepam), psychostimulants [MDMA ecstasy; methamphetamines (ice); amphetamines; and cocaine], ketamine, or gammahydroxybutyrate. Amyl nitrite ('poppers') is popular among the gay population, as is cocaine, which is sometimes together used with heroin ('speed-balling'). Other opioids such as codeine, methadone, and buprenorphine may also be used.

Clinical presentation
The clinical presentation of polydrug use may take different forms. Polysubstance use is often not apparent to the clinician who may focus only on the stated or most obvious substance being used.

Most people with polysubstance use who are seen in medical practice present with symptoms or problems typically seen with single substance use, but often with combinations of other features that are difficult to recognize.

Patients may present to their general practitioner with drug-seeking behaviour and a variety of symptoms including anxiety, insomnia, pain, or loss of scripts. Drugs most commonly sought are benzodiazepines and opioids.

Polysubstance users may also present to a hospital emergency department with accidents, intoxication, or overdose, coma, withdrawal syndromes, including withdrawal seizures, or from other medical or psychosocial complications of multiple substance use.

At times persons who use multiple drugs may present with psychiatric symptoms, such as anxiety, depression, suicidality, agitation, delirium, paranoia, or full-blown psychosis.

Assessment

Where the patient is lucid, a comprehensive drug and alcohol history, as well as a medical, psychiatric and psychosocial history is taken applying the principles and approaches outlined in Chapter 2 pp. 37–53. Persistence and patience are often needed to elicit all the relevant substances being used.

Clinical examination should include inspection for needle track marks and signs of drug intoxication or withdrawal. Relatively specific signs such as pupil constriction in the case of opioid intoxication may give a clue to the nature of at least one of the drugs used.

Laboratory tests should include a urine, blood or salivary drug screen, and breath or blood alcohol concentration. Results of a urine drug screen provide only semi-quantitative levels. However, the assays are sensitive and accurate, and much valuable (and unexpected) information can be obtained, which helps to establish the diagnosis of polysubstance use or abuse. This can be of great assistance for ongoing management of subsequent presentations.

Diagnosis

When a patient is using multiple substances, it is important to note each of these and the associated diagnosis for each, in accordance with the recommendations of DSM-IV and ICD10. It is important to differentiate whether the patient is dependent on a particular drug, or whether the drug is used intermittently in a non-dependent hazardous or harmful manner, or alternatively low risk manner.

However, in some cases substance use is so indiscriminate that polysubstance use, abuse, or dependence is the most appropriate diagnostic term. The diagnosis of polysubstance abuse or dependence is reserved for patients whose pattern of multiple drug use is so indiscriminate or variable that no one drug use disorder can be identified.

Management

A management plan should determine which substance, or substances, is causing major problems and which the patient wishes to cease using, or will agree to cease using. The patient and clinician can reach an agreement on which drugs will be tackled first or whether all drugs will be addressed simultaneously.

When a diagnosis of polysubstance dependence is made, detoxification either as an in-patient or out-patient may be necessary as a first step (See sections on individual drugs). Inpatient detoxification units can be of great assistance in complex cases where the patient's life may be too chaotic to allow out-patient detoxification, or where there is possibility of severe withdrawal syndromes.

Detoxification units vary in their staffing and may vary in their willingness to accept patients with polysubstance abuse or dependence. Patients may become medically unwell and it may not be easy to implicate a particular drug as the cause of the clinical condition. Similarly, some units offer selective detoxification for individuals on opioid maintenance treatment who want to cease benzodiazepine use, while others do not have the nursing staffing to provide ongoing opioid maintenance treatment. Developing an understanding of services in the local area or contacting a person with such understanding, will save considerable time and maximize the appropriateness of referrals.

Polydrug users with psychiatric co-morbidity have a poorer outcome unless their underlying psychiatric problem is appropriately addressed. Detoxification followed by a period of abstinence of 2–4 weeks is particularly important in order to make a correct psychiatric diagnosis.

Because of the complexity, cases of multiple substance use are typically best managed by specialist drug and alcohol facilities. Typically, such services can provide on-going treatment, including pharmacotherapies where indicated, psychological treatments (including specific psychological treatments, as well as supportive counselling and assistance on social issues), and generally apply a range of relapse prevention strategies. Patients with chronic pain syndromes may alternatively be referred to a specialist pain clinic.

Further reading

Curry K, Theodorou S. The poly drug user. In: Hulse G, White J & Cape G (Eds) *Management of Alcohol and Drug Problems*. Oxford: Oxford University Press, 2002.

Marshall EJ. Multiple substance use. *Psychiatry* 2007; **5**(12): 461–463.

Zador D, Sunjic S, Darke S. Heroin related deaths in New South Wales, 1992: toxicological findings and circumstances. *Medical Journal of Australia* 1992; **164**: 204–212.

Kava

Kava is an intoxicating drink prepared from crushed roots of *Piper methysticum*. It is traditionally widely used in south Pacific countries and was also brought to Arnhem Land Aboriginal communities in Australia's Northern Territory in 1982. It is postulated that kava use became more widespread in Arnhem Land because its use is not subject to the strict social controls seen in Pacific countries.

Kava's pharmacological actions include sedation, analgesia, and anxiolytic, muscle relaxant and anticonvulsant effects.

Kava lactones, the psychoactive constituents, are found in the resinous plant components and are a group of mostly lipid soluble pyrones (of the sesquiterpine group of lactones) with a chemical structure characterized by a 5,6-dihydro-α-pyrone ring. Kava's potency has been attributed to the six main lactones found in the lipid soluble fraction namely: kawain, dihydrokawain, methysticin, dihydromethysticin, yangonin, and desmethoxy-yangonin.

Reported adverse health effects of kava include

- A characteristic scaly skin *rash*, described as 'ichthyosis' in heavy regular users. Up to 45% of kava users who had used kava in the month before interview in one study exhibited this rash
- Heavy users may have a reduced mean body mass index, body fat and skin-fold thickness, similar in extent to that seen in anorexia nervosa
- Increases in GGT and alkaline phosphatase, which reverse with abstinence or moderation.

In those who drink kava mixed with water these changes appear to be reversible with no firm evidence for long-term liver damage. However, clinical surveillance is warranted as fulminant hepatitis, and irreversible liver injury have been reported in users of some manufactured remedies containing kava compounds.

- Lymphopaenia: in an Australian study 51% of kava drinkers had lymphocyte counts below the reference range even after controlling for any confounding effects of alcohol
- Risk of infections, such as pneumonia and melioidosis is reported to be increased
- Increased HDL-, LDL-, and total cholesterol and immunoglobulin E levels have been documented in heavy kava users in Australia, together with a lower serum osmolarity
- While there are high rates of coincident renal disease in Aboriginal Australians in the Northern Territory there is no firm evidence that kava causes haematuria, albuminuria or renal injury
- No evidence for long-term neurological damage was found in those who had, in some cases, used kava continuously for up to 18 years

- Heavy kava use has been reported to increase the risks for sudden cardiac deaths in Arnhem Land populations, possibly due to enhanced thrombosis and dehydration and prolonged QT interval. These, and other Arnhem Land studies, controlled for the effects of high levels of co-morbidity with alcohol. No comparative studies have been conducted in Pacific island populations where the population might be healthier and have a lower prevalence of alcohol problems
- In some Aboriginal communities, heavy kava use is said to interfere with involvement in community and family life, and takes a significant toll on family and community finance.

Currently, no specific treatment has been recommended for heavy kava users. Supply control has been the main preventive measure adopted.

Further reading

Clough AR, Jacups SP, Wang Z, *et al.* Health effects of kava use in an eastern Arnhem Land community. *Internal Medicine Journal* 2003; **33**(8): 336–340.

Khat (Qat)

This perennial shrub is indigenous to The Yemen, Ethiopia, and surrounding areas. Like other culture-bound substances it frequently accompanies its users when they migrate from their place of origin. Outside its area of propagation, khat is most commonly used among immigrant Somali communities in the UK, and elsewhere in Europe and the United States. In recent years, concern has grown regarding the possible adverse effects of Khat upon both individuals and their societies. For a recent review, see Cox and Ramses 2003.

Preparation and mode of administration Only the fresh leaves retain their psychoactive potency. Fresh bitter leaves are usually chewed for their stimulant effect (though the leaves may be smoked or infusions prepared), with the extracted juices swallowed and the residue kept within the cheek for some time after. This is a relatively slow mode of administration requiring prolonged chewing to provide a relatively mild stimulant effect.

Psychological effects and contextual use of the drug Like other culture bound substance use such as areca nut, the use of khat has its origins in social, ceremonial, and religious activities. Its mild stimulant effects may promote social interaction, with users reporting increased talkativeness, disinhibition, improved concentration, loss of appetite and improved stamina. Predominately used by men, its increasing use by women is sometimes frowned upon.

Pharmacological effects of the drugs

Khat is a central stimulant, considerably less potent than amphetamine though its mechanism of action through the release of presynaptically stored catecholamines is similar. The main stimulant psychoactive components, cathine, and the more potent cathinone (both phenylpropylamines), are found in combination with a number of other alkaloids and tannins. Cathinone is a very unstable compound that necessitates importation of fresh leaves within a day or two of harvesting, before the active components degrade. Cathinone is classified as a Class 1 drug.

Adverse effects of use

Particularly in its countries of origin, the assessment of the adverse health effects of khat are complicated by poor socio-economic status of many users. Adverse physical effects reported include oral, gastrointestinal (constipation), hepatic, and cardiac disturbances, as well as those related to accidents whilst intoxicated. Cardiac effects appear related to increases in pulse and blood pressure that may compromise cardiac function in those with underlying disease. Compulsive patterns of use consistent with a dependence syndrome have been described, but there does not appear to be a distinct withdrawal syndrome.

Chronic khat use is associated with an increased risk of hepatic cirrhosis. Use among most users does not appear to be associated with the increased risk of psychological symptoms. However, there have been several case reports of short-lived amphetamine-like psychoses among users of khat, although there is little to suggest longer-term psychiatric morbidity among users. Khat use may also exacerbate pre-existing psychotic disorders. Treatment should include cessation drug use and short-term symptomatic treatment with benzodiazepines and less commonly antipsychotics. Culturally appropriate variation on motivational interviewing and relapse prevention may be useful, although addressing the significant social role that khat use has for individuals will be more challenging.

Further reading

Cox G, Ramses H. Adverse effects of khat: a review. *Advances in Psychiatric Treatment* 2003; **9**: 456–463.

Numan N. Exploration of adverse psychological symptoms in Yemeni khat users by the Symptoms Checklist-90 (SCL-90). *Addiction* 2004; **99**(1): 61–65.

Williams T and Nutt DJ, 2005. Khat (qat): assessment of risk to the individual and communities in the UK–Home Office on-line publication. http://drugs.homeoffice.gov.uk.

Areca nut (Betel/Pan)

Epidemiology

The areca nut, often incorrectly referred to as betel nut (betel refers to the leaf that the nut is often wrapped in) and its products are the fourth most commonly used psychoactive substance in the world after tobacco, alcohol, and caffeine. It is used most commonly within the Indian sub-continent, but also prevalent in Taiwan and South East Asia, and southern China. Historically, areca use has its origins in religious, ceremonial, and social activities, and is purported to having many desirable effects. The nut reportedly assists digestion and may be used regularly (daily) by habitués or a social lubricant at social gatherings by occasional users. The nut is typically sliced into thin shards and rolled in a betel leaf with slaked lime and a variety of other additives, such as catechu and cardamoms to enhance the flavour. Commonly tobacco is added to this mix. The folded leaf package ('quid') is then chewed. In recent years the nut has been marketed in a packaged form as a refined areca product containing a variety of mixtures with and without tobacco, commonly known as pan masala. This appears to be the form of areca use most commonly used by Asian immigrants living in the UK and is popular among children. As a gateway to tobacco use, this practice is potentially significant.

Pharmacology and pathophysiology

The areca nut contains a number of psychoactive alkaloids, with arecoline being the one present in the greatest quantity. Anecdotally, the nut and arecoline have significant medicinal properties ranging from an anti-helminthic and astringent to an aphrodisiac, digestive enhancement, and psychomotor stimulant. Research suggests it has complex effects upon both parasympathetic and sympathetic nervous systems, reflected in the subjective experience of a mixed of stimulant and anxiolytic effect not unlike tobacco.

Complications and treatment

Often chewed with tobacco, areca poses significant health risks to long-term chewers, most notably leukoplakia, and sub-mucosal fibrosis, a progressive scarring condition of the oral mucosa with a high risk (50%) of oral squamous cell carcinoma development. Dental practitioners should be alert to this practice and advise on the risk of continued chewing on the ability to maintain health and adequate nutrition. Concurrent tobacco use should be addressed with nicotine replacement and motivational interviewing. A behavioural approach and replacement of the masticatory process with gum may be helpful. Dependence may be seen in chronic users and may be associated with a mild withdrawal syndrome requiring only symptomatic relief.

Further reading

Burton-Bradley B. Betel Nut Chewing in Retrospect. *Papua New Guinea Medical Journal* 1978; **21**(3) Sept: 236–240.

Trivedy C, Johnson NW. Oral cancer in South Asia [letter] *Br Dent J* 1997; **182**(6):206.

Warnakulasuriya S, Trivedy C, Peters T. Areca nut use: an independent risk factor for oral cancer. *BMJ* 2002; **324**(7341): 799–800, Apr 6.

Volatile solvent misuse

Volatile solvent misuse (VSM) refers to the deliberate inhalation of liquid that vaporizes at room temperature/pressure to induce a mental state change.

The substances most often misused are simple hydrocarbons (acetone, toluene, butane, etc.). These may include gases (e.g. butane), aerosols (e.g. air freshener, 'poppers'), glues, and 'others' (e.g. fire extinguishers, correction fluid, petrol, etc.). Over 30 different substances have been implicated in solvent misuse fatalities (80% butane in UK; the majority involve 'gasoline' in USA). Internationally, solvent misuse is responsible for more fatalities among 10–14-year-olds than is 'drug abuse'.

Delivery methods ('huffing', 'sniffing', 'bagging', 'tooting', 'buzzing'):
• Placed in mouth
• Sniff container/sleeve/cloth/plastic bag
• Bag/padding over head/face.

Epidemiology

Volatiles are widely available, relatively cheap, largely legal, easily concealed, and have low perceived dependence risk. The prevalence of VSM is 1–2% of UK 13–15-year-olds (females = males by self-report, but males predominate in treatment populations and fatalities). Sniffing generally occurs in those aged <30 years with declining use with age. As many as 12% of UK adults have misused volatile solvents at some time in their life, with prevalence varying geographically (e.g. lowest in the SE of the UK increasing moving NW). In the USA prevalence is higher in rural than urban populations. In Australia petrol sniffing has been a major problem in some rural or remote, disadvantaged Aboriginal communities.

Mortality: In 2005 there were 45 UK deaths related to VSM (2198 cumulative since 1971; St George's Hospital ongoing study). Of these 20% left a suicide note (previously <10%). Mechanisms for death included direct toxic effects (60% post-1971), vomit inhalation (14%), plastic bag asphyxia (11%), and accidental trauma (11%). More males than females died from solvent misuse, and the age range for these deaths was 7 to >75 years (the older deaths were mainly suicide).

Associations: Include crime, antisocial behaviour, polysubstance misuse, homelessness, poverty, poor education, gangs, family disruption (low cohesiveness/support, poor relationships, especially with father), and social exclusion. In the UK the 'principal' associations are with the criminal justice system, and 'looked after' children.

Natural history Some young people may experiment with VSM, but never progress to harmful use or meet DSM criteria for abuse or the criteria for dependence; 1/5 of volatile solvent misusers develop 'dependence'; many combine/'progress to' other substances (16% versus 7% non-VSM peers use Class A drugs). Among younger teens, VSM is more socially acceptable; among the middle teens VSM tends to be an isolated/solitary activity.

Neurobiology

VSM causes increased permeability of nerve cell membranes, and results in positive GABA-A modulation, NMDA receptor effects and increased serotonin. Toluene increases mesolimbic dopamine. Volatiles are highly lipophilic (and so cross blood–brain barrier easily) leading to rapid onset of effects. Volatiles have an anticonvulsant, anxiolytic and CNS depressant effect (like alcohol, barbiturates, etc.). A withdrawal syndrome similar to alcohol withdrawal may occur after cessation of regular, heavy use.

Effects

- **'Sudden death sniffing syndrome'** (released catecholamines on startling causes sudden death).
- **Immediate (<45 min):** euphoria, disinhibition, disorientation, 'drunken-ness', blurred vision, dizziness, slurring, drowsiness, hallucinations, black-outs (see ICD-10 research criteria for intoxication)
- **Later effects:** hangover, drowsiness, headaches, spots/rashes in the oronasal area, black-outs
- **Longer-term risks:** Medical
  - Neurological
    - permanent neurological damage (progressive cognitive decline, e.g. petrol sniffing)
    - ataxia, cerebral atrophy, encephalopathy, Parkinsonism, peripheral/sensorimotor neuropathy, speech problems, trigeminal neuropathy, tremor
  - Damaged endocrine, GI, reproductive systems, and eyes/ears
  - Skin (burns, dermatitis, hypothermic injury, eczema)
  - Cardiovascular (arrhythmia, fibrosis, ischaemia, VF)
  - Pulmonary (coughing, wheezing, emphysema, pneumonia)
  - Liver and kidney (toxic damage, failure, hepatorenal syndrome, Fanconi's syndrome)
  - Bone marrow (suppression, anaemia, leukaemia)
- **Psychiatric:**
  - Mood disorder/anxiety—45% of VSMs are estimated to have a lifetime history of mood disorder, 36% anxiety
  - Personality disorder (45% of VSMs in one sample, with ASPD in 36% of male VSMs; Wu and Howard, 2007)
  - Apathy, inattention, insomnia
  - Memory loss, psychosis
  - Delirium, dementia, suicide.

Management

- Treat medical and psychiatric symptoms and associations as needed
- No specific drug treatments for harmful solvent use, solvent (inhalant') abuse or dependence itself
- Where leaded petrol has been sniffed, chelating agents can be used to treat lead toxicity
- Education
- For those aged under 16, in many countries there are legal obligations to report the problem to the relevant child protection authority.

Given age ranges and psychiatric co-morbidity involved, principles for treating children and adolescents with solvent misuse and other psychological disorders apply, including family assessment and intervention. Organizations are available, which can offer support and help (e.g. in UK Re-Solv, SOLVE IT).

Prevention

Community-wide efforts have been made at prohibition, prevention, and education.

These vary by country and region, but the following examples give an overview of some of the measures that have been applied:

- **Legal measures**: in UK law, the Intoxicating Substances (Supply) Act 1985 prohibits sale to under 18s if perceived as for misuse. The Consumer Protection Act (supplement 1999) prohibits selling gas lighter fuel to under 18s (maximum £5000 fine/6-month sentence)—inspectors can 'test' vendors by sending in minors. Intoxication with volatile solvents comes under the general law (e.g. breach of peace). Under the Solvent Abuse Scotland Act (1983)/Children (Scotland) Act 1995 it is necessary to notify the Children's Reporter, but no criminality is involved.
- **Other supply control**: in several remote communities in Australia the community has agreed to switch from petrol to a non-sniffable fuel. This in the past has been aviation gas, but more recently a modified petrol known as 'OPAL' has been introduced. Some evaluations have shown promising results for such fuels in reducing prevalence of sniffing. In some centres, supply control has been combined with providing alternative activities, which engage young people.

Further reading

Harris D. Volatile substance abuse. *Archives of Diseases of Childhood Education Practices* 2006; **91**: ep93–ep100.

Orr KS, Shewan D. *Review of evidence relating to volatile substance abuse in Scotland.* Scottish Executive, September, 2006.

Wu Li-Tzy, Howard MO. Psychiatric disorders in inhalant users: results from the National Epidemiologic Survey on Alcohol and Related conditions. *Drug and Alcohol Dependence* 2007; **88**: 146–155.

Psychiatric co-morbidity

Epidemiology

The presence of co-existing mental illness and substance use disorders is common in the general population, and more common in psychiatric settings and addiction medicine settings.

Studies show that over 50% of psychiatric in-patients will have a substance use disorder, though in over half of these the psychiatric syndrome may be secondary to the substance use. Similarly, over half of those with a drug use disorder will have another form of mental disorder, and they are 4.5 times more likely (Odds Ratio = 4.5) to have a mental disorder than those individuals with no lifetime history of a drug use disorder. In comparison, close to 40% of those with an alcohol use disorder will have a coexisting mental disorder.

Alcohol and drug misuse most commonly co-occur with anxiety and depression. The Epidemiological Catchment Area study found that, among individuals with an alcohol disorder, the most prevalent co-morbid mental disorders were: anxiety disorders (19%), antisocial personality disorders (14%), affective disorders (13%), and schizophrenia (4%). Among individuals with any form of drug disorder, the most prevalent co-morbid mental disorders were: anxiety disorders (28%), affective disorders (26%), antisocial personality disorders (18%), and schizophrenia (7%).

Table 11.1 The rates of those experiencing a substance use disorder in those with a psychiatric condition

Psychiatric disorder	% with a substance use disorder
Phobic disorder	25%
Anxiety disorder	30%
Depressive disorder	30%
Bipolar disorder	50%
Schizophrenia	50%
Antisocial personality disorder	80%

Only a minority of individuals with co-occurring disorders in the community are treated, while those with more severe disorders, multiple co-morbid disorders and high levels of distress are more likely to receive treatment from specialist services. Co-existing disorders provide difficult diagnostic and treatment dilemmas for the health professionals involved in their care.

This chapter provides an overview of the type of psychiatric syndromes commonly seen secondary to substance use. Because anxiety disorders and depression are the most common co-occurring disorders with substance misuse, these disorders and some of their treatment strategies are described in detail.

Features of psychiatric co-morbidity

Co-morbid psychiatric symptoms

Co-morbid psychiatric symptoms fit broadly into 5 categories:

- Depressive symptoms
- Anxiety symptoms
- Psychotic symptoms (delusions, hallucinations, thought disorder)
- Organic brain syndromes (e.g. cognitive impairment, delirium, dementia, amnestic syndrome)
- Flashbacks.

Major depressive disorder

Depressive episodes in the community occur twice as frequently in women compared with men, with lifetime prevalence from 10–26% for women and 5–12% for men. These rates are elevated in individuals with co-morbid substance use disorders. Being able to diagnose and effectively treat a co-morbid depressive illness is an important skill for an addiction specialist to develop.

The diagnosis of major depressive episode (DSM-IV) involves the following:

The presence of depressed mood and loss of interest or pleasure for at least 2 weeks associated with at least three of the following symptoms:

- Significant appetite or weight loss or gain
- Insomnia or hypersomnia
- Psychomotor retardation or agitation
- Fatigue or loss of energy
- Feelings of worthlessness or excessive guilt
- Impaired thinking or concentration: indecisiveness
- Suicidal thoughts/thoughts of death.

A major depressive episode is different in quality and duration to brief periods of unhappiness related to difficult life circumstances. The mood disturbance of a major depression is pervasive in nature, so that the person feels down, flat, depressed (and often irritable) most of the day every day for at least 2 weeks or more with loss of interest in pleasurable activities. The mood disturbance is associated with a range of biological (or neuro-vegetative symptoms) including:

- A change in sleep and appetite (either increased or decreased)
- Impaired concentration and memory
- Impaired energy levels and motivation
- Impaired libido.

Psychomotor agitation or retardation may be present in more severe cases. Depressed mood may be associated with depressive thought content, including thoughts that life is no longer worth living and thoughts of suicide. There may be thoughts of hopelessness (there is no way out and no future ahead); worthlessness, excessive guilt, and helplessness (there is nothing anyone can do to improve the situation). More severe forms of major depression result in significant impairment in functioning, so that the patient struggles to manage the everyday tasks they need to complete. Suicidal thoughts may occur with severe major depression and may result in the formation of a suicide plan, with suicide attempts.

Depression may be substance induced, related to periods of intoxication or withdrawal, e.g. significant depressive symptoms are common with heavy drinking, opioid dependence, amphetamine withdrawal. The depression usually resolves with treatment of the substance use disorder. However, some individuals remain significantly depressed despite active treatment of substance use. This depression requires treatment in its own right.

General indicators that depression is not substance related are:

• The patient remains significantly depressed despite a period of abstinence of a month or more
• The patient has a past history of depressive symptoms during a period of abstinence of a month or more
• There may be a positive family history of depression.

Anxiety disorders

The lifetime prevalence of primary anxiety disorders (anxiety that is not due to substance misuse or some form of physical illness) is around 25%, with the lifetime rates for individual disorders is as follows:

• Specific phobia (e.g. fear of spiders, fear of lifts, fear of planes etc) 6–10%
• Generalized anxiety disorder (GAD) 5%
• Panic disorder 1–4%
• Agoraphobia 3–6%
• Social phobia or social anxiety disorder (SAD) 3–13%
• Post-traumatic stress disorder (PTSD) 1–14%
• Obsessive compulsive disorder (OCD) 2–3%

Individuals with substance use disorders have high rates of anxiety symptoms, and it is important to be able to distinguish independent anxiety disorders from substance-induced anxiety states.

Panic disorder

With panic disorder, the individual experiences recurrent, unexpected panic attacks for a period of a month or more, often associated with the fear of having further attacks. A panic attack is a discrete period of intense fear or discomfort, in which four or more of the following symptoms develop abruptly and peak within 10 min:

• Palpitations, pounding heart
• Sweating
• Shortness of breath
• Chest pain or discomfort
• Feeling dizzy, unsteady, light-headed, or faint
• Numbness or tingling sensations
• Derealization or depersonalization
• Fear of dying
• Trembling or shaking
• Sensations of choking
• Nausea or abdominal pain
• Chills or hot flushes
• Fear of losing control or going crazy.

While panic attacks initially occur 'out of the blue' with no clear precipitant, they may become linked to specific events or situations in the individuals mind, creating phobic avoidance of that situation. For example, if a patient experiences panic attacks when in a bus, he may avoid getting on buses for fear of further panic attacks.

Agoraphobia may develop in which the individual avoids places or situations from which escape may be difficult or help unavailable in the event of a panic attack (e.g. wide open spaces, crowded public places).

Social phobia (Social Anxiety Disorder) This involves an excessive or unreasonable fear of social situations, the individual being afraid they will embarrass or humiliate themselves. The individual is aware the fear is excessive or unreasonable, but feels unable to control it, and may experience high levels of anxiety or panic attacks in certain social situations. SAD leads to significant distress or impairment and the individual may avoid social situations or endure them with intense anxiety.

Commonly feared social phobia situations include:
• Parties
• Conversations
• Meeting new people, especially those of higher social standing,
  e.g. doctors, bank managers
• Using public bathrooms
• Eating or drinking in front of others
• Meetings
• Dating
• Performing: music, sports, public speaking
• Writing in front of others.
Symptoms include blushing, tremor, sweating and difficulties in speaking.

Obsessive compulsive disorder (OCD) Involves intrusive, distressing thoughts, impulses or images which the individual recognizes as irrational and tries to manage by suppressing them or neutralizing them with some other thought or action. Compulsions are repetitive behaviours often used to try to reduce and manage the anxiety related to obsessions (e.g. compulsive hand washing to try to cope with fearful thoughts of contamination in the environment).

Generalized anxiety disorder (GAD) Involves excessive anxiety and worry that is difficult to control and occurs more days than not for at least 6 months. The anxiety is pervasive, unreasonable, and involves worrying excessively about many situations, not just specific events. It involves three or more associated symptoms:
• Restlessness/feeling keyed up/on edge
• Easily fatigued
• Difficulty concentrating/mind going blank
• Irritability
• Muscle tension
• Insomnia.

The anxiety causes significant distress or impairment for the individual.

For example, TK had been a 'worrier' since childhood. These days he was frequently preoccupied with the thought that one of his parents would die of cancer, even though there was no family history of cancer. He also worried that the family cat would get lost, would be found dead and he would be blamed. He didn't want to leave his home in case someone broke in, even though he was in a very secure building. He worried that if there was a break-in the neighbours would blame him for not fixing the security lights properly, even though it wasn't his responsibility. While he knew all these anxieties were unrealistic, he couldn't stop thinking about them day after day and this made him feel constantly tense and unhappy.

Post-traumatic stress disorder (PTSD)

The key features of this disorder can be remembered using the mnemonic 'TRAP', namely:

- Trauma
- Re-experiencing
- Avoidance
- Physiological arousal.

Trauma involves exposure to a traumatic event in which:

- The person experienced or witnessed events involving death or threatened death, serious injury, or threat to the physical integrity of self or others
- Response involved intense fear, helplessness or horror
- The threat was physical not emotional.

For example, while losing a job because of work-place conflict may create anxiety and distress, the symptoms experienced would not constitute PTSD, because there is no physical threat involved. In contrast, PTSD occurs in about 80% of women who have been raped, where physical violence and often fear of death are involved.

With PTSD there is persistent *re-experiencing* of the traumatic event in one (or more) of the following ways:

- Recurrent, intrusive distressing recollections
- Flashbacks, nightmares
- Acting or feeling as if the traumatic event were occurring again
- Exposure to cues that symbolize or resemble an aspect of the event can trigger flashbacks and intense psychological distress.

Because any re-experiencing of the trauma can cause intense fear and distress, there is often *avoidance* of any stimuli associated with the trauma and numbing of general responsiveness. This can include:

- Avoidance of thoughts, feelings, conversations associated with the trauma
- Avoidance of activities, places or people that arouse recollections of the trauma
- Inability to recall an important aspect of the trauma
- Markedly reduced interest or participation in significant activities

- Feeling of detachment or estrangement from others
- Restricted range of affect (e.g. unable to have loving feelings)
- Sense of foreshortened future (e.g. does not expect to have a career, marriage, children or normal life span).

A state of high *physiological arousal* is common and can include:
- Difficulty falling or staying asleep
- Irritability or outbursts of anger
- Difficulty concentrating
- Hypervigilance (e.g. scanning the environment to ensure there is no threat close by)
- An exaggerated startle response (e.g. jumping with fright at minor noises in the environment).

> For example, JG's truck crashed into two vehicles, setting one of them alight. A child was trapped in one of the cars and burned to death. For months after the accident, JG could not get into a vehicle without having an anxiety attack. He avoided using any form of transport and walked everywhere. Seeing trucks on the road or on television would trigger terrifying images of the accident, which were so vivid that he felt as if he was back at the scene of the accident. Whenever he heard a loud bang he would jump and become tremulous.

Situational anxiety (adjustment disorder with anxiety)

This is an anxiety state that occurs in relation to a specific stressful situation, but the anxiety is excessive in nature or causes significant impairment in functioning. The main features are nervousness, worry, jitteriness and often somatic symptoms of anxiety. The anxiety disorder often abates as the stressful event resolves.

Treatment for co-existing anxiety and depression

Treatment for problematic co-existing depression or anxiety that is not secondary to the substance use disorder or some other medical or psychiatric disorder generally involves a combination of medication and cognitive behaviour therapy (CBT).

Most antidepressant medications are also effective anti-anxiety drugs. Medication may take 2–4 weeks before the onset of an effect and may need considerably longer (up to 3 months) for full effect. Antidepressant medication given for anxiety disorders may exacerbate the anxiety at the start of treatment, so it is advisable to start with a low dose and titrate the dose upwards gradually, as tolerated by the patient.

Benzodiazepines

While benzodiazepines are highly efficacious for the treatment of anxiety and agitation, there are significant risks using benzodiazepines in individuals with a substance use disorder.

The risks associated with prescribing benzodiazepines for anxiety in-patients with a history of substance misuse include:
- Dose escalation
- Diversion
- Doctor shopping
- Drug affected presentations
- Significant risk of interaction with other CNS depressants.
- The usual risks of using any benzodiazepine including dependence, negative impact on mental acuity, impaired psychomotor performance and subtle changes in mood including depressive symptoms. Drugs with short half-lives have a higher risk of dependence and problematic withdrawal symptoms with inter-dose and early morning anxiety. Drugs with long half-lives have more residual drowsiness and cognitive impairment.

Table 11.2 Medications for anxiety and depression

Medication for anxiety and depression	
SSRI's	Mirtazapine
Venlafaxine	MAOIs (moclobemide)
Reboxetine	Tricyclic antidepressants
Benzodiazepines (but considerable care required in-patients with substance use disorders)	
Other medication for anxiety	
Benzodiazepines	Buspirone
Beta-blockers: very limited evidence base	
Atypical antipsychotics	

Because of these risks, benzodiazepines should be avoided in patients with a history of substance misuse unless:

- A compelling indication exists to use them
- There is no good alternative (e.g. failed treatment with CBT and other medication options)
- Close follow-up and supervision is provided
- Monitoring for misuse is in place.

If benzodiazepines are used, the following guidelines should apply:

- Short-term use only: 2–4 weeks
- Use lowest possible dose
- Give limited supplies
- Intermittent rather than daily use if possible
- Provide supervised administration
- Ensure close monitoring and follow-up
- Explore alternative treatment options: non-benzodiazepine medications and CBT.

Selective serotonin reuptake inhibitors (SSRI'S) are effective for both anxiety disorders and major depression. They are often used as first-line medication because they are generally well-tolerated, improving compliance rates, and rarely lethal in overdose. Anxiety levels can sometimes increase in the early stages of treatment with an SSRI, because of the side effects of the medication, and the anxiety and apprehension of the patient. It is therefore advisable to start with a lower dose if an anxiety state is present, and gradually titrate the dose upwards as tolerated by the patient. An adequate therapeutic trial of SSRI medication for depression is usually 8–12 weeks, but often longer for OCD.

If there is only a partial response to an adequate dose of an SSRI and it is well-tolerated by the patient, a trial of higher dose should be considered. If the patient has a poor response to an SSRI (because of problematic side effects or a limited treatment response), try another SSRI or look at switching to another class of antidepressant.

Doses that are generally effective for anxiety and depression are as follows:

- Citalopram 20–60 mg
- Escitalopram 10–20 mg
- Fluoxetine 20–40 mg
- Paroxetine 20–50 mg
- Sertraline 50–200 mg
- Fluvoxamine 100–300 mg.

Higher doses are required to treat obsessive compulsive disorder and should be overseen by a psychiatrist.

Drug interactions include

- Some SSRIs [paroxetine, fluoxetine] increase tricyclic levels if combined with tricyclic antidepressants through CYP2D6 interactions
- Can cause a fatal 'serotonin syndrome' in combination with MAOI's (tranylcypromine and phenelzine)
- May displace highly protein bound drugs, e.g. warfarin
- Tramadol increases the seizure risk and risk of serotonin syndrome

- Via CYP450 2D6 inhibition, sertraline, fluoxetine, paroxetine and citalopram could theoretically:
  - Interfere with the analgesic effects of codeine; and
    increase the plasma levels of atomoxetine and some beta blockers
- Via CYP450 3A4 inhibition:

Sertraline, fluvoxamine and fluoxetine could increase plasma levels of alprazolam and triazolam; could theoretically increase concentrations of some cholesterol lowering HMG CoA reductase inhibitors (simvastatin, atorvastatin and lovastatin) and could theoretically increase the levels of pimozide with increased risk of QTc prolongation. Paroxetine can also increase pimozide levels

Fluvoxamine can result in toxic blood levels of methadone because it is a potent 3A4 inhibitor. While fluoxetine, paroxetine, and sertraline inhibit 3A4, and theoretically have the potential to increase methadone levels, they are not as potent an inhibitor as fluvoxamine and, in practice, don't appear to be problematic in combination with methadone (however watch the patient's response closely)

- Fluoxetine may reduce the clearance of diazepam or trazodone, increasing their levels
- Paroxetine and fluvoxamine may increase theophylline levels requiring closer monitoring and it has been postulated that paroxetine may increase the anticholinergic effects of other drugs with anticholinergic properties
- Fluvoxamine (through CYP450 1A2) can markedly reduce the clearance of clozapine resulting in increased blood levels, which need to be monitored closely.

Common adverse side effects of SSRI's include:
- Gastrointestinal disturbance: nausea, diarrhoea, constipation, dry mouth, reduced appetite
- Central nervous system side effects: insomnia, agitation, tremors, dizziness, headache. Sedation can also occur and generally follows this order: fluvoxamine > paroxetine > citalopram > sertraline > fluoxetine
- Sexual dysfunction occurs in up to 30% (in men: delayed ejaculation; erectile dysfunction; in men and women: anorgasmia, reduced sexual desire)
- Sweating.

Uncommon adverse side effects include:
- Bruising and rare bleeding
- Hyponaetremia (mostly in elderly patients; reversible on discontinuation of the drug)
- Hypotension
- Seizures: caution advised in-patients with a history of seizures
- Rarely triggers mania in bipolar patients; caution advised in bipolar patients not on a mood stabilizer

- **Activation of suicidal ideation**: patients who are already suicidal and develop agitation as a side effect of an SSRI could be more at risk of an increase in suicidal ideation. This should be monitored closely when any suicidal patient starts an SSRI, even though all the evidence points to SSRIs reducing population suicide risks.

Problematic side effects often improve with time, apart from the sexual side effects. Strategies to deal with side effects include wait for improvement, reduce the dose or switch to another SSRI.

Discontinuation syndrome

While SSRIs are not habit-forming, they can have some short-lived withdrawal effects if stopped abruptly, also called a discontinuation syndrome. It is worse with those SSRIs with a short half-life. The severity for different SSRI's is generally as follows: fluvoxamine, paroxetine > citalopram, sertraline > fluoxetine. The severity of symptoms for fluvoxamine and paroxetine is similar to that for venlafaxine.

The symptoms can be summarized using the acronym 'FLUSH':

- Flu-like: fatigue, myalgia, loose stools, nausea
- Light-headedness/dizziness
- Uneasiness/restlessness
- Sleep and sensory disturbances
- Headache.

With restarting the SSRI, the syndrome usually remits within 12–24 h, but can sometimes last for up to 2 weeks. In order to prevent it occurring, it is best to taper the dose of the SSRI. For example, with paroxetine, many patients tolerate a 50% reduction in dose for 3 days, followed by a further 50% reduction for 3 days then cessation of the drug. However, other patients will need to taper an SSRI over 2–4 weeks. If withdrawal symptoms emerge, raise the dose to alleviate them and then withdraw the drug much more slowly. If symptoms remain problematic, switching to fluoxetine with its long half-life can be helpful, with a gradual taper of the dose of fluoxetine.

Venlafaxine is a serotonin and noradrenaline reuptake inhibitor (SNRI), which acts like an SSRI at lower doses (less than 150 mg) and has more noradrenergic properties at higher doses. It is comparable with the SSRI's for the treatment of anxiety disorders.

Effective doses for anxiety and depression are in the range of 75–225 mg, but sometimes higher doses may be used for more difficult-to-treat depression.

Side effects are similar to SSRIs at doses <150 mg. It is not anticholinergic and generally not sedating. Blood pressure needs to be monitored at higher doses, with around 5% of patients getting hypertension at doses over 225 mg. It has few significant drug interactions. Concomitant use with cimetidine can reduce the clearance of venlafaxine raising blood levels. A discontinuation syndrome is often problematic when the drug is stopped suddenly and patients should be warned about this. As for SSRI's, gradually tapering the dose can help minimize the risk of a significant discontinuation syndrome.

Tricyclic antidepressants (TCAs) are effective for both anxiety disorders and depressive disorders but are generally not used first-line because of problematic side effects, significant drug interactions, and high lethality in overdose.

Common side effects include sedation, anticholinergic effects (blurred vision, dry mouth, constipation), weight gain, and hypotension; these are due to blockade of histamine H1, noradrenaline A1 and cholinergic muscarine receptors. The noradrenaline selective TCAs nortriptyline and desipramine generally have more tolerable levels of side effects than other TCA's.

Because of their sedative properties, TCA's potentiate other CNS depressants, which is potentially problematic in those using alcohol, benzodiazepines and opioids. They cause cardiotoxicity in overdose and as little as 1 g of medication (a week's supply) can be fatal. It is, therefore, inadvisable to give these medications to patients who are prone to take excessive doses of any prescribed medication with a sedative effect or those with suicidal ideation.

A discontinuation syndrome can occur if TCA's are stopped abruptly. The symptoms are mainly of cholinergic rebound, and they include GI distress, headache, malaise, chills, muscle aches, insomnia and agitation.

Because side effects are significant for many patients, starting doses should be low (25–50 mg daily) and the dose gradually titrated upwards. The usual dosage range is 75–150 mg once daily (usually at night because of sedation) or in divided doses.

Mirtazapine is a noradrenaline and specific serotonergic agent (NaSSA). It is reported to have a faster onset than SSRI's, it has minimal anticholinergic effects, no adverse cardiac effects and it is rarely lethal in overdose. Common side effects include increased appetite, weight gain, and sedation. Sedation is useful for insomnia and relief of anxiety. Any residual day time sedation of is often short-term. Patients should have their weight and BMI monitored during treatment. Monitoring for diabetes should occur in any overweight patients pre-treatment, and in those who gain >5% of their initial weight during treatment. Severe neutropenia is a very rare side effect, occurring in less than 1 in 1000. Patients should be advised that if they experience fever and infection while on mirtazapine, they should get their doctor to check their full blood count.

The usual therapeutic dose is 30–45 mg daily, but it is not uncommon to increase the dose to 60 mg daily. SSRI's and venlafaxine can be safely combined with mirtazapine to reduce insomnia related to using either of these medications.

Reboxetine is classified as a selective noradrenaline reuptake inhibitor. Reboxetine is a pure noradrenaline uptake blocker which therefore has a rather different profile of adverse effects to the SSRIs. The main ones are pseudo-anticholinergic in nature especially dry mouth constipation and urinary hesitancy sometime leading to retention. It also can cause sexual dysfunction and insomnia. Benefits are said to include improved energy, social interaction and motivation. Dosing is usually 8 mg/day in divided doses. It appears to have lower rates (about 2%) sexual dysfunction compared with the SSRIs.

Reboxetine can be used in anxiety disorders that are refractory to other treatment. Because is can be activating and has anxiety as a known side effect, the starting dose should be deliberately low, e.g. in 2 mg every few days as tolerated, aiming for 4 mg twice daily. If there is an incomplete response after 3 weeks, move to 10 mg daily. If the patient develops insomnia, the dose can be given in the morning and lunch time rather than morning and night. Once on a stable dose, reboxetine can be switched to once a day if tolerated by the patient.

Other medication options for anxiety

Beta-blockers may be useful for performance anxiety (e.g. giving speeches, playing music in front of an audience) by reducing tremor and tachycardia. A trial dose should be taken well in advance of any performance, to ensure there are no problematic side effects from taking the drug. Otherwise beta-blockers should be taken 30–60 min prior to any performance. Usual doses are:

- Propranolol 20–40 mg prn.
- Atenolol 25–50 mg prn.

Potential side effects include: nausea, diarrhoea, bronchospasm, dyspnoea, cold extremities, exacerbation of Raynaud's syndrome, bradycardia, hypotension, heart failure, heart block, fatigue, dizziness, abnormal vision, decreased concentration, hallucinations, insomnia, nightmares, depression, alteration of glucose, and lipid metabolism.

These medications should be avoided in anyone with reversible airways disease (asthma, COPD), bradycardia, heart block, severe hypotension, angle-closure glaucoma, and diabetes.

Buspirone is a non-sedating, non-benzodiazepine anti-anxiety medication useful for the treatment of generalized anxiety disorder. Higher doses may also have antidepressant effects especially in combination with the SSRIs. Unlike benzodiazepines, tolerance and dependence are not a problem with buspirone, and it does not have a discontinuation syndrome. Starting dose is 5 mg tds, with a maintenance dose of 30–45 mg in three divided doses. The onset of effects is 1–2 weeks with 4–6 weeks for full effect. The medication is not subsidized in some countries, which can make the costs to the patient prohibitive.

Notable side effects include dizziness, headache, nervousness, sedation, excitement, nausea, and restlessness.

Atypical antipsychotics

While randomized controlled trials are awaited to assess the efficacy of atypical antipsychotics for anxiety disorders, it is common clinical practice to use them for treatment-refractory anxiety in low doses, often as an adjunct to other medication, instead of benzodiazepines. Unlike benzodiazepines, tolerance and dependence are not a feature. The risk of developing tardive dyskinesia appears low when used sporadically in low doses.

Atypical antipsychotics used include quetiapine, olanzapine, risperidone and aripiprazole. Doses used are much lower than those used to treat psychosis, e.g. quetiapine 25–50 mg bd or tds. They can also be effective in treating insomnia with anxiety.

Monoamine Oxidase Inhibitors (MAOIs) include:
- Moclobemide
- Tranylcypromine
- Phenelzine

Tranylcypromine and phenelzine irreversibly block monoamine oxidase (MAO) from breaking down noradrenaline, serotonin, and dopamine, presumably increasing the levels of transmission of these monoamines. They are complex and potentially dangerous medications to use because of the dietary and medication restrictions involved. They have a limited placed in treatment when other medication options have failed, and should be prescribed by psychiatrists. Hypertensive crisis with intracranial bleeding, headache and death can occur if these medications are combined with tyramine-rich foods or some contraindicated medications. Foods rich in tyramine need to be avoided, particularly high protein food that has undergone protein breakdown by pickling, aging, smoking, fermentation or bacterial contamination including cheese, pickled herring, yeast extract (e.g. vegemite), salami, pepperoni, soy bean extracts (tofu, miso), and some alcoholic drinks. A detailed list of possible food interactions needs to be provided to patients. Hypertensive crisis can occur when used in combination with opioid drugs and drugs with psychostimulant properties (including over-the-counter cough and cold medications).

Usual doses of these medications are:
- Tranylcypromine 30 mg daily in divided doses; maximum 60 mg daily
- Phenelzine 45–90 mg daily in divided doses.

Moclobemide is a reversible inhibitor of monoamine oxidase A (RIMA), reversibly blocking the effects of MAO-A so that if tyramine is taken this can displace the moclobemide from the active site of the enzyme and become metabolized. It is a well-tolerated medication, which is relatively non-toxic in overdose and less likely to cause sexual dysfunction than SSRI's. Common side effects are nausea, insomnia, anxiety, restlessness, dizziness, which are usually transient and resolve with time. Starting with a lower dose, gradually titrating the dose upwards and taking it with food are useful strategies to minimize side effects. The usual therapeutic dose range is 450–600 mg daily, usually in two divided doses.

Potential drug interactions include a fatal serotonin syndrome in combination with SSRI's, hypertensive crisis in combination with sympathomimetic drugs (be cautious of over-the-counter cough and cold preparations containing these), enhancement of the effects of NSAID's. A low tyramine diet is not usually required below the maximum dose of 600 mg daily.

Anticonvulsants

Some anticonvulsants may be effective in the treatment of anxiety disorders. Sodium valproate may be useful in treatment resistant panic disorder, although the drug may be limited by its side effect profile in this patient group. Sodium valproate and carbamazepine may cause thrombocytopaenia and liver toxicity which could be problematic in those with alcohol related disease, drug related hepatitis or hepatitis C in injecting drug users.

Newer agents with fewer side effects show promise, but are not subsidized on the PBS for anxiety disorders in Australia.

Gabapentin shows some promise as a treatment for social anxiety disorder and as an adjunct to other anti-anxiety medication.

Topiramate and lamotrigine have shown promise in the treatment of PTSD.

Further Reading

Anderson IM, Ferrier IN, Baldwin RC et al. Evidence-based guidelines for treating depressive disorders with antidepressants: a revision of the 2000 British Association for psychopharmacology guidelines. *Journal of Psychopharmacology* 2008; **22**: 343–396.

Andrews G, Oakley-Browne M, Castle D, Judd F, Baillie A. Summary of guideline for the treatment of panic disorder and agoraphobia. *RNAZCP Clinical Practice Guidelines.* Australasian Psychiatry 2003; **11**: 29–33.

Angrist B, Lee HK, Gershon S. The antagonism of amphetamine-induced symptomatology by a neuroleptic. *American Journal of Psychiatry* 1974; **131**: 817–819.

Baker A, Lee NK, Jenner L. *Models of intervention and care for psychostimulant users,* 2nd edn. National Drug Strategy Monograph series, No. 51. Canberra: Commonwealth of Australia, 2004.

Baldwin DS et al. Evidence-based guidelines for the pharmacological treatment of anxiety disorders: recommendations from the British Association of Psychopharmacology. *Journal of Psychopharmacology* 2005; **19**: 567–596.

Lingford-Hughes AR, Welsch S, Nutt DJ. Evidence based guidelines for the pharmacological management of substance misuse, addiction and co-morbidity: recommendations from the British Association for Psychopharmacology. *Journal of Psychopharmacology* 2004; **18**: 293–335.

McIntosh C, Ritson B. Treating depression complicated by substance misuse. *Advances in Psychiatric Treatment* 2001; **7**: 357–364.

Myrick H, Wright T. Co-morbid anxiety and substance use disorders: Diagnostic and Treatment considerations. *Journal of Dual Diagnosis* 2005; **1**(4): 9–27.

Nutt DJ. Death and dependence: current controversies over the selective serotonin reuptake inhibitors. *Journal of Psychopharmacology* 2003; **17**: 355–364.

Nutt DJ. Death by tricyclic: the real antidepressant scandal? *Journal of Psychopharmacology* 2005; **19**: 123.

Special populations

Some sectors of the community need special attention. In this chapter we discuss drug and alcohol use among pregnant women, adolescents, indigenous people, migrants, and elderly people. In the following chapters we address special topics such as pain and opioid dependence, sleeplessness, and oral complications of drug use, and difficult and emergency situations.

Pregnancy

The number of women misusing drugs has increased considerably and a significant number of women in the UK presenting to drug misuse services for treatment are of child-bearing age. Every woman suspected of a positive pregnancy test requires appropriate history-taking, assessment and screening for alcohol and other drug use (see assessment section). Drug and alcohol use during pregnancy is associated with both maternal and foetal/neonatal outcomes. Maternal outcomes include not receiving adequate prenatal care and foetal outcomes relate to a failure to thrive (see Box 12.1). Women of child-bearing age who smoke, consume more than two standard drinks a day, or use other drugs, should be informed of the potential risks to both themselves and the foetus, and offered advice and if necessary told where to get help.

Pregnancy offers clinicians a window of opportunity to help women quit smoking, and to reduce harm associated with problematic alcohol and other drug use. Although pregnancy may act as a catalyst for change, drug misusers often fail to use general health services until late into pregnancy and are, therefore, more vulnerable to medical and obstetrical complications. It is important that obstetric care is organized once pregnancy is confirmed. Where harmful, hazardous or dependent use is suspected or confirmed, a specialist Drug and Alcohol service should be involved.

In collaboration with the Antenatal team, the Drug and Alcohol team can provide specific guidance on treatment and will monitor the patient's alcohol and other drug use during pregnancy. This is particularly important at 12, 18–20, 25 and 26 weeks.

Following the birth of the baby, monitoring is continued by the neonatal team and the Drug and Alcohol teams. If the infant, or an older child, is considered to be at risk, involvement with child protection agencies or departments is mandatory.

Effects on the foetus/infant

The development of the foetus will be affected by factors such as quantity and frequency of use, and gestational stage and drug or alcohol use may lead to:

- Prematurity
- Low birth weight
- Withdrawal syndromes
- Perinatal mortality
- Sudden infant death syndrome: increased 4–5 fold in infants born to pregnant drug users
- Respiratory distress
- Convulsions
- Teratogenic effects.

General complications of alcohol and other drug use during pregnancy

> ### Box 12.1 Effects on the mother
>
> *Pharmacological effects of the drug*
> Chaotic use may lead to:
> - Overdose/intoxication
> - Withdrawal syndromes (alcohol, benzodiazepines, stimulants, cannabis).
>
> If injecting drugs, *complications of injecting*
> - Bacterial infections:
>   - Septicaemia
>   - Subacute bacterial endocarditis, septic thrombophlebitis
> - Viral infections: Hepatitis B, C, HIV (see Box 12.2)
> - Fungal infections:
>   - Candidiasis.
>
> *Other medical complications*
> - Poor nutrition
> - Vitamin deficiencies
> - Anaemia.
>   (For alcohol and specific drugs see tables.)
>
> *Emotional/Psychiatric complications*
> - Anxiety
> - Depression
> - Insomnia.
>
> *Obstetric complications*
> - Placental insufficiency, abruptio placentae, placenta previa
> - Intrauterine growth retardation/death
> - Premature rupture of membranes/premature labour
> - Pre-eclampsia/eclampsia
> - Chorioamnionitis
> - Premature delivery
> - Postpartum haemorrhage.
>
> *Psychosocial issues*
> - Involvement with Child Protection Agencies
> - Domestic violence
> - Financial problems
> - Prostitution
> - Criminal activity.

In general, risk of damage is greatest in the first trimester of pregnancy (especially the first 8 weeks) but caution should be exercised during the second and third trimesters. Transport of drugs across the placenta is greatest in late gestation when placental blood flow is greatest. Women who misuse drugs and alcohol during pregnancy should receive education and advice about safe sex and risk reduction strategies, and be screened for blood-borne viruses and sexually transmitted infections that are spread by vertical transmission. It is advisable that tests are conducted for blood-borne viruses (hepatitis C, B, and HIV) early in pregnancy (see Box 12.2). All testing should be conducted in conjunction with pre- and post-test counselling (see pp. 220, 371). Patient confidentiality must be maintained at all times.

Box 12.2 Blood-borne viruses: hepatitis C, B and HIV in pregnant injecting drug users

All pregnant mothers should be offered screening for hepatitis B, C, and in select cases HIV.

Hepatitis C: Up to 10% of mothers with chronic hepatitis C infection who are HCV RNA (PCR) positive can transmit hepatitis C virus to the foetus. Caesarean section has not been shown to reduce the risk of vertical transmission.

Ideally, the infant should be tested for HCV RNA PCR at 4–6 months and after 18 months when transplacental antibodies have disappeared. However, follow up is often difficult and infants are not tested.

If HCV RNA PCR is positive after 6–18 months—refer to Paediatric Hepatologist or Infectious Disease Specialist.

Hepatitis B: Women who are HBsAb negative should be offered hepatitis B vaccination after birth. All newborn infants in Australia receive hepatitis B immunization. In addition babies of HBsAg positive mothers are given immunoglobulin within 12 h and a total of four doses of hepatitis B vaccination-at birth, 2, 4, and 6 months. Caesarean section is not justified.

HIV: The risk of vertical transmission of HIV is greatest during the last week of pregnancy and during birth. The risk can be reduced by elective caesarean section and intravenous antiretroviral therapy before birth. Zidovudine therapy reduces the risk of vertical transmission from 25% to 8%. It is further reduced by combination therapy. Refer to appropriate Infectious Diseases Specialist and Obstetrician for appropriate advice and treatment.

Effects of specific drugs

Nicotine (see Chapter Five): The vasoconstrictor effects of nicotine impair placental blood supply, while carbon monoxide reduces availability of oxygen to the foetus. The risk of harmful effects is greater in older mothers who smoke. Smoking cessation in early pregnancy will give the greatest benefit, although quitting smoking at any time during pregnancy is beneficial for both the mother and foetus.

Maternal risks: Higher risks of complications during pregnancy.

Foetal/infant risks
- Low birth weight (the risk increases in mothers who continue to smoke during pregnancy)
- Congenital malformation (cleft palate, microcephalus, club foot)

- Increased risk of perinatal mortality
- Sudden infant death syndrome.

Nicotine replacement therapy: As yet there is only limited evidence regarding the safety of nicotine replacement therapy or bupropion during pregnancy and lactation.

Alcohol

There are no internationally agreed guidelines regarding safe limits of alcohol consumption during pregnancy. The UK Department of Health recommends not more than 1–2 units of alcohol once or twice a week. Many countries follow similar guidelines as the US which advise total abstinence during pregnancy or in women who are considering pregnancy.

Foetal Alcohol Syndrome (FAS) is the result of harmful exposure to alcohol early in pregnancy and FAS is reported to be the leading preventable cause of mental retardation in western civilization (see Box 12.3). In North America, estimates for alcohol-related neurodevelopment disorder (ARND) are 10-fold those for FAS. Drinking during pregnancy results in a 30–50% increased risk of delivering a foetus with FAE, particularly in older women >30 years of age. The detrimental effects of alcohol are greatest during the first trimester of pregnancy, often before the woman knows that she is pregnant. Thus, all women of child-bearing age should also be advised of the risks of drinking and restrict their drinking to a minimum if they are likely to become pregnant.

The common pathway of alcohol teratogenesis appears to be its deleterious effects on the developing brain and nervous system. The times of greatest sensitivity of the foetal brain to maternal alcohol consumption are the first and third trimesters. The terms foetal alcohol effects (FAE) and foetal alcohol spectrum disorders (FASD) have also been used to describe less severe foetal effects of drinking.

Sudden cessation of alcohol consumption in pregnant alcohol dependent women is associated with a high risk of seizures. Alcohol detoxification should not be conducted in the community, and needs very careful supervision by obstetricians and alcohol treatment specialists.

Box 12.3 Foetal Alcohol Syndrome

The teratogenetic effects of alcohol cause developmental delay and birth defects

- Characteristic facial abnormalities with underdevelopment of the middle of the face—depressed bridge of nose, thin upper lip, absent philtrum, flattened maxilla; also 'bulls eyes' and low set ears
- Growth retardation (prenatal or postnatal)
- Cardiac abnormalities
- Behavioural disturbances
- Learning disability
- Prematurity, low birth weight; small for gestational age
- Foetal or neonatal death.

Heroin

The incidence of opioid misuse is still increasing in many European countries, with most addicts seeking treatment for the first time between the ages of 20 and 30 years. It has been estimated that around one in every thousand women in Great Britain is opioid dependent, of which a significant proportion are women of child-bearing age. Despite some efforts to address the lack of guidance on managing the pregnant opioid user, an optimal methadone-dosing strategy has yet to be established. The National Treatment Agency for Substance Misuse, which promotes quality, efficiency and effectiveness in drug misuse treatment services in England has highlighted pregnant opioid users as a vulnerable group.

It is better for opioid dependent women to continue using opioids while pregnant than to attempt abstinence. Conversion of heroin to methadone has been found to be the most effective treatment for opioid dependent pregnant women, although in some countries buprenorphine may be preferred. Enrolment of the opiate-addicted gravida in a methadone maintenance programme gives the medical community an opportunity to intervene and optimize neonatal outcome in these high-risk pregnancies. It has been demonstrated that methadone improves prenatal care, neonatal outcome, reduced illicit substance use and improves the overall health of pregnant women. However, the benefits can be negated if inadequate methadone dose is prescribed and heroin is used 'on top'. The dose of methadone may need to be increased in the third trimester of pregnancy.

Pregnant intravenous drug users often have poor antenatal attendance, chaotic lifestyles and poor nutrition, and detoxification of pregnant heroin dependent women is risky. Maternal abstinence may result in foetal distress that may be more harmful than passive dependence, and induce abortion or premature labour. The highest risk period is before the 14th week and after the 32nd week of gestation.

Methadone maintenance treatment in conjunction with a comprehensive drug and alcohol and prenatal programme is the treatment of choice to maintain the patient in a comfortable state (average dose of methadone: 30–80 mg daily). Although neonatal opioid dependence as well as neonatal abstinence syndrome (see Box 12.4) may occur, this is not life threatening and can be managed easily in Special Care Baby Units. Babies born to opioid dependent mothers should be monitored for the neonatal abstinence syndrome (Box 12.4).

Box 12.4 Features and management of neonatal abstinence syndrome

Neonatal heroin abstinence syndrome
- Onset following last illicit use: 24–36 h after delivery. Duration: >1–2 weeks.

Signs and symptoms
- **CNS**: high pitched cry, tremor, sleep disturbance, increased muscle tone, myoclonic jerks, convulsions
- **Respiratory**: sneezing, yawning, nasal flaring and stuffiness, tachypnoea, respiratory distress.
- **Gastrointestinal tract**: poor feeding, excessive sucking, regurgitation, projectile vomiting, diarrhoea.

Neonatal methadone withdrawal syndrome (may be reduced if breast fed)
- Onset: 5–15 days after delivery (i.e. following last dose). Duration: >1–2 weeks

Signs and symptoms
- **CNS**: high pitched cry, tremor, sleep disturbance, increased muscle tone, myoclonic jerks, convulsions
- **Respiratory**: sneezing, yawning, nasal flaring and stuffiness, tachypnoea, respiratory distress
- **Gastrointestinal tract**: poor feeding, excessive sucking, regurgitation, projectile vomiting, diarrhoea.

Treatment
- Place on neonatal abstinence syndrome scale (p. 440)
- Nurse in a quiet environment and minimize stimuli
- If withdrawal symptoms are severe, administer morphine 0.5 mg/mL solution (0.5–0.9 mg/Kg/day in four divided doses) and reduce slowly by 0.1 mg 6 hourly every 4 days or longer.

NB: Administer morphine with caution and only after seeking advice from the specialist neonatologist.
- Discharge planning is important
- Consider the safety of the child. In many regions there is an obligation to notify the Child Protection Services if the child is considered to be at risk.

Box 12.5 Neonatal benzodiazepine withdrawal syndrome

- **'Floppy infant syndrome'**: hypotonia, sucking difficulties, hypothermia or impaired temperature control
- Tremor
- Irritability
- Hyperactivity
- Cyanosis.

Benzodiazepines

The use of benzodiazepines, particularly during the first trimester of pregnancy, is thought to be associated with decreased foetal growth, CNS abnormalities and dysmorphic features resembling FAS (see Box 12.5). However, studies have produced contradictory results, thus arousing controversy about the prescribing of benzodiazepines during pregnancy. Examination of pooled data from cohort studies found no association between foetal exposure to benzodiazepines during the first trimester and risk of major malformations or malformations of the oral cleft alone (cleft lip and cleft palate). However, analysis of pooled data from case-control studies showed a small but significant increased risk for major malformations or oral cleft palate alone. Foetal ultrasonography should be used to screen for cleft lip/palate when problematic benzodiazepine use is suspected or when dependent use is observed.

Cocaine/crack cocaine

Cocaine causes vasoconstriction, thus reducing the blood flow to the placenta and increasing the risk of placental abruption. It also increases uterine contractility, thus increasing the risk of spontaneous abortion and premature delivery. The use of cocaine during pregnancy is associated with an increased risk of Sudden Infant Death Syndrome (SIDS) in the baby.

Multiple substance use

Multiple drug use during pregnancy is common and associated with increased rates of prematurity and intra-uterine growth retardation (IUGR), and also with increased rates of problems during labour including premature rupture of the membranes, meconium stained liquor and foetal distress. Women using cocaine and multiple substances are at particular risk.

Substance use is not necessarily attenuated during pregnancy. An Irish study showed that 2.8% of urines from a sample of 504 pregnant women screened positive for illicit substances at their first antenatal visit, whereas 5.6% of urines from a separate sample of 515 women screened positive 6 weeks post-delivery. The substances identified included benzo-diazepines, cannabis, amphetamines, opiates and cocaine. Less than 2% tested positive for alcohol. Positive screens were associated with women being single, unemployed and having had a previous pregnancy.

Breast feeding

Breast milk is generally regarded as the best nutrition for the child.

In general, mothers should not be discouraged from breast feeding but should be given full information of the risks associated with continued use of alcohol and other substances. See Box 12.6.

Box 12.6 Excretion of substances in breast milk

Tobacco
- Minimal amounts are excreted into the breast milk.
- Offer the mother nicotine patches to reduce the risks associated with passive smoking.

Alcohol
- Alcohol passes through the breast milk so drinking during breast feeding is not recommended
- If the mother insists on drinking, consumption should not exceed one standard drink (10 g) per day and then only after breast feeding.

Opioids
- Mothers who are stable on methadone maintenance treatment may breast feed, but those who are unstable should not be encouraged to do so
- The safety of buprenorphine has not yet been established but the amount in the breast milk is considered to be clinically insignificant.

Psychostimulants
- Advise regular and unstable users against breast feeding
- Inform intermittent users of the risks associated with breast feeding

Cannabis
- Some cannabis is excreted in the breast milk, but the effects on the infant are unknown.

Further reading

Cook J. Biochemical markers of alcohol use in pregnant women. *Clinical Biochemistry* 2003; **36**: 9–19.

Finnegan LP. Treatment issues for opioid dependent women during the perinatal period. *Journal of Psychoactive Drugs* 1991; **23**: 191–201.

Flannery W, Wolff K, Marshall EJ. Substance use disorders in pregnancy. Psychiatric disorders and pregnancy obstetric and psychiatric care. Ed. V O'Kane, T Seneviratne, M Marsh. Taylor and Francis, London, July 2005.

Floyd R, O'Connor M, Skol RJ, Bertrand J, Cordero J. Recognition and prevention of Foetal Alcohol Syndrome. *Obstetrics and Gynaecology* 2005; **106**: 1059–1064.

National clinical guidelines for the management of drug use during pregnancy, birth and the early development years of the newborn. NSW Department of Health (2006). www.health.nsw.gov.au

Adolescents

Outline
- Developmental perspective
- Differentiating significant problems from experimental or occasional use
- How to assess substance use in young people
  - Psychosocial assessment
  - Confidentiality
  - Important details to obtain relating to adolescents' drug use
  - Mental health assessment.

Developmental perspective

The nature of adolescence

Adolescence is an important developmental period during which the transition from childhood to adulthood occurs. Adolescent development is more than the physical phenomenon of puberty. Cognitive maturation and psychosocial development are also important aspects of adolescence.

Physical development commences with the onset of puberty, and is characterized by physical growth and the development of secondary sexual characteristics and reproductive capability.

Cognitive development progresses until the young adult years (around 20 years of age). During this time cognitive capabilities move from concrete thinking in early adolescence to abstract thinking by late adolescence. For instance, talking about the long-term effects of alcohol, such as liver disease rarely has impact on the early adolescent. It is better to talk with the young adolescent about how heavy drinking contributes to difficulties in their relationships with peers or family, or difficulties performing at school.

Psychosocial development includes the development of a stable and independent identity, relationships beyond family to peers, a moral and value system, an understanding of sexuality and acquisition of skills for a future vocation.

Substance use and adolescent development

Regular or heavy substance use frequently inhibits adolescent development by delaying the time that psychosocial milestones are reached, impairing cognitive maturation, reducing educational achievements, impairing the development of healthy relationships and increasing the likelihood of mental health problems in adolescence and adulthood.

Differentiating significant problems from experimental or occasional use. Adolescent substance use fits a spectrum (see Fig 12.1).

> When consulting with an adolescent, it is important for the health professional to discern where the adolescent is in the spectrum of adolescent substance use.

Table 12.2 Developmental stages of early, mid- and late adolescence

Early adolescence (approximately 11–13 years)	Early adolescence is characterized by the physical and physiological changes of puberty.
	Adolescents are frequently concerned at this time about whether their development is 'normal' and in keeping with their peers.
	In early adolescence, teenagers are usually still dependent on family, but peers (usually of the same sex) become increasingly important.
	Early adolescence is characterized by concrete thinking.
Middle adolescence (approximately 14–16 years)	Middle adolescence is characterized by the increasing development of autonomy.
	At this time, identity becomes very important to the young person. Attachment to peer groups takes place and being attractive, accepted and popular are often a focus of this stage of development.
	Experimentation and risk taking are very common. This may include experimentation with alcohol and other substances.
Late adolescence (approximately 17–20 years)	In late adolescence more mature intellectual abilities have developed.
	Independence and a sense of identity and self-worth are usually evident, and plans and aspirations for the future, including employment and relationships are characteristic.

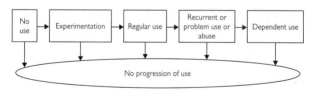

Fig. 12.1 Spectrum of substance use.

'Experimentation' with substances by young people is much more common than progression to regular use. Sometimes adolescents use drugs only in specific situations, for instance, only when attending parties or when socializing with certain peers. This is sometimes referred to as 'situational' or 'recreational' use. Other adolescents use drugs to self-medicate difficulties with sleep or emotional difficulties (this may sometimes be referred to as 'habitual use').

'Abuse' of alcohol or a drug usually refers to situations when it is resulting in recurrent problems. Examples of problems include difficulties with family or friends, failure to fulfil study requirements, or even attend school because of substance use.

'Dependence' on a substance usually refers to compulsive drug-seeking behaviour despite negative consequences.

Research continues to explore what the determinants are of progression from experimentation to abuse or dependence.

> Patterns of substance use that influence progression to problems include:
> * Onset of alcohol or other drug use in early adolescence
> * Heavy use (both in terms of dose and frequency).

Risk factors for substance use

Understanding how adolescent drug use comes about is often explained in terms of a risk factor and protective factor framework. This framework helps to understand why some adolescents follow trajectories that lead to substance use problems while others, even in the face of severe psychosocial stressors and substantial adversity, do not develop drug or alcohol, or other problems. Resilience refers to the ability to be well adjusted and interpersonally effective despite an adverse environment. Factors that counter risk factors and help people deal positively with life changes are referred to as protective factors. Protective factors may be events, circumstances or life experiences.

> Approaches to managing adolescent substance use aim to reduce risk factors and strengthen protective factors where possible.

There is no one single risk factor that can be attributed to adolescent drug use. Psychosocial risk factors tend to 'cluster'. That is, individuals tend to have several risk factors that impact on their development. This explains why many health-risk behaviours (alcohol abuse, heavy tobacco use, other substance use, unprotected sex, delinquency) often co-occur.

Specific details in the substance use history

Polysubstance use. In contrast to many adults, polysubstance use is common among adolescents. Therefore, when obtaining a drug use history from young people, it is important to specifically ask about each substance. Most young people often don't consider alcohol and tobacco to be drugs, and so these need to be specifically asked about.

For any given substance, gather information on:
* How often they take that substance
* The dose used (i.e. how many drinks on a given occasion, how many cigarettes a day, how many times they use marijuana in a given week or on a given day)

Whether episodic binge use occurs and if so, how often.

Table 12.3 Some risk and protective factors for substance misuse in adolescents

Biological factors	Genetic, physiological factors
Temperament and personality traits	Antisocial personality disorder, sensation seeking trait
Familial factors	Familial attitudes that are favourable to substance use, parental modelling of substance use, poor or inconsistent parenting practices
Early onset of substance use	Alcohol or drug use before age 15 years
Emotional and behavioural problems	Conduct disorder, depression, attention deficit/hyperactivity disorder, anxiety
Poor social connections	To school and community groups
Peer use of substances	Attitudes and behaviour favourable to substance use

Table 12.4 Principles of engaging adolescents

Confidentiality	Confidentiality is extremely important in the relationship between a young person and a health professional. Adolescents frequently will not disclose the details of their substance use if they are concerned that confidentiality will not be maintained by the health professional.
Take a broad psychosocial history	Adolescents respond well to a holistic approach, rather than a focus on their substance use.
Screen for mental health problems	Mental health problems often emerge in adolescence and should be screened for regularly.
Avoid judgement	Any perception of judgement about the adolescent's substance use on the part of the health professional impedes engagement with the young person.

Differentiating problematic from experimental use: In addition to the extent of use, it is helpful to find out whether the young person has experienced problems (physical, emotional, social, or legal) with their substance use, e.g. Do things happen when you use drugs/drink heavily that you later regret/wish didn't happen?

Where there is a history of heavy substance use obtained, ask the young person whether they experience:
- Difficulty controlling use of the substance
- Withdrawal symptoms when they do not use a substance (e.g. 'if you don't' use marijuana, how do you feel?').

There is increasing evidence to suggest that these features of physical drug dependence may commence in adolescence, rather than later in adulthood.

Box 12.7 Warning signs of substance use in adolescents

- Drop in school grades
- Behavioural changes—change of friends, lack of interaction with family
- Changes in appearance—red eyes (cannabis), thin (amphetamines)
- Loss of interest in hobbies, sport, activities
- Changes in eating pattern (cannabis increased, amphetamines reduced)
- Changes in sleeping pattern
- Lethargy, loss of motivation
- Mood swings ('uppers and downers')
- Problems with the law (drink driving, assault, break enter and steal, criminal activity).

Management of substance use disorders in adolescents

The Young Person. Management of substance use disorders in adolescents requires a multi-prong approach, which takes into account the adolescent's stage of development and includes behavioural strategies, intervention for mental health and well-being and in some cases, medication.

Cannabis use is particularly common among adolescents and young people. Adolescents should be advised that:

- There is now sufficient evidence that in certain vulnerable individuals with a genetic predisposition, cannabis could increase their risk of developing a psychotic illness later in life. (see p. 194, further reading Moore et al 2007)
- Because there is a great deal of variability in the potency of cannabis, previous exposure to cannabis without apparent ill effect does not mean that subsequent exposure will be equally harmless.

With regard to opioid use, pharmacological management (naltrexone, methadone, buprenorphine) of the drug-dependent adolescent is increasingly undergoing evaluation to clarify when adolescents benefit from pharmacotherapy.

The Family: Depression and anxiety often occur in parents of substance abusing adolescents, sometimes reaching clinical levels of severity. Parents frequently describe feelings of helplessness and a lack of confidence about having the appropriate parenting skills to deal with their teenager's drug use. The health professional can help empower parents through:

- Education about substance use
- Advice and/or referral for assistance with parenting strategies
- Management of depression of anxiety.

With more entrenched substance abuse, disengagement with the family may have occurred. Families are an integral part of the adolescent's world and it is therefore important to try to assist the young person to rebuild connection. Depending on the individual circumstance this connection may be achieved through mediation by the health professional or more formally with family counsellors.

Increasing access to treatment
Outreach
Adolescents generally do not engage with alcohol and drug services for adults. They sometimes need specific outreaching and proactive services that cater appropriately for their developmental stage and incorporate a consideration of their cultural background, lifestyle, and in many cases their family.

Opportunistic health care is very important in young people, particularly the homeless, as they tend not to engage with primary care services. This includes attending to screening and management of blood-borne viruses and sexually transmitted infections, addressing intercurrent health problems (chest infections, skin rashes, etc.).

Mental health problems should always be monitored in young people. Substance use may complicate depression and anxiety that are common in adolescence, but these conditions may not be articulated as such by the young person. Psychosis (drug induced or otherwise) can also occur with heavy substance use.

Transition from adolescent to adult drug treatment services
The transition from developmentally focused youth drug treatment services to more independently orientated adult services can be challenging for young people. The aims of successful transition of young people to adult-orientated health services are to optimize both their health and their ability to adapt to adult roles. The ultimate aim is to promote the young person's capacity for self-management and to improve their life chances. The transition process needs to include the co-ordination of primary and specialty health services, as well as the development of up-to-date detailed written transition plans, in collaboration with young people and their families. Confidentiality and informed consent must be maintained for the adolescent or young person as they traverse systems and engage with different health professionals. This usually means discussing with the young person what information is clinically relevant for the adult health service to be aware of.

Harm reduction in the adolescent context
As for adults, principles of harm reduction apply to the adolescents, although they need to be appropriately modified for young people of differing developmental stages and they also need to take into account the adolescent's context. For example, advice on the less harmful methods of using drugs may be appropriate in adolescents whose substance abuse is unlikely to cease for some time.

Prevention of substance use disorders in adolescence
Resilience in adolescence can help protect against substance use. There is evidence that resilience can be promoted by increasing a sense of connectedness of the adolescent, e.g. to family, school, or to sporting, religious or cultural groups.

> **Box 12.8 Tips for parents in preventing adolescent substance use problems**
>
> - Spend time with young people, communicate with them, be involved in their lives
> - Get to know their friends, and their friend's parents
> - Set a good example—good role modelling is important
> - Be alert to early warning signs of drug use
> - Do not over react, be calm, avoid conflict
> - Do not nag or lecture—reason honestly with them
> - Set sensible ground rules and boundaries
> - Ensure adult supervision at parties, plan how they and their friends get home
> - Seek professional help—from GPs, psychologists, addiction specialists, psychiatrists—if problems arise.

Summary

Management of adolescent substance use requires consideration of:

- Stage of adolescent development
- Risk factor/protective factor framework
- Spectrum of adolescent substance use
- Mental health screening
- Youth specific models of care—outreach, harm reduction, opportunistic health care
- Transition processes from adolescent to adult drug treatment services.

Further reading

Moore THM, Zammit S, Lingford-Hughes A, Barnes TE, Jones PB, Burke M, Lewis G. Cannabis use and risk of psychotic or affective mental health outcomes: a systematic review. *Lancet* 2007; **370**: 317–319.

The elderly

Epidemiology of substance use in the elderly

People aged 65 years and over are the fastest growing group in the populations of Western countries. In 1990, 13% of the US population was over 65 years. It is estimated that by 2030, 21% of the US population will be over 65 years of age.

Community surveys indicate that older people drink less alcohol and have fewer alcohol-related problems than younger people. However, the elderly population of today may be drinking more heavily than previous generations. Between 6 and 10% of elderly people admitted to hospital have signs and symptoms of alcohol dependence. The figures are higher for older people in emergency room settings (14%), psychiatric wards (20%), and nursing homes. Levels of drinking found in cross-sectional surveys may disguise a gradual increase in drinking in older people, and it is likely that the numbers of older people with alcohol problems will rise and become a dominant issue for healthcare budgets in the 21st Century.

The UK National Psychiatric Morbidity Survey of 2000 estimated that 20% of men and 6% of women between the ages of 65 and 74 years, living at home, had AUDIT score is greater than or equal to 8, suggesting an alcohol use disorder.

Reasons for drinking

A number of factors contribute to increased alcohol consumption as people get older. Retirement and decreased social mobility are important factors, as are isolation, loneliness, physical illness, and pain. Bereavement is another key factor. Older people often develop insomnia and use alcohol as a hypnotic (as a night-cap on its own or in a cup of tea or coffee).

Effects of alcohol on the older person

- As people get older they become more sensitive to the effects of alcohol. This is due, at least in part, to an age-related decrease in body water which leads to higher blood alcohol concentrations (BACs) than younger people for the same amount of alcohol.
- Ageing also interferes with the ability of the body to tolerate alcohol, a result of decreased hepatic blood flow, inefficient liver enzymes and reduced renal clearance. Older people become unsteady on their feet at lower levels of alcohol than younger people, and are at an increased risk of falls.
- The ageing brain appears to be more vulnerable to the effects of alcohol than the younger brain. Alcohol depresses brain function, causing memory problems and incoordination, which in turn can lead to falls and confusion. It also heightens emotions leading to arousal and irritability.
- Alcohol interacts with prescribed medication. About one third of older people take four or more different preparations per day.

Consequences of drinking in the older person

- Increased falls and accidents in the home. The risk of elderly people sustaining a hip fracture increases with alcohol consumption. This can be explained in part by the increased risk of falls while intoxicated, but also by the fact that bone density is reduced in elderly drinkers.
- The elderly are also at increased risk of being involved in road traffic accidents (RTAs). The crash risk per mile increases from the age of 55 years and older people are more likely to be injured. Alcohol contributes independently to the increased risk of having an RTA.
- Elderly people are more likely to take prescription medication than younger people. Alcohol interacts with this medication, causing untoward side-effects. Benzodiazepines, often used by the elderly as hypnotics, depress the breakdown of alcohol, thus increasing its effect.
- Although alcohol promotes sleep, it reduces Rapid Eye Movement (REM) sleep and thus the quality of sleep.
- The effects of alcohol on cerebral function can contribute to acute and chronic confusional states, memory impairment, and alcohol-related dementia. Alcohol can also cause or exacerbate family quarrels.
- Incontinence is a common problem in the elderly and can be caused or exacerbated by alcohol use.
- Older people who are drinking heavily are at risk of self-neglect and poor dietary intake. This group may present to emergency services with an organic brain syndrome or in a state of hypothermia.
- Psychiatric co-morbidity is a major problem in older people with alcohol use disorders. They can present with depression, complicated withdrawal states with alcoholic hallucinations, morbid jealousy, and paranoid states.

The elderly problem drinker

Elderly drinkers have been classified as follows:
- Lifelong heavy drinkers: depression and anxiety are more common in this group. Younger people with alcohol use disorders are at elevated risk of becoming older people with alcohol problems.
- Late onset heavy drinkers: this group is more likely to be of higher socio-economic status and to comprise women. It also includes people coping with bereavement, retirement, loneliness, physical infirmity, and marital stress. This group tends to be more psychologically stable and to have better prognosis than the early onset group.
- People who move in and out of problem drinking throughout their lives.

Detection

Drinking in the elderly often goes undetected, and if older people are found to have an alcohol problem they are often not adequately assessed. Assessment is an important part of the successful management of drinking problems in older people.

Detection of alcohol problems in older people may require a different approach from that in younger people. Screening instruments may be of help in detection, but their performance is likely to vary according to the screening setting. In the United States the Michigan Alcoholism Screening Test-Geriatric Version (SMAST-G) appears to perform well, but the

AUDIT less well. UK-based studies show the opposite, with the AUDIT being effective and the SMAST-G performing poorly. In older people the most effective cut-off point for the AUDIT appears to be lower than in younger samples, and to differ for older men (5/6) and older women (3/4).

Healthcare professionals should employ a healthy degree of suspicion when assessing elderly patients in all settings. Alcohol-related problems in the elderly can be mistaken for medical or psychiatric conditions, such as:

• Depression
• Insomnia
• Poor nutrition
• Congestive cardiac failure.

As many as 60% of elderly people admitted to hospital because of confusion, repeated falls at home, recurrent chest infections, and heart failure, may have unrecognized alcohol problems.

Alcohol problems may be disguised by non-specific disorders such as:

• Insomnia
• Gastrointestinal problems
• Depression
• Dementia.

Assessing the elderly patient

Alcohol problems in the elderly often go undiagnosed and untreated. Health care providers, especially emergency room personnel and physicians should consider alcohol as a contributing factor when elderly people present. A comprehensive assessment of the elderly drinker should include:

• An alcohol and drug history. History taking may be difficult in confused patients. so it is sensible to take a collateral history from family, friends or neighbours
• A psychosocial history
• A social support history
• Physical examination
• Laboratory testing.

Managing substance use in the elderly

Some professionals may have a misguided belief that older people should be allowed to continue drinking in an 'at risk fashion' even if it is affecting their physical or emotional health. Only a small proportion of older drinkers are referred to specialist services and yet the evidence clearly indicates that treatment outcomes are good.

Box 12.9 Reasons why older people drink

- Loneliness
- Isolation
- Retirement
- Decreased social mobility
- Bereavement
- Depression
- Physical illness
- Pain
- Insomnia.

'I usually have a glass of sherry at night to help me sleep'
'I drink because I am isolated and lonely'
'Drink sends me off to sleep quick'

Further reading

Johnson I. Alcohol problems in old age: a review of recent epidemiological research. *International Journal of Geriatric Psychiatry* 2000; **15**: 575–581.

Philpot M, Pearson N, Petratou V, *et al.* Screening for problem drinking in older people referred to an older people referred to a mental health service: a comparison of CAGE and AUDIT. *Aging and Mental Health* 2003; **7**: 171–175.

Roberts AM, Marshall EJ, Macdonald JD. Which screening test for alcohol consumption is best associated with 'at risk' drinking in older primary care attenders? *Primary Mental Health Care* 2005; **3**: 131–138.

Singleton N, Bumpstead R, O'Brien M, Lee A, Meltzer M. *Psychiatric Morbidity Among Adults Living in Private Households,* 2000. London: Stationery Office, 2001.

Substance use in disadvantaged populations

Who are the disadvantaged?

Disadvantaged populations include a broad range of individuals, some of whom started life with disadvantage, others of whom have lost everything through substance misuse, mental health disorders, or gambling. The disadvantaged includes those who are alienated from their family and community, the homeless, many of those living in boarding houses or transient accommodation, street kids, those reliant on public housing, and many of those marginalized from mainstream society, such as sex workers. Disparities in health are increasing worldwide.

The association between disadvantage and substance misuse

Where disadvantage exists alongside wealth in a community, the disadvantaged are at increased risk of substance use disorders. In the case of alcohol, disadvantaged communities, or subpopulations are more likely to have a polarization of drinking, with more people abstaining totally, but those who do drink are more likely to drink heavily. Episodic heavy drinking may be common. The disadvantaged are also more likely to be smokers, have a greater prevalence of illicit drug use, particularly polysubstance use, often of a relatively indiscriminate manner.

Where there is a high prevalence of heavy drinking, smoking or illicit drug use, there is an increased likelihood of young people commencing problematic substance use. For those who want to stop substance use there may be regular cues to drug use in everyday life, for example, when they see other people, sometimes including friends and relatives, using drugs or alcohol.

While relative disadvantage is a risk factor for substance use disorders, problem alcohol or drug use in turn tends to cause or exacerbate disadvantage. This is often accompanied by social marginalization and considerable stigma. There may be loss of employment, incarceration, breakdown in marriage and other important relationships, secondary psychiatric conditions and often a combination of these consequences. In the most severe cases, homelessness can occur. Once homeless, engagement with treatment becomes far more difficult, and the peer group may include many other individuals with substance use disorders. In addition, homelessness exposes the individual to further ongoing stress, and to increased risk of major traumas such as assault.

Treatment for substance use disorders among the disadvantaged

The disadvantaged typically have reduced access to treatment and may present later for help, for either their substance use disorder, or a range of complications or co-morbid conditions. Simple tasks such as phoning for an appointment or finding money for a bus fare to attend a clinic may become significant hurdles. Purchase of medications may also be delayed due to lack of available funds.

Outreach services can offer increased access both to primary health care and to treatment services for substance use disorders. Because the disadvantaged are more likely to present late for treatment, systematic screening and early intervention services are particularly important, for example in a primary health care setting.

Integrated care, incorporating primary health care, and facilitated referral or treatment for physical, psychiatric, and/or social needs can be valuable. Attending to housing needs and other pressing social concerns can greatly increase the chance of success with treatment of substance use disorders. The health practitioner can have a role in providing letters of support for public housing, or other advocacy as needed. Screening for co-existing mental health and social problems, including domestic violence, is valuable. Addressing these issues, again is likely to improve the outcome of treatment for substance use disorders. A multidisciplinary team, with good relationships with outside relevant agencies can be of great assistance in providing integrated care.

Prevention of substance misuse related to disadvantage

Clearly government and other agency attempts to reduce disadvantage, and increase access to employment, quality education, support services, and safe and appropriate housing and environment for all citizens are important. Connectedness to society has been shown to be important in providing resilience against substance misuse. Studies of methods to increase connectedness, for example, among young people, have shown promise in reducing the prevalence of substance misuse.

Providing early childhood support or other intervention can improve the outcome for children in troubled families, and is likely to reduce the transgenerational transmission of substance use disorders. Ensuring access to quality mental health services is also important to reduce substance misuse among those with mental health disorders and their offspring.

Prisons

Epidemiology

The rate of incarceration throughout the world varies from 29 per 100,000 adults in Liechtenstein to 750 per 100,000 adults in the United States of America. The variability in incarceration is strongly linked to drug-law policies, and to health and social welfare indicators linked to poverty and social dislocation.

A high proportion of prisoners have a history of alcohol or drug misuse.

Psychiatric co-morbidity: Individuals who misuse drugs disproportionately suffer from mental disorders. Either condition can precipitate non-compliance with treatment and this, in turn, strongly predicts interaction with the criminal justice system. Many prisoners also have adult ADHD which is often primary to their addiction. The appropriate treatment of this e.g. methylphenidate can be useful.

Drugs and Crime: The following crime classification has been developed to provide the criminal justice sector a health paradigm for the interactions between substance misuse and crime:

- **Psychopharmacological crimes**: crimes committed under the influence of a psychoactive substance, as a consequence of its acute or chronic use
- **Economic-compulsive crimes**: crimes committed in order to obtain the means to support drug use
- **Systemic crimes**: crimes committed within illicit drug markets—drug supply, distribution and abuse
- **Drug law offences**: crimes committed in violation of drug and other related legislations.

Box 12.10 Substance misuse in the prison population in New South Wales, Australia

Approximately half both male and female prisoners drank in the harmful range (by AUDIT score) immediately prior to coming into prison.

Approximately three-quarters of female prisoners and two-thirds of male prisoners had used at least one illegal drug at some time prior to incarceration—approximately 40% were using illicit drugs at the time of arrest.

One-third of females and one-fifth of males injected drugs while in prison. Of those who inject in prison, 70% shared injecting equipment. An estimated one in thirty prisoners inject for the first time while in prison.

New South Wales Inmate Health Survey, 1997.

Avoiding imprisonment

Attempts to re-engage clients with substance use disorders with community health and welfare services, through low-level courts, is the subject of a number of diversion programmes being trialled in different jurisdictions. 'Drug Courts' are just one example.

Prevention of drug and alcohol use in the prisoner population (prison setting)

Alcohol: Controlled in prison reasonably well, as the quantities required make it difficult to conceal, and easy to detect. Also, because of the disinhibitory effects of alcohol, with consequent disruption to a closed and overcrowded community, tolerance by both custodial authorities and inmates is low, and when tolerated, short-lived.

Other drugs: Supply is constrained through regulation and physical barriers, but the success of supply reduction has never been supported with evidence. Random urine testing of prisoners confirms that drugs, licit and illicit, available in the community, are being brought through to prisoners—either through corrupt staff or contractors, or by coercion of families and friends.

Diversion of prescribed medications is minimized through supervision of almost all medications by health service staff.

Management of drug and alcohol use in the prisoner population (prison setting)

Transition from the community may involve:
- Catastrophic interruption of substance use (transfer to a coercive, non-therapeutic environment), or
- Continuation of interrupted therapeutic associations, or
- Opportunity to address substance use disorder in a relatively controlled environment (particularly, polydrug misuse).

Prison-based opioid pharmacotherapy programmes include:
- Maintenance (some systems impose low fixed-dose regimes, while others restrict the particular correctional centres that 'allow' opioid pharmacotherapies through the prison classification system)
- Reduction (clients from community programmes are withdrawn from their treatment, in a non-consensual manner)
- Enforced withdrawal (in jurisdictions where no opioid pharmacotherapies are sanctioned).

Harm reduction in the prison environment, despite extreme risks of blood-borne virus transmission often receives inadequate attention.
- Undue priority is given to supply reduction (e.g. surveillance, interdiction)
- Demand reduction—psychological approaches are favoured by custodial authorities; therapeutic approaches are constrained; most experience is with methadone, and little with buprenorphine and naltrexone
- Harm reduction is limited to immunization programmes and rarely extends to education about bleach and making bleach available for cleaning injecting equipment. Outside of 11 countries worldwide, there is no access to regulated exchange of injecting equipment.

Management of psychiatric co-morbidity

Imprisonment may provide an opportunity for management of psychiatric co-morbidity including sometimes undiagnosed primary psychiatric conditions. In some prisons ADHD is increasingly being diagnosed and treated.

Transition to the community

Transfer to a community treatment programme is organized.

Post-release mortality: The period immediately after release from prison is a very dangerous one. Often tolerance to drugs such as opioids or benzodiazepines is reduced due to enforced abstinence, but the desire to use a substance is high. Australian male prisoners were nearly four times more likely to die soon after release than their non incarcerated peers, [all-cause Standard Mortality Rate (SMR) 3.7] and women on release from prison were nearly 8 times more likely to die (SMR 7.8). Drug-related causes of death were the most common.

Efforts to reduce post-release mortality include education, offering increased doses of opioid maintenance pharmacotherapy just prior to release, and ensuring a smooth transition to community-based treatment and support services.

Summary

Despite some improvements in recent years, there remains an overwhelming need for enhanced responses to mental health and substance use disorders for people who are or have been in prison. The inconsistencies between prison systems, and sometimes even within the system, make the transition from community to prison and back to community difficult for service providers, and dangerous for clients.

Further reading

Butler T, Kariminia A, Levy M, Kaldor J. Prisoners are at risk for hepatitis C transmission. *European Journal of Epidemiology* 2004; **19**: 1119–1122.

Drugs in Focus: *Drugs and Crime—a complex relationship*. Lisbon: European Monitoring Centre for Drugs and Drug Addiction (EMCDDA), 2007. Available at: http://www.emcdda.europa.eu/attachements.cfm/att_33064_EN_2007_2721_EN_WEB.pdf (accessed 26 January, 2008).

Kariminia A, Butler TG, Corben SP, Levy MH, Grant L, Kaldor JM, Law MG. Extreme cause-specific mortality in a cohort of adult prisoners—1988 to 2002: a data-linkage study. *International Journal of Epidemiology* 2007; **36**: 310–316.

Substance use in different cultural contexts

Cultural issues in clinical practice

Many studies point to the influence of culture, gender, and ethnicity on the clinical manifestations and courses of psychiatric illnesses, as well as substance and alcohol use disorders. In numerous countries, patients with alcohol or substance use disorders are from diverse cultural and linguistic backgrounds, with differences in their practices and beliefs; they live in different community settings (urban or rural) and may have varied life experiences. Socio-economic contexts, living conditions, physical environments, and access to education and health care resources can affect peoples' choices, use of alcohol or other substances, and subsequent problems. Health care professionals need to ensure that these patients are treated with fairness and dignity. Effective communication is important in understanding and managing alcohol and substance use problems, and clinicians need to be aware of some specific factors that may impact on the patients and their families. Although the use of standardized screening and diagnostic instruments and well-defined diagnostic criteria have provided a substantial improvement in assessment and treatment in clinical practice, some issues are still a problem.

Quantification of the level of alcohol or substance intake

The level of consumption is an important determinant of the likelihood of alcohol or substance withdrawal, its severity and other related problems, which influences the choice and effectiveness of clinical interventions. However, many situations influenced by the cultural practice of the community make the quantification of the substance intake difficult.

People in many countries are not familiar with a standard drink or they may not even use a standard container to drink alcohol. For example, in some rural villages in Thailand and Malaysia where homemade alcohol is produced from the sugar-palm juice, the alcoholic beverage is put in a bamboo shoot, the size of which varies. In addition, it is a custom in some areas that drinkers share the same container when they drink together in a closed group. Again, alcohol served at a party is often a determinant of the host's socio-economic status and generosity, so the host keeps on filling up the guest's glass. Therefore, it is difficult to quantify an individual level of intake.

This issue also exists with other substances, for example marijuana, where users report their amount of consumption using the unit familiar in their community, and with methamphetamine, when users sit in a circle and share, smoking the fumes from the same vessel. Different street names are often known only among people from the same community. Some substances are only used or popular in some areas; often they are local plants or products. For example, mitragynine speciosa, kroth, or krathom is an addictive plant commonly used in southern part of Thailand and Malaysia. Quantification of illicit substances is also difficult as they are often mixed with other ingredients, for example, heroin and methamphetamine are sometimes mixed with benzodiazepines and the users of codeine-cough suppressant syrup tend to mix it with cola.

It is therefore necessary to inquire about the method of administration, the so-called unit and size of the container, the street names of the substances, the form of the substance used—whether it is a leaf, liquid, or powder—and the places or the situations where the substances are used. It is sometimes helpful to ask in terms of money the person spends each day on the substance and the number of associates who join the group. In order to obtain this information effectively, the clinician needs to be knowledgeable about the common type and patterns of alcohol or substance use in their community and incorporate it into the assessment of the patient.

Taboo and stigmatization

Alcohol and substance use may be taboo in some cultures, families or religions. In Muslim countries, alcohol consumption is strictly prohibited. In Buddhism, lay people are taught to conform to the Five Precepts, the fifth of which is to refrain from using distilled or fermented intoxicants, including alcohol, tobacco, and other addictive substances, which often lead to undesirable behaviours. In surveying patterns of alcohol consumption among Thai Buddhists, the rate of response to a question on whether a respondent feels guilt or remorse after drinking is high, as people always feel that they violate a religious rule when they drink. In some countries it is thought that alcohol use is a man's behaviour, and there is a greater stigma attached to drinking by women than by men.

The perception of causes or explanatory models of illnesses also differ among ethnic groups. The biological model is predominant in the Western world; alcohol or substance dependence is viewed as a disease instead of a social problem. Some cultures, however, still regard alcohol or substance use as a moral issue. Many people are therefore too embarrassed to report that they or their relatives need help with their alcohol- or substance-related problems. They may also feel ashamed that they will be judged as a bad person or even a criminal. Responses may also depend on the individuals' social expectations; e.g. marital or family problems, perhaps resulting from a drinking husband, may be kept secret as women are taught not to discuss such things outside the family. Symptoms such as tremors and sweating from alcohol withdrawal may be considered as caused by breaking a taboo.

The patient may also seek treatment from both a traditional healer and a physician. The physician in this case needs to accept the patient's explanation of his illness and allow him to continue receiving traditional treatment as long as it causes no further harm.

Many people may feel that substance misuse is other people's problem or it is the problem of people from other ethnic communities and cannot accept that it is their own problem. Clinicians need to recognize that people from any communities can and may use substances, licit or illicit, and anyone can experience harms associated with intoxication, overdose, or dependence. It is important to find the most comfortable way to help people to talk about their alcohol or substance use and related issues.

Clinicians need to show respect and provide an atmosphere in which the patient can reveal and discuss sensitive issues by ensuring that their experiences are listened to in a non-judgmental manner, validated, and kept confidential. In some cases, clinicians may need to seek advice from cultural consultants, other liaison staff, or a patient's family member or friend, if available. Some patients may feel more comfortable to talk with a clinician of the same gender or with someone older so the clinicians should be open minded and allow them to do so if possible. It is also helpful to spend time talking about general health issues or the patient's immediate concern before asking about sensitive issues. Explain why you are asking about these personal issues and that such information will be used to help the patient.

Communication problems in different cultures

It is important to recognize if the patient's symptoms are normal or abnormal within the cultural context. In a community where drinking often occurs in groups and drinkers drink from the same container until the supply is depleted, someone may spend a long time in a drinking group, but does not drink a lot. Therefore, when asking if he spends a lot of time drinking, being high, or being hung over, he may give an affirmative answer, leading to mistakes in diagnosis. Clinicians may have difficulty in exploring clinical symptoms, which are culturally specific, when they are not familiar with the patterns of behaviour within a particular social group.

In performing a psychiatric interview, a clinician not only elicits symptoms and signs from verbal communication, but also from observing patient's general appearance and non-verbal behaviour, including hygiene, dress and grooming, psychomotor activity, eye contact, affect and quality of expression. In some cultures activities such as hand shaking and touching, especially with someone of the opposite sex, and eye contact may be restrained or avoided. The clinician may misinterpret the patient's normal social behaviour as abnormal or may respond inappropriately. The norms for expression of emotion also vary in different cultures. In most eastern cultures, the open expression of emotion, whether elation or depression, is not encouraged. Some may even deny these emotional symptoms; hostile psychotic patients may appear shy and quiet when participating in a group activity. Clinicians may, therefore, miss a diagnosis of co-morbid psychiatric disorder if they are not aware of this cultural restriction.

The patient's language can also influence how symptoms are reported. They may not speak English well, or the language of the country they are living in, and may appear anxious, agitated, disturbed, or restricted when interviewed. They may not comprehend some psychiatric terms which describe their mood or affect, such as feeling depressed or anxious, and respond to the interview incorrectly or deny the symptoms. Clinicians need to explain the meanings of the terms they use or use non-technical terms. In taking patient's history, clinicians should listen carefully and pay close attention to what is described by the patients; they should not too hastily interpret what the patients have said, as this may be based on the observer's own cultural background rather than on what is actually meant.

People from some ethnic groups may fear hospitalization, talking with people outside their group or who speak a different language, and separation from their families and community. Family members or trusted friends will be good mediators, but if they are not available, health care staff, social workers, or someone from the patients' community would be an alternative source of support. It is important to understand that when people are under stress, sick or under some medications, alcohol or substances, their ability to adjust to the new environment or speak a different language is even more difficult.

Some issues in management

In traditional Asian culture, family plays a very important role in daily living, as well as in anyone's decision to seek and maintain a treatment programme. Families are largely close-knit and extended, and members are taught to respect authority, and take care of their parents and senior relatives. Direct family members, such as parents, children and siblings are usually the patient's main source of support. Collateral information from family members about patient's patterns and consequences of substance use may sometimes be more reliable than direct information from the patient and may be a sole source of information in some cases, in particular in intoxicated, withdrawing, or disturbed patients. Family members should be encouraged to participate in the treatment programme, and be educated about the nature of illness and plan of management. If clinicians and treatment team are sensitive to the importance of family and can communicate with them directly, this will help to keep them all engaged in the treatment programme and reduce the occurrence of relapses. Patients may prefer to have a family member, relative, or a trusted friend present when talking with the healthcare staff or stay with them while they are admitted in the hospital. However, some may not want their family to know that they use a substance; therefore, the patient's wishes should be ascertained before contacting others.

There are some religious rituals that people need to practice, for example, Muslim prayers 5 times per day, a special diet, or the Ramadan month of fasting. Hospital staff should respect these rituals and allow in-patients to practice them wherever possible.

Adherence to treatment and medication is often a problem. Among some ethnic groups whose beliefs and concepts about the causes and course of psychiatric illnesses, as well as substance use disorders are not of the biological model, non-compliance to treatment, and medication can be very high. This is particularly true when they believe it to be a moral problem. Failure to control use may be viewed as ethical inadequacy or weakness of mind and they may not value modern treatment. As stigmatization is very strong in some cultures, the need for treatment or long-term medications may be interpreted as severity of their problem. A more complicated issue can arise when patients do not disclose a lack of adherence to medication because they do not want to upset the doctors. It is helpful for the health care team to use an active educational approach, discuss the bio-psycho-social explanatory model of substance use disorders, and describe pathological patterns of dependence such as a repeated desire to cut down, or using substance for a longer time and a larger amount than intended as behavioural symptoms of a disease, not a moral weakness. Treatment, both pharmacotherapy and psychosocial intervention, should be explained as a means to relieve these troubling symptoms. Responsibility for change always lies with them, thus the success of treatment does depends on their 'mind', if that is their belief.

There is a variety of herbal anti-abusive drugs for alcohol; some may act on the metabolism of alcohol and cause physically distressing symptoms similar to those caused by disulfiram. Many herbal medicine remedies are also available that help to relieve alcohol hangovers or are believed to prevent alcohol-induced liver damage. If the patient believes in herbal medicine, a detailed medication history should be taken to prevent untoward side effects that may cause further non-compliance.

Box 12.11 Some useful principles in approaching patients with diverse cultural backgrounds

- Listen to the patient carefully, emphasize his/her description of symptoms, cause and course of illness rather than interpreting this information
- Show empathy, non-judgmental attitude and respect by treating the patient and family members as persons equal to yourself
- Show your interest in the patient as a whole not just his/her symptoms, illness, or problem
- Build a friendly, but professional and reliable therapeutic atmosphere. Ensure privacy and confidentiality when discussing sensitive personal issues
- Be aware of culturally specific taboo, stigma, belief, or normative perception of the illness, including its cause, explanatory model, course and treatment. Be sensitive to the patient's embarrassment when discussing certain issues
- Be aware that people from some ethnic groups may adhere to the cultural practices within their group. Some issues may be considered as personal, sensitive or irrelevant and they may feel offended if you discuss those issues directly
- Ask if the patient would like to have a family member or friend present when being interviewed or otherwise. Do not assume anything based on your own experience or cultural background.
- If the patient seeks a family member's opinion before making a decision about treatment, welcome and encourage family involvement in the process of management if it helps maximize compliance to treatment and support for the patient
- Avoid using technical terms and explain what you mean clearly and gently in a simple way. Check if the patient understands what you have said correctly
- Use appropriate verbal and non-verbal approaches. Be careful with some physical manners that may not be acceptable in some cultures
- Consult a cultural consultant, interpreter or patient's family member or friend if you are not sure how to approach a patient from a different culture.

In summary, this section has provided some insights about cultural factors, which may influence the clinical manifestations and health care seeking behaviours of patients with alcohol and substance use disorders. The content is not comprehensive as there are many other cultural issues that have not been discussed in this section which are worthy of further exploration. Examples are given to illustrate that there is variability across cultures in the ways that how substance use disorders are perceived, experienced and expressed. It is necessary for a clinician to be sensitive to and acknowledge the cultural factors that determine the patient's presentation of illness and at the same time understand and respect their right to adhere to their cultural beliefs and practices, in order to assess and treat them effectively.

Mental health and substance use disorders in immigrants and refugees

Mental disorder is the product of the complex interplay between biological vulnerability, psychological factors that are shaped by personal life history, and a person's environment, particularly the local world in which the person lives. This local world includes, but is not limited to, issues such as pattern of relationships, social and economic circumstances, access to education, employment, housing and other necessities of life, the prevailing cultural context, and access to health care. The prevalence of mental disorders among different immigrant groups is highly variable. Immigrant status, in itself, is not associated with either increased or decreased risk for mental disorder. Among the groups most vulnerable to the development of mental health problems are refugees and asylum seekers. It is the specific circumstances of pre-migration experience, migration and settlement that are important in influencing risk for mental disorder. Among potentially relevant circumstances are: traumatic experiences or prolonged stress prior to or during migration; being adolescent or elderly at the time of migration; separation from family; inability to speak the language of the host country; prejudice and discrimination in the receiving society; low socio-economic status and, particularly, a drop in personal socio-economic status following migration; non-recognition of occupational qualifications; isolation from persons of a similar cultural background; and extent of acculturation.

A consistent finding in Australia and other English-speaking countries with large immigrant populations is lower levels of utilization of mental health services by immigrant communities, although here also there is wide variation. It is not known whether this is due to lower prevalence of mental disorder among these communities or whether the lower rates of service use may be explained by factors such as conceptions of mental health and illness that do not accord with mainstream views, higher levels of stigma associated with using mental health services, perceptions of inappropriateness of services, or simply lack of awareness of what services are available. There is little research evidence on the question of whether the quality of treatment outcomes for immigrant and refugee patients of mental health service is the same or different to that of majority communities.

Studies of the epidemiology of substance use disorders in immigrant receiving countries show broadly the same pattern of findings as studies of mental illness. The core feature is the great variation in research findings. This reflects the wide variation in the demographic, cultural and migration profiles of the groups being studied and the wide variation in national health service, social support and legal systems, and also the significant methodological and practical challenges to carrying out high quality research in immigrant and refugee communities. The patterns of alcohol use tend to reflect patterns in the home countries of immigrants. To a significant extent this is also the situation with injecting drug use, although the rates of drug use in some young immigrant and second generation groups is of great concern. Socio-economic position and cultural dislocation—local worlds—are important contributors. Co-morbidity is very common, with causality operating in both directions. The presence of a mental disorder increases the risk of alcohol and other forms of drug abuse and dependence, and the presence of drug use disorder increases the incidence of mental disorder, particularly mood disorders, most commonly depression and anxiety.

The existence of culturally appropriate treatment and prevention services for mental and substance use disorders is the exception rather than the rule. Where such services do exist they are almost never rigorously evaluated. In most countries mental health services and drug and alcohol services are separately administered. Given the very high rates of co-morbidity this is generally an unsatisfactory situation. Mental health services are usually not competent to treat drug and alcohol problems, and drug and alcohol services are generally not competent to treat mental disorders. People with both types of problems bounce around between services and, more often than not, receive poor quality care. There is increasing recognition of this system level problem and attempts to integrate mental health and drug and alcohol services are becoming more common, as is the recognition that mental health clinicians require at least basic training in skills relevant to drugs and alcohol, and drug and alcohol clinicians require basic mental health competencies. All clinicians require additional training in effective cross-cultural clinical practice, and health services require assistance in developing effective models of service delivery to cultural minority groups.

A key impediment to understanding mental disorders and substance use disorders among immigrants and refugees is the systematic exclusion from research of communities that do not speak the official language of countries. This occurs for methodological and practical reasons. Recruiting representative samples of immigrant and refugee communities is complex, time-consuming and expensive. Further research difficulties include:

• Lack of consensus on the definition and usefulness of concepts such as ethnicity
• Lack of cross-culturally reliable and valid research instruments
• Problems associated with cross-cultural diagnosis
• Lack of generally acceptable methods for studying culturally derived concepts of mental illness and substance use disorders
• Variations in the nature of clinical presentation across cultural groups and health systems.

These and other research challenges have the unfortunate effect of gradually widening the gap in knowledge—and, therefore, in availability of evidence for successful intervention—between host and immigrant communities. Predictive factors (risk factors for developing disorder, prognostic factors, or predictors of response to intervention) that have been derived from studies of one population (e.g. the dominant host community) may not be sufficient or even relevant to the prediction of disorder in various immigrant groups.

We do have some useful information on the epidemiology of mental and substance use disorders among immigrants and refugees in those countries with a long history of permanent immigrant settlement, although this information is more limited than it should be. In these countries there is generally a policy framework that at least recognizes the cultural and linguistic diversity of populations, and the responsibility of services (variably, and never fully, discharged) to respond effectively to this reality of diversity. However, in countries that have become immigrant receiving countries only in recent decades there is generally both a lack of epidemiological and other necessary information, and little in the way of policy and practical service response to diversity. About the situation of other categories of immigrants we know almost nothing. These include:

- Hundreds of millions of internal, rural to urban, migrants in China, India, Indonesia, Brazil, and other countries
- Temporary labour migrants, most commonly women and almost entirely from poor countries;
- Large numbers of trafficked women;
- Tens of millions of international students;
- Huge numbers of illegal migrants living in countries without the benefits of permanent residency or citizenship and in constant danger of imprisonment and deportation.

These less visible and under-researched groups are likely to be most at risk of developing mental and substance use disorders, and are least likely to have access to effective services.

Indigenous populations

Indigenous populations are those who have inhabited a land for thousands of years as distinct from those who have lived there only a few hundred years. They typically have a strong concept of unification of the people with the natural world. Each has a distinct culture, spirituality, and traditions, and many speak a distinct language or languages.

Indigenous peoples include Aboriginal and Torres Strait Islander Australians, Maori (or 'Tangata Whenua'—'people of the land') in New Zealand, First Nations in North America and Canada (including Indian, Métis, and Inuit) among many others.

In some countries, the indigenous people form the largest population group and holds power (such as in Fiji). However, in many countries indigenous populations have been subject to colonization, and have become economically and socially disadvantaged. In such countries indigenous peoples have typically faced considerable challenges across many generations through loss of individuals' identification with their culture, disempowerment, loss of land, lack of access to quality education, employment, and wealth, as well as challenges to traditional sense of worth, law and identity. All of these factors predispose to increased risk of both substance use disorders and mental health disorders. Furthermore new psycho-active substances were introduced at the time of colonization, in this context of threats to community values and authority.

In several countries, for example, Australia, US and Canada, European authorities for a time encouraged or forced indigenous peoples to leave their traditional lands and live in defined communities, often in mission settlements. In some cases, there was also enforced removal of children from their parents with the intention of hastening assimilation into the mainstream. In some areas this practice occurred as recently as the 1960s. Childhood separation, loss of sense of identity, and in some cases exposure to physical or sexual abuse within institutions have often left psychological scars that may include anxiety, depression, and post-traumatic stress disorder. These mental health disorders further predispose to substance use disorders. As adults, these individuals face major challenges bringing up their own children, having had limited opportunity to observe parenting skills. This can result in transgenerational transmission of substance use and mental health disorders.

Prevalence and impact of substance use disorders in indigenous communities

Data on the prevalence of substance use disorders in indigenous communities is often limited. Available studies generally show higher rates of abstinence from alcohol, but among those who do drink, higher rates of problem drinking. For example, in a household survey of urban Aboriginal Australians in 1994, respondents were more likely to be non-drinkers than non-Aboriginal Australians, but in those who did consume any alcohol 70% drank above recommended limits. Similarly, Maori are more likely to be non-drinkers than are other New Zealanders, but the average consumption per drinking occasion for those who do drink is 40% higher. Smoking rates in indigenous communities are typically double that of the non-indigenous population. There may be a higher prevalence of cannabis and other illicit substance use. Some Aboriginal and Torres Strait Islander communities, for example, in Northern Australia, report significant problems from cannabis, including high financial outlays, psychiatric complications, and stress or even violence when cannabis is not available. There may be higher rates of solvent misuse, including glue and paint sniffing in urban settings, and petrol sniffing, particularly in rural and remote settings.

Other health disorders and substance use

In many disadvantaged indigenous communities there is a high prevalence of other physical disease. For example Aboriginal and Torres Strait Islander communities in Australia have a high prevalence of diabetes, renal failure, and rheumatic heart disease. Coping with one's own chronic medical condition or with recurrent premature deaths in the community, may encourage escaping through drinking or drug use. Alcohol or drug use itself impacts significantly on the ability of the individual to manage their chronic disease, and adherence to medication regimes may be low or unpredictable. Alcohol use may also have a direct effect on glycaemic control in diabetes. Acute alcohol consumption may precipitate hypoglycaemia, while chronic heavy consumption may increase insulin resistance. Any experience of alcohol withdrawal may be more severe in persons with multiple medical disorders. Any pharmacotherapy advised for alcohol dependence needs to recognize the challenges the individual will face with compliance if they are living in a troubled setting. For example, the acamprosate regime of two tablets three times per day may not be feasible, whereas once a day naltrexone or, in carefully selected and informed individuals, disulfiram may be possible.

Treatment for indigenous persons with substance misuse

There is a pressing need for further evidence on specific approaches likely to be successful when working with indigenous patients. In the meantime clinical practice is informed by a small number of evaluations, by case studies, by clinical experience, and by consultation with indigenous communities.

The concept of 'cultural competence' is used to describe the set of attitudes, knowledge and skills that allows the health care professional to care effectively for a person from another culture (see also pp. 336–341 on cross-cultural care). This typically incorporates not only awareness of and respect for the culture of the patient, but also awareness of the clinician's own culture and how it can affect their approach. The ability to develop relationships that engender trust and respect is critical.

Communication and engagement with indigenous clients can be assisted by:
- Taking ample time for effective communication
- Willingness to learn about the patient's culture and environment, including understandings of causation of mental and physical illness
- An awareness that one's own culture influences one's beliefs and interactions

- Indigenous health professionals or clinical aides can typically achieve enhanced quality of communication and engagement, and help ensure a welcoming and culturally secure environment
- Where language differences impair communication, quality translation is essential.

Some indigenous communities may have fundamental differences from European cultures in basic concepts, such as time, cause and effect, and individualism. Western logic often compartmentalizes and classifies, and follows a linear, temporal flow. In contrast, some indigenous cultures take a far more holistic view of time and the world, and may have very different approaches to logic and order. In these cases, less structured 'yarning' and allowing the patient to tell their story can be more effective in obtaining a history and engaging the patient than a series of directed questions. This can be followed up by 'filling in the gaps' with more structured questions, linked where possible to the story you have already elicited. A holistic approach to medical, psychological and social needs is recommended.

There is currently still little evidence on how standard psychological techniques should be adapted to indigenous cultures. Certainly, it is particularly important with the indigenous client to consider the home, family and community context, as extended family and kinship or community ties, and responsibilities can be particularly strong. These ties can bring both challenges and resources. If close kin are also problem drinkers, it can be challenging for a dependent drinker to avoid cues to drinking. On the other hand, non-drinking relatives may provide great support. An awareness that for every patient (indigenous or non-indigenous) cultural and spiritual beliefs influence behaviour is important.

Indigenous peoples have their own cultural beliefs regarding health and treating sickness, which must be acknowledged and respected. In some indigenous communities specific traditional approaches to healing have been utilized in treatment of substance use disorders. For example, in North America sweat lodges have been used in rehabilitation for alcohol dependence. Efforts need to be made to ensure that treatment respects the patient's culture, but also includes access to the full range of modern therapies, including pharmacotherapies. In many countries health services run by indigenous communities provide an alternative to mainstream services or work in collaboration with mainstream services.

Box 12.12 Principles for improving a treatment service for indigenous peoples

- Consultation with indigenous community representatives—to identify and address any barriers to treatment access
- Collaboration and consultation with indigenous-specific services where available
- Cultural awareness training
- Employment of indigenous staff, including translators where necessary, and their involvement in service planning
- Particular attention to a friendly, welcoming, flexible atmosphere
- A visually appealing service and printed materials
- Health care that integrates services for mental, physical, psychological and social needs as far as possible
- keeping in mind the individual as part of the family, extended kinship and community.

The patient in the context of the community

At times, whole communities may be seriously affected by alcohol or drug use disorders. This tends to normalize heavy substance use, and also provide a traumatic and sometimes violent environment for children and adults alike. In communities such as these, where an individual seeks to stop drinking they can face immense challenges, with constant cue exposure and stressors. It can be challenging for communities to tackle these problems, given the threats to cultural values and traditional authority systems with colonization, and current social disruption. Support of community efforts to address drinking is likely to increase the chance of success of any one individual. Some remote communities afflicted by widespread alcohol misuse have successfully embraced a range of supply controls, including regional alcohol bans, restrictions to the amount or time, or location of alcohol sales, restriction of sales to low alcohol beer, or a system of individual permits to buy alcohol, where a permit is lost in the case of alcohol-related violence. These measures have had documented success.

In efforts to reduce volatile substance misuse in Australia, good results have been obtained by supply control (switch to non-sniffable fuel) combined with increasing opportunities for young people and for general community members to be productively engaged with work or community life.

Further reading

Gray D, Saggers S, Sputore B, Bourbon D. What works? A review of evaluated alcohol misuse interventions among Aboriginal Australians. *Addiction* 2000; **95**: 11–22.

Kirmayer LJ, Brass GM, Tait CL. The mental health of Aboriginal peoples: transformations of identity and community. *Canadian Journal of Psychiatry—Revue Canadienne de Psychiatrie*, 2000; **45**: 607–616.

Saggers S, Gray D, eds. *Dealing with alcohol: indigenous usage in Australia, New Zealand and Canada.* Cambridge: Cambridge University Press 1998.

Addicted physicians

The prevalence of substance use disorders among medical practitioners is overall similar to that in the general community. However there are some distinct differences: doctors smoke tobacco far less than the general population in many countries (e.g. Australia, UK). Rates of dependence on opioids, particularly pethidine and fentanyl are higher than the general community, indicating availability to be a relevant aetiological factor. Approximately 43% of doctors used opioids before being detected and 15% listed depression as a trigger for their substance use.

Within the medical profession, there are great variations in prevalence. High risk groups among physicians are anaesthetists, emergency medicine physicians, psychiatrists, rural general practitioners and practitioners in solo practices. Male doctors are at greater risk than female doctors. Younger men with an average age 30–39 years are more likely to be polydrug users. Among doctors over the age of 45 years, there is a high prevalence of co-morbid depression.

Risk factors include family history of addictions, co-morbid psychiatric illness, concurrent physical illness, marital problems, poor coping skills with stress, particularly work-related stresses. Education and intelligence are not protective factors.

Addiction in medical practitioners emphasizes the positive reinforcement of wanting to use, as well as the reinforcement of avoiding withdrawal. Once addicted to pethidine, previously obsessional doctors will break the law, lie outrageously, ignore relationships, compromise patient care and defy authority, long before they have begun to exhibit clear withdrawal features.

Barriers to treatment

Because of fear of stigma, loss of registration or of loss of omnipotence, impaired physicians rationalize, deny, or minimize their alcohol or drug use. They tend to avoid the patient role and continue to self diagnose and self medicate.

Box 12.13 Substance using doctors—work related stresses

- Overwork
- Sleep deprivation
- Exposure to trauma and death
- Ethical and diagnostic dilemmas
- Treatment failures
- Inadequate resources and support
- Medical and legal concerns
- Conflict work/life balance.

Box 12.14 Pointers to the possibility of substance use disorder

Behavioural changes
- Change of personality
- Mood changes
- Decreased efficiency and decisiveness
- Poor compliance with required documentation
- Inappropriate prescribing
- Increase in sick days
- Patient complaints—attitude and behaviour, inadequate pain relief.
- Collecting patient medication from pharmacy.

Evidence of advanced disease
- Smells of alcohol at work
- Intoxicated/drug affected at work, work functions
- Dishevelled appearance at work
- Evidence of drug use—track marks, drowsy, tremulous

Box 12.15 Dealing with an addicted colleague

- 'Take action or make sure someone does'
- Seek advice/inform senior colleagues
- Consider impact on clinical work
- Encourage self -reporting
- Inform the relevant Medical Board—not mandatory in all regions, but may have ethical and professional responsibility to do so.

Colleagues of impaired physicians, even when they eventually identify alcohol or drug use generally do not know what to do. They do not want to create waves and hope that someone else will act. They fear legal action and feel intimidated.

The treating doctor tends to treat the impaired physician as a colleague and not as a patient. Over-identification, collusion, denial, avoidance, minimization, and rescuing all act as barriers to appropriate treatment.

Consequences of not taking action

The impaired physician is a threat not only to him/her self, but to patients and to the family. Lives can be ruined and careers destroyed without the phenomenon of withdrawal. Once addicted to pethidine or other drugs, previously obsessional doctors will break the law, lie outrageously, ignore relationships, compromise patient care, and defy authority long before they have begun to exhibit clear withdrawal features.

Management

Effective physician health programmes provide a combination of treatment and monitoring.

Monitoring

Workplace monitoring may involve anything from an occasional chat with peers or employers to regular use of a breathalyser. Chemical monitoring is most commonly undertaken by drug urinalysis, but may also include carbohydrate deficient transferrin for the alcohol dependent and liver function tests for those in whom hepatic damage has already been established.

Treatment is provided completely separately from this monitoring programme.

Treatment

- Individual case management, with regular appointments with a counsellor
- Group supervision, where peers also under supervision are able to give feedback and support, facilitated by a clinician with group work skills.

Comprehensive assessment and treatment are required components and are assured given the intensity of this monitoring. Consistent application of behavioural principles means that restrictions on hours of work, prescribing and intensity of monitoring can be relaxed in a stepwise fashion as longevity of abstinence is established. Thus, very real markers of progress, such as going from three times weekly urinalysis to random fortnightly urines reinforce recovery. Any return to substance use results in negative consequences, such as restricted working hours or even suspension of registration. Monitoring typically persists till participants have 3–5 years of continuous abstinence, after which relapse rates are quite low.

Given the success of this approach, one would think that the only issue was how to propagate it. Politics often intervene. More punitive programmes necessarily receive lower referral rates, but may erroneously be able to reassure the unwary that it is illness rates not referral rates that are lower than those jurisdictions with more permissive policies and consequent higher rates of involvement in monitoring. Medical boards are entrusted to act in the best interests of the public. More progressive boards have decided that this goal is served by having the overt aim of returning addicted doctors to work, thereby decreasing barriers to involvement in the programme and exposing more of the iceberg of medical addiction.

Box 12.16 Treating the substance using doctor

- Treat as a patient not as a colleague
- Assess as for any patient: history, clinical examination
- Do not assume knowledge of the problem
- Do not expect to take more responsibility for their own management
- Provide information as for any other patient
- Be directive about follow-up
- Never allow to prescribe or procure their own medication.

When under close supervision of a medical board or physician health programme, wonderful outcomes have been achieved that are unthinkable in the rest of addiction medicine. Programmes like the one in Ontario claim to have results as good as 75% remaining continuously abstinent for 5 years and another 17% responding to treatment after initial relapses. The Tennessee programme is remarkable for the fact that its supervisees are regarded as good risks by the local indemnifying organization.

The person who has developed a persistent pattern of irrational behaviour will characteristically excuse, obfuscate, or minimize their behaviour and so it is with recently identified medical addicts. There is often focus on the 'outrageous excesses' of the medical board or monitoring programme. But as time allows greater distance, and longevity of abstinence increases, awareness dawns that they could have been managed much more harshly and gratitude usually replaces the previous hostility towards those who acted as their external conscience when their own had failed them. This illustrates the evolution of ego defence mechanisms from more primitive to more mature during the recovery process.

Recovery is further clarified by the alacrity with which so many (though certainly not all) addicted doctors bond to 12-step groups. Many of the harsher stereotypes of AA/NA members are broken when these men and women of science with high intellect and intact professions happily and productively incorporate a spiritual dimension into their recovery lives.

Once committed to the altruistic 12-step path, physicians will form groups with considerable power. An example of this process is the recovery specific groups in North America—International Doctors in Alcoholics Anonymous (www.idaa.org), the United Kingdom—the British Doctors and Dentists Group (http://www.medicouncilalcol.demon.co.uk/bddg.htm) and Australia—Australian Doctors in Recovery (www.ausdocsinrecovery). Equally, recovery has allowed many to make contributions to addiction medicine and to the general community.

Further reading

Cadman M, Bell J. Doctors detected self-administering opioids in New South Wales, 1985–1994: characteristics and outcomes.[see comment]. *Medical Journal of Australia*. 1998; **169**(8): 419–421.

Weir E. Substance abuse among physicians. *Canadian Medical Association Journal* 2000; **162**: 1730.

Specific clinical situations

The sleepless patient

The subjective experience of insomnia, with difficulty getting off to sleep, frequent and prolonged awakenings during the night and early morning wakening are very common in substance-abusing patients who are abstinent. In fact, about 60% of alcohol-dependent patients suffer from insomnia before they stop drinking, and have probably self-medicated with alcohol to get to sleep, and opiate dependent individuals with sleep problems use benzodiazepines or alcohol to help initiate sleep. Co-morbidity of substance abuse and depression is common, and the effects of both conditions on sleep are additive.

In non-dependent drinkers, alcohol promotes sleep, both by shortening the time to fall asleep (sleep onset latency) and by increasing deep restorative sleep in the first part of the night, although later in the night sleep is worse than without alcohol. However, in heavy and dependent daily drinkers the opposite occurs, so that sleep is difficult to initiate, lighter and more interrupted than normal, probably because of changes in brain GABA-A and glutamate receptors. This fragmented pattern persists into abstinence, with subjective complaints of frequent awakenings and difficulty getting off to sleep at night.

Opioid-dependent individuals maintained on adequate doses of methadone, and without sleep complaints may be satisfied with their sleep on admission for detoxification, but as methadone is tapered about 70–80% of patients will complain of sleeplessness, usually with a peak 5–10 days after taper is started. This often continues for weeks after detoxification and can persist for months in some patients. The mechanism for this is unknown—insomnia after heroin withdrawal is short-lived and, although methadone has a longer duration of action in the brain, this alone does not account for its detrimental effects on sleep. One possibility is that because methadone has some activity at glutamate receptors, adaptive changes in these may lead to the withdrawal syndrome. Buprenorphine, used more commonly now in opiate addiction, has been reported to give rise to fewer sleep problems on withdrawal but this is based on very few studies.

Why should we be taking these sleep complaints seriously and treating them?

First, sleep difficulty has a tremendous impact on quality of life in general, as we all know from just one or two disturbed nights. Persistent insomnia often leads to tiredness, difficulties in concentrating, irritability, and sometimes low mood. Secondly, sleep problems are not only distressing but also predict relapse in abstinent alcohol-dependent patients, and often in opiate addiction too. In a study by Drummond et al. (1998) sleep problems 5 months after stopping drinking predicted relapse at 14 months. Brower et al. (2001) similarly reported that patients who had had insomnia while drinking were twice as likely to relapse. Therefore, treating insomnia in these patients is a key element in primary goal of preventing relapse.

Treating the sleepless patient

Early abstinence: alcohol

Prescription of traditional hypnotic medication, such as benzodiazepines, is usually not appropriate in this group because of concerns about misuse, although to treat other symptoms early in abstinence these patients generally receive a long-acting benzodiazepine, such as chlordiazepoxide. Giving part of the daily dose at night will help sleep, as well as withdrawal the next day. Other drugs such as antidepressants are also known to improve sleep, particularly those blocking 5HT2 receptors, such as mirtazapine and trazodone, and may be considered in those patients with depression.

Detoxification: opioid dependence

Both clonidine and lofexidine, a similar compound, improve agitation during opiate detox, and also seem to help sleep. Zopiclone is occasionally prescribed at night, as are antihistamines which induce drowsiness and decrease anxiety.

Maximizing the chances of good sleep

During the difficult time of early abstinence there is a lot to think about in terms of lifestyle reorganization, but the impact of insomnia is so great that we believe that it is worth emphasizing and addressing any sleep problems. For instance, a sleep diary could replace a drink diary in alcoholics.

Strengthening the processes that initiate and maintain nightly sleep is very important, both during early abstinence and also during the weeks and months following, when a stable sleep-wake pattern will help patients adapt to the changes in their lives.

Three processes that contribute to good sleep

The homeostatic or recovery drive to sleep

The longer the time without sleep the higher this drive to sleep becomes, and during sleep it declines. The ideal time from one period of sleep to the next is about 16 h, so if someone is used to getting up at 08:30, then the maximum sleep drive on this process will be at about 00:30. Taking a nap in the afternoon will delay the sleep drive, so sleep will be more difficult to initiate then.

The circadian process

A large number of physical processes follow a circadian variation that is they show a regular pattern which repeats every day. The timing of this circadian rhythm is controlled within the brain by a few cells in the hypothalamus, which function as the body's biological clock, controlling many bodily processes, including the sleep-wake cycle. This clock is reset by light and other stimuli each day, thus making the circadian rhythm stronger. Exposure to daylight in the morning (even on overcast days) resets the body clock via a neural pathway directly from the eyes to the hypothalamus. Other influences on the clock are routines such as activity in the day and eating and drinking. Irregular routines of any kind decrease the strength of the circadian sleep-wake rhythm, and make sleeping (or being wide awake) at the desired time more difficult.

One common disruption happens in people without a fixed routine, like recovering addicts. They get into a habit of staying up late at night and sleeping late the next morning. Their innate rhythm is shifted through the day, so that on a day when they have an appointment say at 9 am their body clock is still 'switched' to sleep, and if they try to go to bed earlier at night the clock is still in the awake phase.

Arousal level—influence on sleep

Although it seems obvious, this aspect of sleep propensity is extremely important, particularly when insomnia is a problem. Maintaining a high level of arousal during the day, both physically with exercise and activity, and mentally with interesting or demanding tasks, and decreasing this level as bedtime approaches, is as important for sleep as the other 2 processes above. It is also the process which most commonly goes wrong. Boredom and inactivity during the day results in unwanted naps, and high levels of mental arousal late in the evening leaves us in lying in bed with the mind racing, unable to get to sleep.

All 3 of the processes above are commonly disrupted in early abstinence from alcohol, with the chaotic lifestyle which has often become established during drinking, taking a long time to settle down to a regular pattern.

To address sleep difficulties, advice to clients should ideally include the following

Homeostatic
- No naps in the day
- Schedule enough time for sleep at night.

Circadian
- Stick to a regular routine, particularly a regular getting-up time, even on weekends
- Get some daylight in the morning
- Take some exercise every day, in the morning or early evening (not after 20.00 h).

Arousal
- Keep the bedroom for sleeping or sex, no TV in bed
- Wind down towards bedtime
- Deal with problems early in the evening, write them down, no worrying about bills in bed.

Synthesis

Sleep problems in early abstinence are similar to those experienced by other groups of patients with insomnia, and can lead to relapse if not taken seriously and treated appropriately. Many aspects of good sleep habits may need to be reinforced. The best approach may lie in making healthy life style changes and reinforcing sleep hygiene. We recommend making these an integral part of a treatment programme for alcohol and drug dependent patients in abstinence, particularly in the first few days to weeks.

Further reading

Beswick T, Best D, Rees S, Bearn J, Gossop M, Strang J. Major disruptions of sleep during treatment of the opiate withdrawal syndrome: differences between methadone and lofexidine detoxification treatments. *Addiction Biology* 2003; **8**: 49–57.

Brower KJ. Insomnia, alcoholism and relapse. *Sleep Medical Review* 2003; **7**: 523–539.

Brower KJ, Aldrich MS, Robinson EA, Zucker RA, Greden JF. Insomnia, self-medication, and relapse to alcoholism. *American Journal of Psychiatry* 2001; **158**: 399–404.

Drummond SP, Gillin JC, Smith TL, DeModena A. The sleep of abstinent pure primary alcoholic patients: natural course and relationship to relapse. *Alcohol Clinical Experimental Research* 1998; **22**: 1796–1802.

Insomnia: A Clinical Guide to Assessment and Treatment. Charles Morin and Colin Espie Kluwer, 2003.

The Consultation-Liaison Service

Consultation-Liaison (C-L) Services in Addiction Medicine originated in the 1970s in several countries and now form an important component of service provision. The most common setting in which they operate is within general hospitals. C-L services in general hospitals were developed in recognition of the high proportion of patients who are admitted with disorders caused by the use of alcohol, tobacco, addictive medications and illicit drugs. Other C-L services have been established more recently, such as those provided to police detention facilities and prisons. A variant of these services involves outreach to high risk populations such as homeless and transient people, the mentally ill, and former prisoners.

The principal aims of consultation-liaison services are two-fold:
- To provide advice on the clinical management of patients or other persons who are known or considered possibly to have an alcohol, tobacco, medication or illicit drug problem, with the goal of optimizing their treatment
- To increase the knowledge, skills, familiarity, and professional practice standards of staff in hospital wards and other facilities where persons with the substance disorders are present.

The justification for such services is optimization of in-patient treatment regimes, and many studies have shown that they are very cost effective through the minimization of admission duration.

The scope of clinical management

Consultation-Liaison services are very diverse in terms of the clinical management that they provide. At a very basic level, the service may be confined to the provision of information material about substance use and its attendant disorders, and on telephone help lines, counselling agencies, self-help groups, and other relevant local services. At a more well-formed level, the service may provide assessment and brief therapy for hazardous substance use or substance dependence, which might include a session of counselling on the ward or arrangements made for the person to attend a self-help group.

More comprehensive C-L services provide specialist assessment of the patient's substance use and related disorders in the context of their presenting condition and psychosocial background. Such consultation-liaison services are typically multidisciplinary. The initial assessment may be undertaken by a specialist consultation-liaison nurse, with training in addiction, psychiatric or medical nursing, a medical resident, a postgraduate medical trainee in addiction medicine, psychiatry or general medicine, or a medical addiction specialist. Typically, there would be regular meetings of the multidisciplinary team to confer, update team members and establish a management plan for the patient from a multidisciplinary perspective.

The most common forms of assessment and management such a team would provide include:

- Assessment of the risk of withdrawal syndrome and advice on its treatment
- Management of detoxification from alcohol, tobacco, prescribed medication or illicit drugs
- Comprehensive assessment of substance use where the history has been difficult to elicit or is inconsistent, to identify the aetiological significance of substance use for the presenting disease
- The management of acute, e.g. post-operative pain in a person with known or suspected substance (particularly opioid) dependence
- The assessment and management of a person with chronic pain, and known or suspected drug (particularly opioid dependence)
- The management of drug-seeking behaviour particularly in a hospital setting
- The differential diagnosis of post-operative delirium in a patient with known or suspected substance dependence
- The linking of patients to continuing therapy for their substance use disorder following discharge from hospital
- Contribution to the discharge planning process from a substance use disorder perspective.

Enhancing the skills of hospital staff

The second and equally important objective of C-L services is to enhance the knowledge, skills and professional practice of staff who have not been specifically trained in addiction management. The underlying principle is that of a multiplicative effect: the C-L service contributes to the optimal management of patients with substance use disorders to a greater extent than could be achieved by direct patient management alone. The C-L Service would typically provide in-service training sessions for hospital ward staff in the assessment of substance use and related disorders, the assessment of risk of withdrawal, training in monitoring withdrawal states, and in the nursing and pharmacological management of patients in withdrawal states. Other topics might include the recognition and management of drug-seeking behaviour and the development of policies to manage such patients. The in-service sessions may take the form of case presentations or may adopt a more didactic approach in the form of a lecture or tutorial.

Pain and opioid dependence

Opioid drugs are powerful analgesics, which, in addition to relieving pain, promote a sense of well-being and relaxation. Opioids have a number of **side effects**, including nausea and vomiting, constipation, increased sweating, and decreased sexual function. Side-effects probably contribute to quite high rates of early discontinuation of opioid treatment for chronic pain.

Hyperalgesia

Hyperalgesia describes a syndrome in which pain sensitivity is increased, and analgesic response to opioids is diminished, in association with neuro-adaptation to opioids. For example, patients receiving methadone treatment for heroin dependence tolerate cold-pressor pain only half as long as do matched controls. Treatment with buprenorphine also produces hyperalgesia, although to a lesser degree than methadone.

This phenomenon is not simply a particular genetic or personality vulnerability among people who have been addicted to heroin; individuals who abuse stimulants and those who abuse opioids have been shown to be less tolerant of pain than former drug users who are now drug free.

Tolerance and withdrawal

The repeated administration of opioids can produce **tolerance and withdrawal**. After a period of prolonged exposure, ceasing the opioid may lead to physiological and psychological changes—an 'abstinence' or 'withdrawal syndrome'. Some relevant features are generalized aches and pains, dysphoric mood, and craving for opioids. During withdrawal, patients are more depressed, and more sensitive to pain.

Repeated administration of opioids, in some individuals and in some social contexts, can also produce **dependence**, a pattern of thinking, and behaviour in which drug use and drug-seeking become self-perpetuating, dominant behaviours, displacing other activities, and producing harm to the individual. As described in Chapter 8 opioids, p. 206 dependence is characterized by:

- Tolerance
- Withdrawal
- The substance is often taken in larger amounts over a longer period than was intended
- There is a persistent desire or unsuccessful efforts to cut down or control substance use
- A great deal of time is spent in activities necessary to obtain, use or recover from using the substance
- Important social, occupational or recreational activities are given up or reduced because of substance use
- The substance use is continued despite knowledge of having a persistent or recurrent physical or psychological problem that is likely to have been caused or exacerbated by the substance.

These criteria are cited to illustrate the difficulty in diagnosing drug dependence in the presence of chronic pain. While many people with chronic pain retain active lifestyles and remain socially connected, some patients with chronic pain adopt a very restricted, invalid lifestyle, becoming preoccupied with pain and pain relief. If they request increases in analgesia requirement, clinicians are uncertain whether this reflects tolerance (criterion 1) or simply inadequate pain relief. Once established on opioids, if blood levels fall, resulting withdrawal symptoms are experienced as an increase in pain (criterion 2). Many have unrealistic expectations of cure meaning they frequently find themselves taking medication for longer than planned (criterion 3) or periodically try to cut down on medication and experience associated worsening of pain (criterion 4). Some withdraw from social and occupational roles, (criteria 5 and 6). In short, many people with chronic pain and using opioid drugs have behaviours consistent with dependence or with pain.

Addiction is another term frequently used in association with opioid drugs. There is a readily recognizable 'addict' lifestyle, people habitually using drugs, often involved in crime, a lifestyle characterized by poor social integration, often illegal activity, and a central focus on drug-seeking and drug use. Despite its popular usage and familiar stereotype, 'addiction' is ill-defined. The problem with using the label 'addict' (which is how many drug users identify themselves) is that it is a judgement, rather than a description. The risk is that we can use the label 'addict' to dismiss people's request for analgesia, to 'blame the patient', rather than treating them as complex patients to be managed with care.

The contribution of opioids to pain

Repeated withdrawal symptoms, an increase in somatic focusing, and opioid-induced hyperalgesia may contribute to perpetuating and worsening chronic pain states. About 40% of heroin users entering a US methadone programme reported having chronic pain, confirming that many opioid-dependent people develop chronic pain.

Place of opioids in pain management

In the past, opioids were used sparingly, but doctors now face pressure to offer 'adequate' analgesia for all pain complaints. In this section we review the three critical questions—are opioids effective, what is the risk of dependence, and what is the risk of diversion of prescribed opioids.

Effectiveness of opioids in chronic non-cancer pain

A recent meta-analysis of 41 randomized trials, involving 6019 patients, examined the effectiveness of opioids in chronic, non-cancer pain, and concluded that opioids were more effective than placebo for both pain and functional outcomes. Most studies were short (mean duration 5 weeks (range 1–16), yet dropout rates were high; 33% in the opioid groups, and 38% in the placebo groups. Pooling trials where there were comparisons with naproxen or nortriptyline, although strong opioids produced better pain relief, they did not produce better functional outcomes than naproxen or nortriptyline.

Most trials were sponsored by the pharmaceutical industry, consistent with the rapidly expanding market for opioid drugs.

Risks of dependence

Most efficacy trials are too short for a reliable estimate to be made of the risks of drug dependence and misuse associated with opioids for chronic pain. Despite this, controlled clinical trials of opioids usually report problems of 'non-compliance' with medication in around 10–15% of participants. Such trials usually exclude people with histories of substance misuse, and as a result are likely to under-estimate the frequency with which problems arise. One recent, 'real world' study investigated patients with chronic, non-cancer pain who were referred to a chronic pain disease management programme within an academic internal medicine practice (Ives, 2006). Over the 1-year study period, opioid misuse occurred in 62 (32%) patients. Fifteen patients were found to have repeatedly negative urine drug screens for prescribed opioids, suggesting diversion.

Diversion and misuse of prescribed opioids

A recent US study investigated new entrants to methadone treatment. Thirty-eight per cent of entrants to treatment reported they were primarily dependent on prescription opioids. The most frequent source of prescribed opioids were dealer, friend, or relative, or doctor's prescription. Internet or forged prescriptions were uncommon. Prescription opioid dependence was particularly common in the age group 18–25.

Predictors of opioid misuse

- Age (18–25 years)
- Family history of substance use
- History of cocaine use
- Drug or drink driving convictions
- Low socio-economic status (misuse and diversion).

Pain management in patients dependent on opioids

Patients receiving maintenance methadone are cross-tolerant to the analgesic effects of morphine and pain relief, when obtained, does not last as long as expected.

Management of acute pain

Patients currently dependent on opioids

If a heroin user is hospitalized, it is judicious to commence methadone (to manage opioid withdrawal) and then add opioid analgesia as needed. As with any patient commencing treatment, care is required to avoid respiratory depression during the first week of treatment and naloxone should be readily available.

If a heroin user on methadone maintenance treatment is admitted to hospital and has a condition requiring analgesia, appropriate management is to maintain on the patient's usual dose of methadone (after verifying dose and time of last dose with the methadone prescriber), and administer other analgesics in addition, titrating the dose against the patient's response. Typically, opioids such as morphine or fentanyl are administered for the relief of pain.

Patients on methadone maintenance treatment with acute pain of sufficient severity to warrant opioid analgesia require higher and more frequent doses of opioid analgesics to achieve adequate pain control, even when methadone is continued at the usual dose. If the patient is unable to take methadone orally, and there are no precautions (such as head injury or respiratory compromise), one option is to administer methadone by intramuscular injection, giving one-third of the dose, twice daily, while patient is unable to take medication by mouth.

Pain management of opioid dependent patients on buprenorphine maintenance treatment is more complex. This is because buprenorphine is a partial opioid agonist (or mixed agonist-antagonist) with a high affinity for the mu receptors and slow dissociation from the receptor. This results in a plateau effect both for efficacy and toxicity. There are theoretical reasons why patients maintained on buprenorphine might have little response to opioid analgesics. However, in practice, this does not appear to be a major problem. Patients on buprenorphine should continue on it, and additional opioid analgesia administered, titrated against response.[1]

Patients who were formerly opioid dependent

Managing acute pain in drug-free, formerly opioid-dependent people, is more complex. Although the risk is difficult to quantify, such patients are at risk of relapse to drug dependence if exposed to opioids. However, withholding analgesia if it is clearly needed is not appropriate. In situations opioid analgesia is clearly indicated, it should not be withheld, but patients should be closely monitored. In general, it is preferable to discuss risks with the patient, and explore the use of non-opioid analgesia.

Management of acute pain

- Skilled nursing—reassure patient; monitor regularly for signs of opioid toxicity.
- Continue current opioid maintenance treatment with methadone (or buprenorphine).
- Identify cause and provide adequate pain relief:
- Opioids: morphine with patient controlled analgesia or as required (may require 2–3 times higher than standard doses; careful monitoring). Alternatively fentanyl may be used
- If mild start with non-opioid analgesics—paracetamol, NSAIDs, tramadol
- Tricyclic anti-depressants.
- Non-pharmacological interventions.

---

[1] In the management of acute pain in hospitalized opioid dependent patients who have been maintained on buprenorphine, some centres discontinue buprenorphine and replace it with methadone (starting dose 30–40 mg) to manage opioid withdrawal and add opioid analgesics (morphine or fentanyl) for adequate pain control. However, this may sometimes cause difficulties/complications.

Managing chronic pain, managing dependence

Managing chronic pain in opioid-dependent people is complex, and is a case for specialist assessment and management. Care should be co-ordinated with the doctor delivering methadone treatment. It is usually not appropriate to prescribe other opioids in addition to methadone or buprenorphine.

There is a tendency, particularly in the American literature, to maintain a dichotomy between patients with a valid problem (pain), for which opioids are indicated, and patients with a character flaws (addiction) in whom opioids should be avoided. The irony is that opioids are effective drugs for the management of opioid dependence, but only modestly effective in treatment of chronic pain.

Given the rising problem of diversion of opioids prescribed for pain, it is no longer valid, if it ever was, to make rigid distinctions between pre-scribing opioids for treatment of pain, and prescribing for treatment of dependence. This has led some authors to recommend 'universal precau-tions'—adequate assessment, urine testing, and at times daily dispensing of medication—in prescribing opioids, whether for pain or for treatment of established dependence.

Supervision of administration, monitoring with urine drug screens, regular appointments to review progress—are all parts of the structure of treatment. For people with a sense of loss of control over their pain, their lives, and/or their drug use, externally imposed controls are thera-peutically useful. By minimizing the temptation to divert or misuse pre-scribed medication, it makes treatment safer. The importance of such structures as part of treatment seems to be better appreciated by patients than by clinical staff, who tend to regard structures as imposed by regulatory authorities.

Management of chronic pain in opioid dependent patients

Relieve pain
- Prescribe methadone or buprenorphine in adequate doses
- Non-opioid analgesics: paracetamol, NSAIDs).
Dosing should be on a regular, rather than on a prn basis
- Adjunctive analgesia.
Tricyclic or other mixed action anti-depressants (also relieves neuro-pathic pain).

Non pharmacological interventions
- CBT
- Physiotherapy.

Avoid
- Short-acting, parenteral opioids
- Benzodiazepines.

Precautions
- Always contact the patient's usual methadone or buprenorphine prescriber to verify the current maintenance dose and time of last use before administering methadone or buprenorphine.
- Consult Addiction Specialists during the patient's admission
- The Addiction Specialist and Pain Management team should work in collaboration recognizing the different perspectives that each speciality contributes to the management process
- In opioid dependent patients, buprenorphine (a mixed agonist-antagonist) may:
  - Reduce the effect of opioid agonists or
  - Precipitate withdrawals if given too soon after the last dose of the opioid. For short acting opioids wait at least 8 h before recommencing buprenorphine. For longer acting preparations wait 12–24 h
- Methadone may cause prolongation of the QT interval in high doses
- Although its 'ceiling effect' gives buprenorphine a relatively safe profile, respiratory depression caused by buprenorphine in conjunction with other respiratory depressant drugs is not readily reversed by naloxone
- Drug interactions: (also see pp. 225–226):
  - Fluvoxamine/methadone—increased methadone levels
  - Pethidine or tramadol/MAOIs—adverse effects
  - Risk of serotonin syndrome:
    - pethidine/SSRIs
    - tramadol/SSRIs
  - Risk of CNS depression with a combination of CNS depressants such as opioids, alcohol, benzodiazepines, anaesthetics.

Conclusions: opioid dependence and chronic pain

Many clinicians have had the experience that attempting to wean from opioids people with established opioid dependence and chronic pain can be a very damaging experience. Prescribing oral, long-acting opioids with appropriate monitoring is usually a better strategy. However, it does not follow that long-acting opioids are a good treatment for chronic pain. They are good treatment for opioid dependence.

Data from clinical trials suggests only modest benefits of opioids over placebo in the management of chronic pain. While it may be possible to minimize the risk by careful patient selection, there is considerable data that many people on opioids prescribed for pain have previous or current histories of substance use disorders, and in this group misuse of medication is not rare. The management of chronic pain should involve multiple modalities before consideration of opioid therapy.

Table 13.1 Approximate equi-analgesic doses of various opioids

Opioid	Oral	Parenteral	Duration of action (h)
Morphine	30 mg	10 mg	Injection: 2–3 h
Codeine	180–240 mg		Linctus: 3–4 h
Methadone	Acute dosing 30 mg Chronic dosing 7 mg (methadone accumulates—it takes ~5 half lives, or 5–7 days, to reach steady state levels)	In patients on methadone maintenance treatment, give two-thirds of the usual dose in two split doses IM	Syrup/tablet or injection: 6–8 h initially; increases to >24 hours with long term use
Buprenorphine	0.4 mg	0.1 mg IV or SC	6–8 h
Oxycodone	10 mg	5 mg	3–4 h tabs/injection 12 h SR tab
Pethidine	–	100 mg IM or IV	2–3 h
Tramadol	100–150 mg	50–100 mg IM or IV	3–6 h
Fentanyl		100 micrograms IM, IV, SC	0.5–2 h lozenge/injection 72 h -patch

Adapted from Therapeutic Guidelines 2007.

Further reading

Alford DP, Compton P, Samet JH. Acute pain management for patients receiving maintenance methadone or buprenorphine therapy. *Annals of Internal Medicine* 2006; **144**: 127–134.

Gourlay D, Heit HA, Almahrezi A. Universal precautions in pain medicine: a rational approach to the treatment of chronic pain. *Pain Medicine* 2005; **6**(2): 107–112.

Ives TJ, Cheloninski PR, Hammett–Stabler CA, Malone R, Perhac JS, Potisek NM, Shillday BB, DeNalt DA, Pignone MP, (2006). Predictors of opioid misuse in patients with chronic pain: a prospective cohort study BMC Health Services Research 2006; **6**: 46.

Mao J. Opioid-induced abnormal pain sensitivity: implications in clinical opioid therapy. *Pain* 2002; **100**: 213–217.

Therapeutic Guidelines Analgesic. Version 5, 2007. Therapeutic Guidelines Ltd. http://www.tg.com.au

Medical complications of injecting drug use

Causes of complications

Complications may be due to:

- The pharmacology of the drug
- Contaminants and adulterants
- Unsafe injecting practices
- The associated lifestyle.

Complications related to contaminants and adulterants

Illicit heroin and other injected substances are typically non-sterile and the potency is unknown. The drug may be contaminated or 'cut' with a variety of substances, e.g. starch, talc. The user may experience unexpected allergic reactions, pharmacological effects or toxic effects. Injection of particulate matter may result in microemboli or granulomas.

Complications relating to unsafe injecting practices

Injecting illicit drugs and sharing of injecting equipment places individuals at risk of infections with a variety of agents including blood borne viruses (hepatitis C, B, and HIV), as well as bacteria and fungi. The vasculature and surrounding tissues are also exposed to repeated trauma and sometimes chemical irritation.

Non-infective local complications

- Aseptic thrombophlebitis
- Lymphoedema
- Indurated, thickened skin and soft tissue.

Associated lifestyle

These include complications related to marginalization, involvement in the criminal scene, efforts to obtain money for expensive illicit drugs (e.g. theft, sex work), etc (see p. 41).

Nutrition and self-care may be poor, because of the higher priority given to drug use than to other aspects of life.

Infections

Bacterial infections

Most commonly caused by *Staphylococcus aureus*; also *Streptococcus viridans*, *Pseudomonas*, aerobic Gram-negative rods, anaerobic cocci, clostridium, and rarely, community-acquired MRSA (methicillin-resistant *Staph. aureus*).

Local infections

Infections at the site of injection and surrounding soft tissue—septic thrombophlebitis, abscess, (see p. 44, Fig. 2.2) cellulitis, necrotizing fasciitis (mainly with clostridium following subcutaneous injection), necrotizing ulcers, gas gangrene, and pulsatile pseudo-aneurysms, e.g. in the neck or groin.

Systemic or distant infections
Bacterial infections may become systemic and life threatening. In cases of high unexplained or chronic fever in an injecting drug user always consider endocarditis, septicaemia, or another hidden focus of serious infection.

Bacterial endocarditis: An important problem with injecting drug use. Staphylococcus aureus is the most common organism accounting for 90% of cases. Other causes include *Streptococcus viridans, Pseudomonas aeruginosa*, and rarely candida and other fungal infections.

Although endocarditis typically affects the tricuspid valves it may also affect the mitral or aortic valves, particularly if there is pre-existing valvular disease. In left-sided endocarditis septic embolization may lead to abscesses in other organs such as the brain or spleen. Mycotic aneurysms may also result from systemic emboli.

Endocarditis may be a cause of unexplained fever and weight loss, with or without a murmur or other the typical features of endocarditis. If there is any suspicion of endocarditis the person should be referred urgently to hospital for investigation.

Do blood cultures in all febrile injecting drug users.

Emboli: Thrombo-embolism, metastatic abscesses, mycotic aneurysms.

Viral infections: Injecting drug users are at risk of one or more blood borne virus infections, and in particular hepatitis C, B, and HIV.

Hepatitis C: Injecting drug use is the single most important risk factor for spread of hepatitis C. The worldwide prevalence of hepatitis C among injecting drug users varies from 30 to 90% (e.g. 65–70% in Australia); incidence ranges from 10 to 30% per year. Hepatitis C is associated with a significant burden of chronic liver disease, including cirrhosis and hepatocellular carcinoma.

Hepatitis B is a less common complication than hepatitis C, and may be acquired through unsafe injecting practices or unprotected sex. Only about 15% are actively infected, 30% are HBc antibody positive, and only 50% are immune.

HIV: HIV prevalence rates vary from 1% among injecting drug users in Australia (where needle syringe exchange programs are available) to 20% in many cities in the US. In some countries (e.g. in many parts of Asia) HIV infection in injecting drug users is a relatively common complication, affecting up to 70% of injecting drug users with consequent risk of spread to other segments of the community. Should immunodeficiency develop the individual can present with a range of unusual and/or severe infections.

NB: The relatively limited impact of needle syringe exchange programs in prevention of hepatitis C transmission in contrast to its marked impact on HIV transmission levels suggests the greater efficiency of blood to blood hepatitic C transmission via sharing of injecting equipment and paraphenalia (other than needles), such as spoons, filters, swabs, tourniquets.

Fungal infections: Mainly candida, aspergillus and penicillium. Distant or systemic infection including fungal endocarditis, fungal ophthalmitis.

Candida albicans: Oral, vaginal or systemic candidiasis, particularly in patients with HIV (lemon juice used to dissolve substances may be a source of *Candida albicans*).

Illicit injection of diverted sublingual buprenorphine tablets increases the risk of blood borne of mouth organisms, including candida.

Sexually transmitted infections: chlamydia, syphilis, gonorrhoea and/or HIV may be acquired through unprotected sex, either as part of sex work to raise money for drugs, or when under the disinhibiting influence of alcohol or the influence of other substances (e.g sedated with heroin or benzodiazepines; or increased libido with stimulant use). HIV is more commonly associated with sexual activity than with injecting drug use.

Complications by body system Complications may also be due to the property of the drug, the injecting practices and/or the associated lifestyle. (Also refer to chapters and sections on individual drugs)

Cardiovascular complications
- Cardiomyopathy
- Arrhythmias (stimulants)
- Hypertension (stimulants)
- Myocardial infarction (cocaine)
- Endocarditis (see above)
- Vasculitis, vascular damage
- Vascular spasm due to local trauma of injecting, or injecting of cocaine
- Angiitis (amphetamines)
- Inadvertent or deliberate injecting into arteries with distal ischaemia, gangrene
- Embolism
- Arteriovenous aneurysm
- Mycotic aneurysms.

Pulmonary complications
- Pneumonia—bacterial pneumonia, e.g. as a result of septic embolism from endocarditis, pneumocystis (in HIV patients)
- Aspiration pneumonia
- Tuberculosis—consider in-patients presenting with pneumonia and HIV infection
- Lung abscess
- Atelectasis
- Pulmonary haemorrhage, pulmonary emboli, pulmonary infarction (from septic thrombophlebitis or coincident cocaine use)
- Non-cardiogenic pulmonary oedema (heroin)
- Pulmonary granulomas (from insoluble additives and/or injection of crushed tablets).

Gastrointestinal complications
- **Constipation**: constipation may be a troublesome complication of heroin and other opioid use. Occasionally reduced bowel motility becomes a medically serious complication with gastroparesis or intestinal pseudo-obstruction.
- Bowel infarction (cocaine)

- Hepatic ischaemia (cocaine)
- Hepatitis B, C.

Musculoskeletal complications
- Osteomyelitis
- Septic arthritis
- Rhabdomyolysis: may result from pressure following prolonged unconsciousness with heroin (and/or benzodiazepines, alcohol); also reported with cocaine or amphetamine use. May lead to acute renal failure if not diagnosed and appropriately treated.

Renal complications
- Renal failure secondary to rhabdomyolysis
- Glomerulonephritis, interstitial nephritis or immune mediated in viral hepatitis
- Nephropathy (including HIV associated).

Dental complications: As opioids (illicit or prescribed) dry the mouth, bacteria can reproduce more readily that cause dental decay. Combined with sometimes poor dental hygiene, dental decay is common. This can result in acute or chronic pain, and dental infections (p. 375).

CNS complications
- Overdose/coma or death from respiratory depression (heroin and other CNS depressants)
- Seizures (psychostimulants)
- Cerebrovascular accidents, cerebral infarct, cerebral haemorrhage (psychostimulants).

Neuropsychiatric complications
- Anxiety
- Depression
- Agitation, psychosis (stimulants)
- Altered consciousness, organic brain syndrome.

Physical examination
As described on pp. 42–47.

A systematic examination of the body systems is required.

In particular, look for signs of complications of injecting drug use, such as vein damage, stigmata of liver disease, cardiac murmurs, mental state examination.

Laboratory tests
Routine blood tests
- Full Blood Count (FBC)
- Urea and electrolytes (EUC)
- Liver function tests (LFT; isolated elevation of ALT suggests chronic hepatitis C infection; levels may fluctuate)
- Coagulation tests (INR, APTT).

Tests for sexually transmitted infections
Other investigations as indicated
- Blood cultures (if febrile, three sets to be taken before commencing treatment with antibiotics)
- Creatine phosphokinase (CPK, rhabdomyolysis; CK-MB; chest pain after cocaine use)
- Urine drug screen
- Chest X-ray
- Cardiac ECHO (suspected endocarditis)
- CT head/MRI when indicated (e.g. suspected cerebral abscess).

Assessment of blood borne viral infections
Assessment of blood borne viral infections should be undertaken at the drug and alcohol clinic or general practice as these patients will often not attend another speciality service, whilst still having problems with injecting drug use.

> Offer serological testing for hepatitis C and B and HIV to all patients with a history of injecting drug use and, where appropriate, tests for sexually transmitted infections.

Serological investigations for blood borne viruses
- **Hepatitis C**: Anti-HCV
  - If Hep C Ab positive, can periodically test HCV RNA (PCR) to assess if viral replication is occurring
- **Hepatitis B**: HBsAg, HBsAb, HBcAb (see below).
- **HIV**: Anti-HIV.

Pre- and post-test counselling is important, not only to avoid stress, but as an opportunity for raising awareness of the risks of blood-borne virus infection associated with injecting drug use and for ongoing monitoring should hepatitis be present.

> ### Interpretation of hepatitis C serology
>
> - **Hep C Ab positive**: current or past infection (60–70% of injecting drug users are Anti-HVC positive)
> - **HCV RNA (PCR) positive**: active replication of virus, infectivity (if positive, encourage patients to consider treatment)
> - **Hepatitis C** genotype and viral load (if treatment is being considered)
>
> Effective treatment of chronic hepatitis C is now available with pegylated interferon and ribavirin. All HCV RNA positive patient should be informed of the availability and efficacy of treatment.
> Treatment effectiveness varies for different genotypes.

Interpretation of hepatitis B serology

- **Hep B sAg positive**: acute or chronic infection with hepatitis B
  - If Hep BeAg is also positive there is a high level of viral replication, higher level of infectivity, higher risk of progression of HBV liver disease
- **Hep B cAb positive**:
  - Where HBsAg is negative, core antibody (IgG) represents past exposure to hepatitis B
  - Where HBsAg is positive, core antibody (IgM) may reflect acute infection or recent flare in chronic infection
- **Hep B sAb positive**: reflects immune state secondary to either vaccination or past infection.

Injecting drug users who are not immune to Hepatitis B should be offered vaccination.

Hepatitis B antigen positive patients with abnormal LFTs should be referred for possible treatment and their contacts followed up and tested.

Hepatitis B serology is complex and patients may, at times, revert from Ab +ve status to Ag +ve status, particularly in relation to eAg.

HBV DNA testing provides much more specific information about viral replication.

HBV genotyping is not currently routine, but may be used in future to provide information on disease severity and treatment responsiveness.

Serology for HIV

Anti-HIV positive: probable HIV infection, confirm with HIV RNA PCR or western blot.

If positive, refer for specialist care.

In some cases, liver ultrasound or CT scan may be indicated to assess the severity of viral hepatitis, or the presence of a complication such as hepatic carcinoma.

Treatment of complications

Bacterial endocarditis: Do three sets of blood cultures in all febrile injecting drug users before commencing treatment. Treat with intravenous antibiotics for at least 6 weeks. The team should involve addiction specialists, cardiologists, microbiologists and infectious disease specialists. A cardiothoracic surgeon should be involved if infection persists, there are repeated emboli or other complications

Blood borne virus infection: All injecting drug users should be advised of the risk of exposure to hepatitis C, hepatitis B and HIV, and should be well educated about the value of monitoring as an early warning system should disease progression occur. Patients should be educated on avoiding spread of hepatitis C , HIV and hepatitis B (e.g. care with blood spills or open wounds, safe disposal of sanitary pads, avoid sharing of toothbrushes, nail scissors or razors, washing hands; avoiding sexual spread of hepatitis B and HIV).

Hepatitis C: Hepatitis C has spread to epidemic proportions among injecting drug users. It is now the commonest reason for liver transplantation in many western countries. Patients with chronic hepatitis C infection are generally asymptomatic and often believe that if they feel well there is no need for testing or treatment. If symptoms occur, the main symptom is tiredness or lethargy.

Any patient who is hepatitis C antibody positive needs regular monitoring of LFTs (usually twice yearly) and testing for HCV RNA (PCR). A negative HCV RNA suggests that the virus has cleared, this happens without treatment in about 20–30% of cases. However, if HCV RNA remains positive it indicates active replication of the virus, as well as infectivity. Such patients should be encouraged to consider treatment to prevent progression of the disease and further spread of hepatitis C viral infection. If treatment is being considered, test for viral load and genotype.

Where there is persistently abnormal LFTs or evidence of reducing liver function (e.g. falling platelets or rising INR, even in the presence of normal LFTs), refer to a liver specialist.

Assessment for treatment will usually include liver ultrasound and/or CT scan. Some centres perform liver biopsy prior to treatment, though, in an attempt to remove barriers to treatment, this is becoming less routine in some countries (e.g. Australia).

Patients with hepatitis C should be advised not to drink alcohol to excess as this aggravates the severity of viral hepatitis. There is no clear evidence as to what level of drinking is safe in this condition. Although abstinence is the ideal goal, this may not be achievable . Some clinicians advise limiting consumption to half the recommended limit for a healthy person and ensuring the consumption is not daily.

Treatment with pegylated interferon and ribavarin is effective and can produce sustained viral response in 40–50% of genotype 1 and 4 infections, and up to 80% of genotype 2 and 3 infections.

Hepatitis B

Injecting drug users who are not immune to hepatitis B (or currently infected) should be offered vaccination.

Hepatitis B antigen-positive patients should be referred for possible treatment, and their contacts followed up and tested. Advice on preventing spread should be provided (e.g. vaccination of key contacts, protected sex with non-immune partners).

In persons with established cirrhosis, regular monitoring will include AFP and hepatic ultrasound, to screen for hepatic carcinoma. Wherever possible, treatment and monitoring will be conducted in association with a liver specialist.

HIV: Patients who are HIV Ab positive should be referred to the appropriate HIV specialist, e.g. immunologist or infectious diseases specialist to assess the need for treatment and for monitoring.

In addition to a multidisciplinary team treating the substance use disorder, treatment of complications of injecting drug use should involve referral to other relevant medical or psychiatric specialists.

Further reading

Beynon RP, Bahl K, Prendergast BD. Infective endocarditis—clinical review. *British Medical Journal* 2006; **333**: 334–339.

Cherubin CE, Sapira JD. The medical complications of drug addiction and the medical assessment of the intravenous drug user 25 years later. *Annals of Internal Medicine* 1993; **119**: 1017–1028.

Dore GJ, Thomas DL. Management and treatment of injecting drug users with hepatitis virus infection and HCV/Human Immunodeficiency Virus co-infection. *Seminars in Liver Disease* 2005; **25**: 18–32.

Gordon RJ, Lowy FD. Bacterial infections in drug users. *New England Journal of Medicine* 2005; **353**: 1945–1954.

The oral complications of drug and alcohol misuse

Epidemiology

Drug abuse and alcohol, combined with tobacco, may be associated with the following oral problems:

- Rampant caries
- Periodontal diseases
- Tooth surface loss
- Oral mucosal lesions.

It should be noted that there are few well controlled epidemiological studies, but many case reports and comparisons of dental health of drug abusers with data from national surveys.

Clinical presentations

Rampant caries

This describes rapidly progressing caries lesions affecting all surfaces of teeth where plaque stagnates. It may involve surfaces of teeth that are usually caries free. It is seen in opioid misuse, including the treatment modality, methadone, stimulant misuse including methamphetamines ('meth mouth'), cocaine, ecstasy, and barbiturate misuse. The rapid progression of caries lesions is due to:

- Xerostomia and salivary hypofunction caused by the drugs
- Poor oral hygiene as a consequence of a general lack of self-care
- Consumption of large amounts of carbonated sugary drinks often taken in an attempt to relieve dry mouth. Those taking opium and amphetamines often crave sugar. The stimulants (e.g. methamphetamine) increase metabolic rate, resulting in physical over-activity, excess perspiration and generalized dehydration
- Methadone is produced in a sugar syrup form and this treatment exacerbates the caries problem. Patients may retain methadone syrup in their mouths in an attempt to increase its absorption.

Periodontal diseases

People who are dependent on alcohol or other drugs tend to have poor oral hygiene, resulting in gingivitis. When teeth are brushed, the gums bleed. Acute ulcerative gingivitis, where gums are ulcerated, bleeding and painful, has also been described. Cannabis users may present with a painful, fiery-red, gingivitis associated with white patches. It is claimed progressive bone loss (adult periodontitis), leading to loosening of teeth, is more prevalent in drug users. This may be due to immunosuppression. However, many drug and alcohol users also smoke tobacco and this is a known risk factor in progressive periodontal disease.

Tooth surface loss

Excessive tooth wear may be caused by:

- Tooth grinding (bruxism), chewing, and clenching, has been reported with opioid dependence and stimulant use. This causes occlusal wear
- Hyposalivation caused by the drugs exacerbates the wear

- Erosive (acidic) drinks taken to relieve xerostomia, cause erosion
- Regurgitation, bulimia, and vomiting deliver stomach acid into the mouth where it erodes teeth.

Alcoholics may show erosive tooth wear, particularly of palatal surfaces of upper incisors and this may be a consequence of vomiting.

Mucosal lesions

Candida infection and angular cheilitis are common in drug users due to:
- Dry mouth and consequent altered oral flora
- Compromised immune response
- Poor denture hygiene.

Premalignant and malignant mucosal lesions are associated with alcohol, tobacco, and betel nut use. Smoking cannabis, may result in leukoplakia and erythroplakia that could progress to neoplasia. The smoke is claimed to be more carcinogenic than tobacco smoke.

Shorting cocaine may lead to nasal septal and palatal perforation due to the vasoconstrictive activity of cocaine, causing ischaemia and necrosis.

Management

The physician should:
- Advise the patient to see a dentist and have names and locations of clinics that may be dedicated to the care of dependent patients
- Advise the patient to brush their teeth with a fluoride-containing dentifrice
- Never prescribe methadone in a sugar base
- Advise the patient and the dentist on relevant medical problems (see below)

The dentist should advise on plaque control and diet and be aware that:
- Patients may have behavioural problems and are not always good attenders or compliant with treatment
- Patients may be carriers of viral hepatitis (C and/or B) and may have HIV or other sexually transmitted infections
- A right-sided endocarditis is common as a result of infection from intravenous drug injection, often caused by *Staphylococcus aureus*. This may damage the tricuspid valve and the physician should be consulted to advise on the need for antibiotic cover for dental procedures likely to cause bacteraemia, although recent guidelines have questioned this need
- Liver damage is common especially in alcohol misuse, and may cause a bleeding tendency and also impair metabolism
- An alcohol dependent patient who is taking disulfiram (Antabuse) should not be prescribed a mouthwash containing alcohol as it is may precipitate headache and vomiting
- Drug users are often malnourished and immunocompromised
- A cannabis user under stress during dental treatment may faint
- Dental treatment on a cannabis intoxicated patient may cause acute anxiety, dysphoria and paranoid thoughts. Local anaesthesia with adrenaline may prolong the acute tachycardia already induced by the acute dose of cannabis
- The chronic opioid user may get an adrenal crisis with surgical stress due to diminished adrenocortical reserve. Contact the physician to discuss steroid cover.

Pain management

- The drug user may be resistant to local anaesthetics
- They may be anxious. It is important to use profound local anaesthesia and to gain the patient's trust
- When a patient stops heroin and starts a methadone maintenance programme, dental pain from carious teeth may become apparent
- Use only non-steroidal anti-inflammatory drugs for pain control because all other analgesics are potentially addictive
- General anaesthesia or sedation can trigger a relapse to drug misuse and should only be considered after consulting the physician
- If methadone has been prescribed by the physician, it should be maintained during treatment.
- Local anaesthetics with adrenaline and adrenaline impregnated cords should not be used where recent use of cocaine is suspected otherwise there may an acute rise in blood pressure.

Behaviour problems of relevance to the dentist

- Patients tend to fail appointments. Discuss this with the patient from the outset and use telephone reminders
- Oral hygiene tends to be poor and sugar intake high
- Cost is a barrier as money has been spent on drugs
- The drug user may not disclose the history of drug use
- The addict may show general anxiety, heightened dental fear and needle phobia.

Dental management

- Keep treatment as simple as possible
- Concentrate on improving oral hygiene with a high fluoride dentifrice (e.g. Duraphat 2800® or 5000® Colgate®)
- Apply fluoride varnish to carious lesions
- Discuss diet concentrating on reducing frequency of sugar intake, selecting safe snacks, drinking water for thirst, and use of sugar substitutes in beverages such as tea and coffee
- Advise use of sugar-free chewing gum to stimulate salivary flow
- Treat Candidal infections with sugar-free topical antifungals
- Extract grossly carious and painful teeth
- Use simple excavation of gross caries and glass ionomer cement to restore cavities the patient cannot clean (the Atraumatic Restorative Technique).

Prognosis

Prognosis may be poor because caries control depends on the efforts of the patient particularly in keeping the mouth clean. When the mouth is dry, even the most compliant patient may have trouble controlling caries lesion progression.

Further reading

Brand HS, Gonggrijps S, Blanksma CJ. Cocaine and oral health. *Brit dent J* 2008, **204**; 365–369.

Cho CM, Hirsch R, Johnstone S. General and oral health implications of cannabis use. *Australian Dental Journal* 2005: **50**: 70–74.

Graham CH, Meecham JG. Dental management of patients taking methadone. *Dental Update* 2005; **32**: 477–485.

Klasser GD, Epstein JB. The methamphetamine epidemic and dentistry. *General Dentistry* 2006; **54**: 431–439.

Petti S, Scully C. The role of the dental team in preventing and diagnosing cancer: 5. Alcohol and the role of the dentist in alcohol cessation. *Dental Update* 2005; **32**: 454–462.

Scheutz F. Five-year evaluation of a dental care delivery system for drug addicts in Denmark. *Community Dental and Oral Epidemiology* 1984; **12**: 29–34.

Scully C, Diz Dios P, Kumar N. *Special Care in Dentistry: Handbook of Oral Healthcare.* Edinburgh: Churchill Livingstone Elsevier, 2007.

Titas A, Ferguson MM. Impact of opioid use on dentistry. *Australian Dental Journal* 2002; **47**: 94–98.

Difficult and urgent situations

The Emergency Department

Managing patients within the Emergency Department is a difficult task. The spectrum of presenting complaints, the variable access to previous medical or collateral history, together with the 'pressure-cooker' work environment combine to make clinical decision making challenging.

Illicit drug users in the Emergency Department

This is particularly the case when caring for or dealing with patients who either have confirmed or suspected substance misuse. At all times senior Emergency Medicine practitioners should manage such cases and consistency of communication with those involved is crucial. The principles of clinical history and examination apply (see Chapter 2), but these are often threatened through variable patient compliance. These patients are a particularly vulnerable group with mixed psychological and physical pathology, as well as having higher tendencies towards social exclusion, domestic violence (as victim or perpetrator), criminal history, and anti-social behaviour. Within this context the treating clinician has the additional consideration of his/her responsibility for the safety of not only the patient, but also others within the department, including other patients and healthcare workers. As in all aspects of clinical medicine the decision needs to be made in the best interests of the patient, while taking into consideration the impact upon those within the department.

Drug causes of acute presentation of agitation

- Intoxication:
  - Alcohol
  - Sedative hypnotics/anxiolytics, in particular benzodiazepines
  - Cannabis
  - Cocaine
  - Amphetamines and derivatives
  - Hallucinogenic agents
- Side effects/interactions/toxicity
  - Antidepressants
  - Salicylate toxicity
  - Serotonin syndrome
  - Neuroleptic malignant syndrome (NMS)
  - Anticholinergic syndrome
  - Antipsychotic reaction
- Withdrawal syndromes.

The use of the multi-disciplinary team is crucial to the successful determination of cause of any altered behaviour as well as the ensuing management. Patients who have a history of substance misuse are likely to have involvement with a range of hospital and community-based services. The early availability of information from these groups will support more informed decision-making, which is crucial to the development of an adequate risk assessment.

Urgent situations within the Emergency Department can be divided into two main groups that can be difficult to manage:

Reduced level of consciousness

Maintenance of an adequate airway and ensuring sufficient ventilation are the key initial steps for clinical care.

Patients must be carefully evaluated to exclude rigorously causes of coma. At the same time preventative steps must be taken to ensure that complications of coma are avoided or minimized. Where opioid overdose is suspected, naloxone is used as an antagonist. If another toxicological cause is confirmed then the early use of an antidote should be provided to reduce any associated morbidity. However, in most cases where the toxin is unknown the care will be supportive with necessary ventilatory and circulatory support, while excluding other possible causes.

It is not the place to list the spectrum of possible causes for coma, but it is important to appreciate that the reduced level of consciousness or coma may be:

- A result of direct toxic effect on the CNS
- Secondary to the effects of CNS depression, e.g. hypoxia, hypoglycaemia, hyponatraemia, hypotension, seizure
- A non-toxin medical issue, e.g. sepsis, meningo-encephalitis, cerebro-vascular accident, space-occupying lesion.

Agitation and aggression

These patients are very challenging as they often require several members of staff in order to gain a measure of control and calm. At the same time they are often extremely unwell, with a range of potential complications ranging from acid-base disturbance, hyperthermia, hypoxia and dehydration.

The patient needs to be cared for in a calm and secure environment, both to minimize external stimuli and ensure everyone's safety. It is imperative that efforts are made to provide repeated reassurance and ongoing explanation as this helps to maintain calm. The use of sedation should be considered early and its necessity reviewed frequently as the situation is likely to change. The presence of dedicated 1:1 nursing, the assistance of consistent allied health staff and security/police are necessary to help ensure control is maintained. If compliance is possible then the use of an oral anti-psychotic may be helpful to maintain calmness. If the situation deteriorates and there is concern in regard to the patient causing harm to him/herself or to other patients or staff, then controlled physical restraint should be used while intravenous sedation is provided.

The role of physical restraint is to provide temporary control while pharmacological control is obtained. It should be provided through trained staff, ensuring that broad control of arms and legs is maintained while a clinician is able to titrate intravenous sedation. It is imperative that the airway is maintained throughout this process. The sedation is titrated until the patient is rousable to voice, but is calm. The suggested agent would be benzodiazepines (diazepam, lorazepam). Second line agents would include antipsychotics, including olanzapine and haloperidol.

Once sedated, general supportive care needs to be provided within the Emergency Department, including airway protection and observation, and suitable monitoring to assess respiratory, ventilatory, and haemodynamic stability. It is at this stage that it may also be possible to complete a physical examination to ensure that there are no stigmata of infection or inflammatory conditions that could explain the level of confusion, as well as obtaining necessary investigations including FBC, EUC, LFT's, septic screen, blood and urine for toxicology screen, ECG, imaging (CXR, ultrasound or CT as required). This process is crucial to ensure that any condition that may contribute to agitation is diagnosed early, allowing for appropriate treatment to be instigated. Examples of such conditions are provided below:

Possible non-toxicological causes of agitation

- Hypoxia
- Hypoglycaemia
- Sepsis
- Hyperthermia
- Auto-immune disease
- Acid-base and electrolyte disturbances
- Trauma (occult brain injury/subdural/subarachnoid haemorrhage)
- Central infection (meningo-encephalitis)
- Cerebro-vascular accidents: TIA through to stroke
- Seizures
- Endocrine disturbance
- Acute alcohol or drug withdrawal
- Organ failure.

Strategy for dealing with agitated patients within the Emergency Department

Any departmental strategy needs to take into consideration the past history of a patient and any known successful preference to maintain control and calm. Any action must keep the clinical needs and the reduction of any associated risks to the patient as a priority. At the same time, it is imperative to decide treatment and actions in the context of the duty of care that needs to be provided not only for the presenting patient, but also for other patients and all staff within the department. The layout and availability of services and support within the facility will all be important factors in determining the appropriate clinical management:

- Early assessment of any patient with agitation or behaving strangely.
- Aim to obtain collateral history/information from medical records
- Staff should avoid confrontation, ensure adequate assistance, defuse tensions, adopt de-escalation strategies, ensure other patient and staff safety

- Clinician needs to establish patient's concerns, reassure patient and any accompanying relatives/friends, encourage reasoning by offering reasonable options through non-threatening actions
- If efforts to de-escalate have succeeded, then there is a need to conduct a medical and mental health assessment. Consider use of oral sedation to assist in maintaining calmness and compliance
- In the situation of increasing urgency or failure of de-escalation efforts, then the role of physical restraint with view to acute sedation should be discussed within the treating team
- At all times frequent monitoring of both the physical and mental state should be provided.

Once patients have been calmed and the situation is under control, there is time to determine the physical ± any associated psychological causes. The need for a period of observation is important and it may be appropriate for the patient to spend an extended period of time within the Emergency Department Observation Unit (EDOU) for further investigations or monitoring of improvement/stability prior to discharge. This EDOU is required to have the necessary medical and nursing staff to ensure safety for all within it. It will require the input of colleagues from psychological medicine/drug and alcohol services/social services, as well as clinical colleagues for any presumed toxicological effects. Its effectiveness relies upon tight guidelines and protocols for admission and clinical review while within the unit. Of particular importance in caring for such agitated patients is that a suitable psychological risk assessment is made prior to any admission to the unit, together with review through community and liaison services as an integral part of a planned discharge.

Dealing with children and adolescents

The practice within the Emergency Department in dealing with children and adolescents is similar in most ways, but has the additional requirement of parental consent. Disturbed children do attend emergency departments and our aim is to reduce the level of agitation so as to make a thorough clinical assessment as soon as possible. This will involve the same principles of crisis prevention, reducing external stimuli, remaining calm and non-confrontational, while working towards keeping the patient calm within a safe and contained environment with the necessary multidisciplinary team support. If the situation escalates or it is not possible to sustain calm then the use of physical restraint and intravenous sedation with benzodiazepines (as first line) needs to be considered.

In regard to consent there are two situations:

- **Parent not present**; in this situation it is appropriate to act in the best interest of the child and/or others within the department
- **Parent present**; if consent is provided then it is possible to proceed with emergency sedation utilizing physical restraint as required. However, if consent is not forthcoming then either the Mental Health Act needs to be invoked (via the child psychiatrist on-call) or through child protection procedures. In either of these situations the involvement of hospital legal opinion and support is beneficial to ensure that all are adequately informed of the process.

Dealing with alcohol within the Emergency Department

Alcohol abuse and dependence are an increasingly evident clinical problem within the Emergency Department. The clinical assessment will be firstly aimed at determining and managing life-threatening complications. Apart from the clearly alcohol intoxicated patients there are numerous alcohol-related presentations, with some studies estimating upwards of 30% of all Emergency Department attendances being alcohol-related.

Within such a context the role of screening and brief intervention is crucial. The Emergency Department provides an ideal opportunity to screen rapidly for possible alcohol-related issues. This needs to be an active and promoted programme of brief intervention within the Emergency Department. Otherwise the ability of clinicians to identify patients with alcohol-related problems falls substantially.

Some of the reasons as to why clinicians are poor at screening for alcohol are listed below:
- Inadequate training regarding substance misuse
- Negative attitudes towards patients presenting with substance misuse
- Scepticism about the effectiveness of any treatment
- A belief that alcohol-related screening is not in the domain of the general Emergency Medicine practitioner
- A concern in relation to the time taken to screen
- A lack of specialist practitioners able to respond to patients identified through any screening programme.

The FLAGS acronym is a useful guide to Emergency clinicians in dealing with this large group of patients and can be used in scenarios where brief intervention may be regarded as beneficial.

FLAGS acronym

Feedback: Review problems caused by alcohol with the patient
Listen: To the patient's response, and readiness to change, past efforts
Advice: Advise to cut down or abstain from alcohol
Goals: Negotiate a goal with the patient
Strategies: Provide options to assist the patient's change in behaviour.

Brief intervention is provided with an empathic approach, and respecting the patient's right and responsibility to make a decision about changing their drinking. Optimism is conveyed that change is possible.

The scope of the problem

Patients with **alcohol use disorders** (AUD) such as alcohol dependence, alcohol abuse or with risky alcohol use are seen about 1.5–3 times more frequently in emergency rooms compared with primary care clinics. For some it might be the only contact with the health care system. Some patients with lifestyle risks are progressing towards severe problems, e.g. from risky alcohol use towards overt dependence. Only a minority of the patients with lifestyle risks seek formal help. This underlines the unique position of the ED physicians in this context.

Many patients with AUD are seen in EDs after trauma. Trauma patients have been characterized as being a group of predominantly younger males with high rate of substance misuse, such as alcohol use disorders (AUD: 25–50%), as well as smoking (up to 60%) and drug use (up to 34%). These patients tend to show more risk-taking behaviour, sensation seeking, and low coping mechanisms. Physical health is in general good, but mental health seems to be impaired in comparison to the general population. Re-trauma rate is also higher compared with patients without AUD. Trauma has, therefore, been described as a recurrent disease.

AUD patients show a 2–5-fold higher rate of post-operative or post-traumatic complications. Chronic alcohol consumption increases morbidity due to the impact on the nervous system, cardiovascular system, liver, musculoskeletal and immune systems. AUDs have been related to psychiatric co-morbidity, including other substance misuse. The alcohol withdrawal syndrome is a potential life-threatening complication in alcohol dependent patients. Alcohol withdrawal often complicates a critical illness. Long term alcohol misuse might lead to cardiac arrhythmias, dilatative cardiomyopathy and hypotonic circulatory dysregulation. Bleeding complications are increased 2-fold during and after surgery. In medical ICUs more than 50% of liver injuries and chronic pancreatitis have been related to chronic alcohol misuse. Alcohol promotes carcinogenesis. This increased morbidity of patients with AUD not only accounts for more frequent ED visits but is also is responsible for prolonged hospital stay.

Important immune functions are suppressed by chronic heavy drinking. Immune suppression results in an increased incidence of infectious complications like pneumonia, wound infection and urinary tract infection. These findings are related to an altered stress response in these patients and are in line with increased postoperative and post-traumatic infectious complications. Nicotine misuse, if found together with alcohol use, also increases the risk of infectious complications.

Stress due to surgery and trauma, infection or withdrawal states might be deleterious and induces a variety other changes in body functions. This includes—along with the above mentioned immune suppression—changes in body fluid composition, electrolytes, catecholamines and hormones, tryptophan metabolism, and even condensation products such as harmans or norharmans. Cognitive impairment in emergency or critically ill patients, such as delirium or 'acute brain dysfunction,' implies a multitude of differential diagnoses. This requires a reliable and fast rule out strategy in order to adjust treatment, e.g. septic encephalopathy is often misinterpreted as alcohol withdrawal syndrome, or the clinical presentation of a patient with a subdural haematoma might be considered intoxication by the ED physician. The clinical presentation of critically ill patients with a history of alcohol and/or drug misuse may differ significantly from other patients. Delayed diagnosis of AUD and related co-morbidity (e.g. alcohol intoxication and head trauma, withdrawal state, vitamin deficiencies, drug use, significant psychiatric disorders, infections, etc.) may have severe consequences. An increased attention to avoid delayed treatment is mandatory.

Accurate and complete diagnosis

Rule out without any delay other medical conditions that resemble conditions frequently found in alcohol and drug misusing patients, using the acronym **I WATCH DEATH**.

Infections
Withdrawal
Acute metabolic
Trauma
CNS
Hypoxia
Deficiencies
Endocrinopathies
Acute vascular
Toxins/drugs
Heavy metals

Diagnosis

As AUD patients show a 2–5-fold higher rate of postoperative complications, they require increased attention to avoid delayed treatment and the development of multiple organ failure. The **diagnosis** of AUD relies on the synopsis of history and collateral information, clinical findings, questionnaires, and biomarkers. Diagnosis of chronic alcohol abuse or dependence is performed by specific medical history, examination, and assisted by validated tests.

For screening purposes, the use of **questionnaires** has been recommended. For ED-screening purposes the AUDIT (including its short version, AUDIT-C) and CAGE variants have been found very useful and are more efficient than routine clinical history (pp. 91–92 Appendix 419–420). The chosen cut-off should not just reflect the scope of the problem, but also the resources of the setting and should therefore be adapted to the needs of the patient group (e.g. males and females, trauma) and the setting (e.g. ED).

Biomarkers are a means of assisting in diagnosis of chronic alcohol dependence in sedated, intubated, and emergency patients (pp. 100–101).

While questionnaires and blood alcohol concentration (BAC) are of great assistance in the diagnosis of an AUD in trauma settings, they are not always applicable, and the BAC value does not always distinguish between acute and chronic consumption. It has been demonstrated that the sensitivity and specificity of clinical detection of acute alcohol intoxication by trauma centre staff are poor.

Between 16 and 39% of trauma victims are blood alcohol (BAC) positive: 55–75% of injured patients who are BAC positive have an alcohol abuse or dependence diagnosis, but a substantial number of trauma patients with AUDs (11–45%) are BAC negative on admission. Especially in the early phase of care in patients with severe trauma, patient history may not be available and the use of questionnaires is limited. In a prospective study of 349 trauma patients aged 16–49 years admitted into a general hospital trauma centre, two-thirds of trauma patients were hazardous drinkers, including 61% frequent binge drinkers. Blood alcohol on admission was an accurate indicator of this in contrast to conventional markers of heavy drinking. However, BAC cannot discriminate between acute and chronic consumption or risky use, abuse, and dependence. The detection time frame of BAC is limited and it cannot detect hangover state. In a research setting, newer markers of recent alcohol consumption such as urinary 5-HTOL/HIAA and ethylglucuronide, with a larger window of detection, may provide additive important information. These markers are currently under evaluation. Hangover might substantially contribute to the incidence of trauma and readily available markers of recent consumption do have the potential to detect hangover state. Another crucial advantage of BAC in contrast to the potential new markers is the fact that it is possible to determine breath alcohol at the 'point of care'.

Markers of chronic consumption (such as GGT, MCV and, where available, CDT) may add valuable information and may be helpful to identify patients at risk of developing complications related to chronic heavy drinking. In patients with multiple severe trauma, CDT showed a sensitivity of 65% in detection of alcohol dependence or abuse. Early venepuncture in the emergency room and before administration of large volumes of fluids or blood in the phase of initial care increased the sensitivity to 74% for CDT. In the ability to detect alcohol dependence or abuse, CDT was superior to GGT and MCV (sensitivities <36%) in that setting. In patients with elevated CDT, intercurrent complications (alcohol withdrawal, tracheo-bronchitis, pneumonia, sepsis, congestive heart failure) were significantly increased after trauma.

However, no biomedical marker with adequate accuracy has been found in screening for heavy alcohol consumption in the general population, especially when the rate of young, hazardous non-continuous, low level, binge pattern consumers is considerable. A stepwise screening procedure, which includes the use of questionnaires such as AUDIT and CAGE variants, has been proposed. However, evidence concerning clinical decision making based on biomedical alcohol markers in respect to relevant outcome is still limited.

Algorithm: detection and management of alcohol use disorders in the ED

Routine clinical assessment
- ± Questionnaire (e.g. AUDIT-C, PAT, FAST, TWEAK)[*]
- ± Marker (BAC, Drug screen, GGT, MCV, CDT)

Consider therapy together with brief intervention, when
- Clinical routine history or examination positive for AUD
- Clinical routine history or examination negative, but AUDIT positive > = 8 or other brief screening questionnaire above cut-off
- Clinical routine history or examination negative, AUDIT or other brief screening questionnaire negative or not applicable, but two markers positive ('chronic' markers: GGT, MCV, CDT).

Perform further evaluation when: Clinical routine history and examination negative and/or AUDIT or other brief screening questionnaire negative or not applicable and one marker (BAC, GGT, MCV, CDT, Drug screen) positive.

Consider brief intervention and further evaluation: Clinical routine history and examination negative but AUDIT ≥ 5 in females.

Additional confirmation tools: Detailed alcohol intake history (including frequency of alcohol intake >60 g/occasion), ICD/DSM criteria for harmful use/abuse and dependence, collateral information, assessment of motivation, assess relevant somatic and psychiatric co-morbidity.

Treatment
Existing therapeutic options are effective, if started early during admission:

Therapeutic options
- Prophylaxis, stress reduction
- Treatment of withdrawal if underlying dependence and of co-morbidities
- Brief interventions/motivational interviewing
- Advice is communicated using the FLAGS acronym: communicating need for abstinence (in dependence) or to cut down
- Consultation with addiction medicine specialist team.

Short-term outcome can be positively influenced by interventions addressing withdrawal and stress prevention. Interventions at the level of the hypothalamic pituitary A axis (morphine or ketoconazole) improve the immune response to surgical stress. These interventions in long-term alcohol-dependent patients were associated with decreased post-operative pneumonia rates and shortened intensive care unit stay together with a decrease in the usual postoperative hypercortisolism and with a prevention of the impairment of the cytotoxic T-lymphocyte type 1:type 2 ratio.

[*] Examples of these brief alcohol screening tests are shown in the appendix (pp. 420–422).

Alcohol withdrawal prophylaxis in dependent patients if applied early and symptom-oriented, can prevent withdrawal or reduce severity. The use of scores for withdrawal rating is recommended. Any delay in the treatment of overt alcohol withdrawal complicates the clinical course.

Prophylaxis and treatment of alcohol withdrawal in surgical ward patients

Prophylaxis: First-line treatment: benzodiazepines and monitor with a withdrawal rating scale (e.g. aim for AWS <5, CIWA-Ar <10); Delirium Detection Scale (DDS) <8 for example

- **Diazepam** po or IV 6-hourly; titrate the dose against withdrawal symptoms, e.g. 5–10 mg (pp. 115–116) OR
- **Chlordiazepoxide** 6-hourly 5–25 mg OR
- **Lorazepam** po or IV; titrate against signs, 0.25–2 mg (older patient, at night) OR

Monitoring: 4-hourly with RASS/DDS or CIWA-Ar for 24 h, reduce frequency of monitoring if stable.

Target: CIWA-Ar =<10, DDS <8; ICU treatment if CIWAr> 20.

Adjust medication as needed according to symptoms (prophylactic therapy)
- Adjust benzodiazepine medication
- **Autonomic signs:** clonidine (start with 0.15–0.3 mg)
- **Hallucinations:** haloperidol (initially 5–10 mg)
- Monitor vital signs (heart rate, blood pressure, temperature)
- Obtain laboratory results (sodium, potassium, magnesium, blood sugar, arterial blood gas analysis, WBC, Hb, Hct).

CIWA-Ar = Revised Clinical Institute Withdrawal Assessment for Alcohol Scale—Mod. Spies & Rommelspacher 1999, Sander et al. 2006.

DDS = Delirium Detection Scale, Otter et al. 2003.

RASS = Richmond Agitation-Sedation Scale; Sessler et al. 2002

Rule out without any delay other medical conditions that resemble conditions frequently found in alcohol and drug misusing patients.

Consider electrolyte, vitamin and mineral needs: e.g. magnesium 10–30 mEq, potassium 60–180 mEq, and phosphate 10–40 mmol/l daily, Vitamin B_1, B_6, and nicotinic acid deficiencies. All hypoglycaemic patients (who are treated with IV glucose) with evidence of chronic alcohol ingestion must be given thiamine replacement immediately because of the risk of acutely precipitating Wernicke's encephalitis (WE).

ED prophylaxis and treatment of Wernicke's (also see pp. 119–120): According to the Royal College of Physicians (2002) thiamine replacement must be given immediately in adequate amounts parenterally (oral thiamine is ineffective) to avoid irreversible brain damage (e.g. Wernicke's encephalopathy)

• In the UK for Wernicke's prophylaxis Pabrinex® ampoules 1 and 2 are given: this contains Vitamin B_1 (thiamine) 250 mg plus Vitamin B_2 (riboflavin) 4 mg, Vitamin B_6 (pyridoxine) 50 mg, nicotinamide 160 mg, Vitamin C (ascorbic acid) 500 mg; administered in 100 mL normal saline over 30 min. In Australia thiamine 100 mg IM or IV is given.

• High-risk patients for WE are poorly nourished patients and all alcoholic patients, e.g. in detoxification, road traffic accident head injuries, and in patients with alcohol misuse with ophthalmoplegia, ataxia, acute confusion, memory disturbance, unexplained hypotension, or hypothermia.

• Treatment dose in established or presumptive diagnosis of WE is much higher (2 pairs of Pabrinex® ampoules tds or at least 100 mg thiamine IV tds), and should be given for 2 consecutive days. If no response observed after this time, discontinue. If a response is observed, then continue with 1 pair of ampoules for another 5 days or longer if improvement continues.

Long-term benefit can potentially be achieved by abstinence or long-term reduction in alcohol intake. There is evidence that in non-dependent drinkers, brief interventions are able to induce long-term behaviour changes in order to reduce harmful alcohol use, alcohol consumption and adherent risks. A directive, but not confrontative, brief counselling style like MI seems to work through strengthening resources, and thus 'compressing' the phase in which the patient is at risk. Motivational interviewing (MI) is a client-centred, directive method for enhancing intrinsic motivation to change (e.g. their risky alcohol use) by exploring and resolving ambivalence (p. 62 and also www.motivationalinterview.org). Reductions in motor-vehicle crashes and related injuries, falls, alcohol-related injuries, and injury emergency visits, hospitalizations, and deaths have been reported after a variety of different brief interventions with reductions of 35% (range: 27% to 65%). One trauma centre study using the MI style was able to show a 50% reduction in repeat trauma from 10 to 5% in the first year of follow-up using regional trauma registry data. Labour-saving approaches, such as computerized interventions have been trialled. Computerized brief tailored advice led to a reduction of alcohol intake in the year after trauma in minimally injured patients in the ED. Results were equivocal across all ED trauma patients. There are several unsolved issues in regard to screening and intervention in the ED including differences in 'Efficacy, Efficiency and Effectiveness', the role of the setting, the mechanism behind the intervention (what works?), when and how long does it work, difficulties and obstacles in the implementation process, and the role of individual socio-demographic and psychological variables on the effect, such as level of education, peer factors, significant others and motivation.

Summary
- Screening and Intervention for AUD is recommended by a variety of national and international guidelines. However, despite some efforts, implementation rate needs considerable improvement
- Prophylaxis in terms of pharmacotherapy, encouraging periods of abstinence, and brief intervention strategies can help to prevent or ease some of the complications of substance misuse, and can decrease the rate of long-term injuries
- US recommendations suggest that screening for AUD should be incorporated into routine care of injured patients. History and physical findings consistent with AUD should be documented and brief intervention should be provided. Care for alcohol-impaired patient(s) should always be provided in a professional and non-judgmental manner. Health professionals should advocate in the community for public education, prevention programmes, public policy, and treatment programmes, and should participate in collaborative research, education, and data gathering to improve the care of patients with AUDs, as well as integrate alcohol screening and alcohol education into curricula, continuing education, and standards for emergency health care professionals.

Further reading

Dinh-Zarr T, Goss C, Heitman E, Roberts I, DiGuiseppi C. Interventions for preventing injuries in problem drinkers. *Cochrane Database System Review* 2004; **3**: CD001857.

D'Onofrio G, Bernstein E, Bernstein J, Woolard RH, Brewer PA, Craig SA, Zink BJ. Patients with alcohol problems in the emergency department, part 1: improving detection. SAEM Substance Abuse Task Force. Society for Academic Emergency Medicine. *Academy of Emergency Medicine* 1998; **5**: 1200–1209.

D'Onofrio G, Degutis LC. Preventive care in the emergency department: screening and brief intervention for alcohol problems in the emergency department: a systematic review. *Academy of Emergency Medicine* 2002; **9**: 27–38.

Runge JW, Hargarten S, Velianoff G, Brewer PA, D'Onofrio G, Soderstrom CA, Gentilello LM, Flaherty L, Fiellin DA, Degutis LC, Pantalon MV. *Recommended best practices of emergency medical care for the alcohol-impaired patient: screening and brief intervention for alcohol problems in the Emergency Department.* Available at: http://www.nhtsa.dot.gov/people/injury/alcohol/EmergCare/recommended.htm.

Urgent situations

The violent patient

Consider psychostimulant use, alcohol intoxication.

As for Suicide Risk Assessment, Violence Risk Assessment involves weighing up the balance of **Risk Factors and Protective Factors**. Risk factors can be static and dynamic in nature. Questions to ask include:

- Have you had any recent thoughts of wanting to lash out at or hurt others?
  - If yes—can you tell me about those thoughts? Do you have a particular person in mind?
- Do you have a specific plan in your mind about how you would hurt this person?
  - If yes—can you tell me about this plan? (ask in detail about the plan, any access to weapons, etc)
- Do you feel it is likely you will try to carry this plan out?
  - If yes—when?
- What are some of the things that are stopping you from harming this person at this time?

Static risk factors include factors in the patient's history and disposition which are generally not able to be modified through treatment or alterations in the patient's environment and social networks. They include:

- **Past history of violence**: past behaviour tends to predict future behaviour
- **Family history of violence**, which may be a risk factor by role modelling aggressive behaviour and providing an increased genetic risk of antisocial behaviour
- **Personality traits and disorder**: those with poor anger control, those with antisocial personality disorder, and those with high levels of impulsivity are more likely to engage in risky behaviours including getting involved in aggressive incidents
- **Sex**: for most types of criminal behaviour, men commit far more violent crime than women
- **Age**: The peak age of offending in the general population is in the mid- to late adolescent years. Mentally ill offenders tend to commit their first offence at a later age
- **Social situation**: lower socio-economic groups are over-represented among violent offenders in the community
- **Neurobiological factors and intellectual function**: some forms of brain disease and damage can predispose to higher risk for violence, e.g. frontal lobe damage causing irritability and disinhibition. There is also an over-representation of people with lower IQ in those who are arrested
- **History of mental illness**: while the links between mental illness and violence are not always clear, some patients (e.g. with bipolar disorder, schizophrenia, depression) are at higher risk of violence during acute exacerbations of illness. While having a mental illness is a static risk factor, the patient's mental state as a consequence of that illness is potentially modifiable and, therefore, a dynamic risk factor

In contrast, *dynamic risk factors* are potentially modifiable with treatment and changes in the patient's environment and social networks. Such risk factors include:

- **Social networks**: a lack of family and social supports may lead to deterioration in the patient's mental state and may increase the risk of violence if other factors are in play
- **Homelessness, unemployment, poverty** are common in the background of mentally ill offenders and should be addressed as part of a treatment plan

Mental state

- **Evidence of psychotic symptoms**: certain psychotic symptoms are more associated with violent events than others, e.g. persecutory beliefs that others want to harm the patient and delusions of infidelity. Patients who respond to command auditory hallucinations telling them to commit dangerous acts are also at higher risk of violence
- **Evidence of mood disorder**: violence may increase for some individuals when they are depressed or in a manic state
- **Thoughts/plan/intention to harm others**: These should always be assessed as part of the MSE. Questions should include: Have you had any recent thoughts of wanting to lash out at or harm others because of their behaviour towards you? What thoughts have you had? Have you put together a plan to try to hurt them? What does that plan involve? (If weapons are involved—Do you have access to weapons that you could use in this plan?) How likely is it that you will try to carry this idea through? What might stop you acting on this plan?
- **Poor insight and judgement**
- **Compliance with medication**: this can be modified through education designed to increase insight, through supervision and the use of the Mental Health Act where appropriate
- **Substance misuse/dependence** can increase risk because of irritability and disinhibited behaviour. Some substances (e.g. amphetamines) increase persecutory beliefs that others want to harm the patient and thereby increase the risk of acting out violently.

Risk factors

Risk factors include past history of violence, untreated schizophrenia with acute psychosis and lack of insight, substance misuse, social and cultural isolation, homelessness, and unemployment. However, with treatment a number of these risk factors (untreated psychosis, insight, substance misuse, homelessness, social isolation) have now been addressed and he currently appears to be at low risk for further violence.

Reducing and managing risks (also known as 'Risk Management') involves carrying out a full risk assessment, and setting up a comprehensive management plan to monitor and manage those risks.

Causes of substance–induced psychoses

- Cannabis, in high doses
- Psychostimulants:
  - Amphetamines and amphetamine-type substances
  - Cocaine
  - MDMA
- Hallucinogens: LSD, psilocybin
- Withdrawal states:
  - Alcohol
  - Benzodiazepines.

Domestic violence

Domestic violence is any behaviour used by one partner in a relationship to gain and maintain control over another person's life.

The most common example of domestic violence is the use of force by men to maintain control over their partners. One in four women is likely to be subjected to domestic violence.

Some forms of domestic violence
- **Physical assault**: punching, hitting, kicking, pushing, slapping, choking or the use of weapons
- **Sexual assault**: being forced to have sex (rape), indecent assault, being forced to look at pornography
- **Psychological abuse**: threats of violence or death, emotional and verbal abuse which threatens, degrades or insults a person
- **Social abuse**: being stopped from seeing family or friends—social or geographical isolation
- **Economic abuse**: having no access to, or control over money or other resources and being forced to live without money.

Domestic violence is often related to use of alcohol and other drugs, in particular psychostimulants, by the perpetrator. The perpetrator may also have underlying psychological/psychiatric problems.

Domestic violence is a crime in most Western countries. Acts of domestic violence and the subsequent outcomes are deemed the sole responsibility of the perpetrator.

Risk factors (in the perpetrator):
- Drug and alcohol use
- Mental illness
- Parental history of abuse.

Some outcomes of domestic violence
- Fear, loss of self confidence by victims
- Increasing risk of psychological and/or physical harm due to worsening of abuse and assaults over time
- Risk of psychological and/or physical harm to children and young people who witness the domestic violence
- Relationship/family break-up
- Assault, homicide, suicide
- Criminal charges, imprisonment.

Clinical assessment

History: Clues that the patient has been a possible victim of domestic violence include:
- Psychological/psychiatric problems
- Social isolation
- Fear, anxiety, panic attacks, depression
- A vague, variable or bizarre history of injuries which are inconsistent with the physical findings
- Alcohol and other substance use problems
- Overdose, suicide attempts.

Physical examination

The victim of domestic violence may show:
- Bruising, lacerations, welts, bites, scratch marks, burns, scalds over the face, neck, head or other parts of the body
- Multiple injuries or bruises, trauma, fractures, head injuries
- Bruising, injuries, tears, or bleeding from the genitalia or anus; genital warts or evidence of sexually transmitted infections.

A perpetrator of domestic violence may:
- Appear overly concerned about the victim
- Speak for partner or children
- Show some signs, e.g. facial scratches and injuries, by the victim fighting back.

What can one do?

In serious cases, medical care for injuries may be needed. It is important to document signs of injury found on clinical examination (a photographic record may be valuable for any later legal action).

The clinician can encourage a victim to report an incident to the police; however, it is important to respect the patient's right to decide whether she or he wishes to take this action. In some cases, the victim is rightly afraid of the consequences to themselves should they speak to the police.

Ensure the victim is aware there may be a range of legal actions open to them including placing criminal charges or (in many regions) seeking a court order designed to protect them. Such a court order may restrain the perpetrator from approaching them (often known as a restraining order or apprehended violence order). In other cases, a magistrate may order the partner not to drink or use substances in the home.

Assist the victim to access other support:
- Subsidized legal aid may be available
- Domestic violence help lines are available in many regions. The patient can call for ongoing advice and support
- Family support services may be able to offer support to children in the family.

Where there are children in the family who are placed at risk from domestic violence, the clinician is legally obliged to report domestic violence to the Government Department responsible for child protection in many countries. Reporting must occur when children and young persons under the age of 18 years are at risk of physical, psychological, or emotional harm as a result of what is done (physical, sexual, or psychological abuse) or not done (neglect) by another person responsible for their care.

The victim may use alcohol or other psychoactive substances to cope with the after effects of domestic violence. Psychotherapy can also target developing more productive responses. In some cases, the victim's own substance use, or disinhibited behaviour as a result of substance use, may be a trigger for domestic violence. While this never excuses the violence, the patient's safety may be enhanced by increasing awareness of the triggers to violence and how to avoid these, and/or other self-protective action that may be effective.

The suicidal patient

The acronym SAD PERSONS can be used to guide an assessment of suicide risk

S **Sex**: males complete suicide 3 times more often than females usually because of using more lethal methods (e.g. guns, hanging)

A **Age**: older and younger individuals are more vulnerable

D **Depression:** a history of depression is evident in around 70% of suicidal individuals

P **Positive family history and past attempts**: a positive family history of suicidality is a risk factor because of role modelling suicide as a way of coping, as well as the likelihood of a genetic vulnerability to depression. Up to 50% of those who have made a past suicide attempt will make a further attempt and up to 10% will succeed in subsequent attempts

E **Ethanol and other drug use** have a disinhibiting effect and make it more likely the individual will lose control and act on their suicidal thoughts

R **Rational thinking loss**: patients who have lost their ability to think rationally (e.g. due to psychosis or an organic brain syndrome) are less likely to be able to control and manage suicidal thoughts and intent

S **Social support**: patients with limited social support are at higher risk than those with good supports around them

O **Organized plan**: patients who not only have suicidal thoughts but have an organized plan and an intention to carry out that plan are at higher risk

N **No hope**: patients who feel hopeless about their situation and see no escape and no future ahead are at greater risk. Hopelessness is one of the main factors bringing together a history of depression and the development of a plan and intention to commit suicide

S **Sickness**: intercurrent medical illness is a further risk factor, e.g. chronic pain, terminal illness

Should the patient be scheduled/compulsorily detained?

Different countries and regions have clear criteria to determine whether a patient can be compulsorily detained (see p. 414).

Legal and ethical issues

Drinking and driving

With a blood alcohol concentration (BAC) of 0.06 g/100 mL, a driver is twice as likely to die in a road crash as one with no alcohol. Risk rises rapidly with further increases in BAC.

In order to comply with a BAC maximum of 0.05 g/100 mL for driving, a general guideline for an average healthy person is that:

- Women drink no more than one standard drink in the first hour, then only one drink per hour thereafter
- Men drink no more than two standard drinks in the first hour, then no more than one standard drink per hour thereafter.

NB: Some people of small build, or who are ill, or who have concurrent medical problems or who are on medication (e.g. sedatives), will need to drink less or not at all.

In some countries/regions a medical practitioner is obliged to report to the Driver Licensing Authority a driver who is repeatedly drinking to the extent that their driving ability is impaired or is unfit to drive. Medical practitioners need to weigh the benefits of patient mobility with the increased risk posed to other road users and make themselves aware of local guidelines.

Drinking-driving

'Drinking-driving' is the favoured term for the criminal conviction of driving a vehicle under the influence of alcohol (WHO, 1994). Drinking-driving accidents are a problem in all countries that make use of motor vehicles for transportation. Drinking-driving countermeasures have been developed and many of these have been evaluated.

In the field of traffic safety, the blood alcohol concentration (BAC) is expressed as the percentage of alcohol in millilitres or decilitres of blood. In the United States and Australia it is expressed as g/dL, e.g. 0.10% or 0.10 g/dL. In the UK it is expressed as mg per 100 mL (mg %). The legal driving limit differs in different countries. In the UK and the United States it is 0.08% (expressed as 80 mg/100 mL in the UK). In Australia and in most of continental Europe it is 0.05%.

The risk of a fatal crash for drivers with a positive BAC compared with other drivers (the relative risk) increases with increasing BAC, and rises more steeply for drivers under the age of 21 years than for older drivers. The table shows that there is a marked deterioration in performance between BACs of 0.05 and 0.09%.

BAC can be measured by taking a blood sample from a driver, but also via analysis of breath alcohol. The invention of the Breathalyser test and other portable devices for collecting samples of drivers' breaths has had a major impact on the enforcement of drinking-driving countermeasures.

Table 15.1 Relative risks for a single-vehicle fatal crash for various BACs

BAC level: g/dL	Relative risk of a single-vehicle fatal crash
0.02–0.04	1.4
0.05–0.09	11.1
0.10–0.14	48
>0.15	380

A number of factors influence alcohol-induced impairment including:

- **Alcohol tolerance**: the repeated performance of a particular task in association with alcohol consumption can lead to a form of adaptation known as 'learned' tolerance. This acts to reduce the alcohol-induced impairment under routine circumstances.
- **Age**: the fatality rate for 16–19-year-old drivers is four times higher than that for their 25–69-year-old counterparts. For male drivers under 21 years, an increase in BAC of 0.02% will more than double the relative risk of a fatal single-vehicle crash. The greater risk in younger people can be explained in part by lack of experience and overconfidence. The risk increases if there are other teenagers in the car.
- **Gender**: women metabolize alcohol differently from men and achieve higher BAC levels for the same 'dose' of alcohol.
- **Medication**: combining certain types of medication with alcohol increases crash risk. This applies particularly to sedatives and tranquillizers (e.g. benzodiazepines), which have an increased crash potential when taken on their own. Other drugs implicated include anti-depressants, codeine and other morphine-like analgesics, antihistamines, also some cardiovascular and anti-psychotic medications.
- **Sleep deprivation**: drowsiness increases crash risk and alcohol consumption increases the adverse effects of sleep deprivation.

Factors influencing blood alcohol concentration levels (BACs)

Different people metabolize alcohol at different rates. As a rule of thumb, one unit of alcohol (10g) will lead to an increase of 15 mg% (0.15%) in the blood alcohol concentration (BAC). The body eliminates about 15 mg% of alcohol per hour.

Listed below are some of the factors that influence the concentration of alcohol in a person's breath or blood (BAC):

- The quantity and concentration of alcohol consumed
- The time since the last drink, and the rate of drinking
- Whether alcohol was consumed on an empty stomach
- The amount of alcohol that remains in the stomach
- The amount of alcohol already metabolized by the liver
- The general condition of the liver
- The person's metabolic rate
- The person's emotional state
- Physical factors, including gender, weight, body size, and lean tissue to body fat ratio
- The volume of water in the tissues of the body, which can be affected by such factors as medication, illness, and the menstrual cycle.

Decline in drinking and driving

Since the early 1980s there has been a general decline in the incidence of drinking-driving in the developed world, where alcohol-related traffic deaths have been cut dramatically as the result of drink driving legislation.

In the United States alcohol was the leading cause of traffic fatalities in the mid 1970s (>60% for all age groups and two-thirds of traffic deaths in 16–20-year-olds). The institution of preventive measures means that alcohol is now involved in 40% of traffic deaths (36% of deaths in 16–20-year-olds). The number of alcohol-related traffic deaths among 16–20-year-olds decreased from 5224 in 1982 to 2115 in 2004 largely as a result of raising the minimum legal age of drinking to 21 years and the passage of Zero Tolerance laws for drivers under 21.

General deterrence as prevention

Lowering BAC limits: The implementation of strict legal alcohol limits (e.g. 0.08% or 0.05% or above for the whole population and 0.02% for young drivers) have been successful in reducing the level of the problem. However, the impact of these measures is eroded over time, and this has led to countries implementing more stringent BAC levels.

Enforcement: Intensification of police enforcement of breath testing reduces accidents in the short-term, but the effects are generally temporary. Highly visible, random breath testing is effective at reducing drinking-driving and the associated crashes, injuries, and deaths.

Severity of punishment: Punishments include fines, suspension of driving licences, court-mandated treatment for alcohol problems, and imprisonment. Licence loss has been shown to be the most consistently effective deterrent.

Repeat offenders

In a number of jurisdictions repeat offenders are subject to more draconian interventions, such as confiscation and loss of their licences for longer periods, and imprisonment. The impact of routine punishments can be enhanced when combined with alcohol treatment. This can range from short-term educational sessions to longer programmes lasting up to 1 year. Victim impact panels are a relatively new type of intervention. Another approach is to use ignition interlock devices that prevent the driver from starting the car until they have passed a breath test. Some states in the USA arrange for vehicle impoundment or immobilization. The evidence supports comprehensive treatment including counselling plus licence suspension.

Restrictions on young or inexperienced drivers

A numbers of prevention strategies have been successfully implemented, as follows:

- **Lower BAC limits**: sometimes called 'zero tolerance laws', set the legal BAC limit for drivers under 21 at 0.00 or 0.02%. They have been successful in reducing the proportion of drinking drivers involved in fatal crashes in the under- 21 year age group in the United States. They also invoke other penalties, such as automatic confiscation of the driving licence.
- **Licensing restrictions**: graduated licensing schemes that include delayed access to a full licence and curfews for young drivers have been well-accepted where implemented and have shown safety benefits.

United Kingdom

In the United Kingdom 3000 people on average are killed or seriously injured per year in drink drive collisions (Department for Transport, 2007). Nearly one in six of all road deaths involve drivers who are over the legal limit. Although drinking and driving occurs across all age groups, young men aged 17–29 years are most often involved, as perpetrators and casualties.

The legal alcohol limit is 80 mg of alcohol per 100 mL of blood, which can also be expressed in terms of levels in the breath (the official measure) or in urine:

- **Breath alcohol**: 35 µg/100 mL or
- **Urinary alcohol**: 107 mg/100 mL.

This is roughly equivalent to 2 pints (4 units) of ordinary strength lager in an average man and less for a woman. Men should therefore consume no more than 4 units and women no more than 3 units if they wish to remain below the legal limit. Just two 175-mL glasses of 12% ABV wine would put the average woman over the legal limit.

Australia

Australian-born single men under the age of 30 years are more likely than any other group to drink and drive. There have been intensive media campaigns and concentrated police efforts, including an increase in random breath testing, to discourage people from drinking and driving.

The legal limit for drivers in all states in Australia is below 0.05%. No alcohol is allowed for drivers on a probationary licence (P plates) or learner drivers (L plates). The laws impose severe penalties for convicted drink drivers, including licence loss, fines, and occasionally imprisonment.

United States

The definition of 'drunk driving' is consistent throughout the United States. Every state and the District of Columbia define impairment as driving with a BAC at or above 0.08%. In addition, they all have zero tolerance laws prohibiting drivers under the age of 21 from drinking and driving. Generally, the BAC in these cases is 0.02.

Drink-driving campaigns target drivers under the age of 21, repeat offenders and 21–34-year-olds, the age group that is responsible for more alcohol-related fatal crashes than any other.

Further reading

Assessing fitness to drive: for commmercial and private vehicle drivers. Austroads Inc. Sydney 2003.

Babor T, Caetano R, Casswell S et al. Alcohol: no ordinary commodity. Oxford: Oxford University Press, 2003.

Driver and Vehicle Licensing Agency (2007). At a Glance Guide to Medical Aspects of Fitness to Drive. Swansea: DVLA.

Is there a safe level of daily consumption of alcohol for men and women? NHMRC 1992.

National Institute on Alcohol Abuse and Alcoholism. Alcohol Alert Number 52. Alcohol and Transportation Safety, 2001.

Zador PL. Alcohol-related relative risk of fatal driver injuries in relation to driver age and sex. J. Stud. Alcohol 1991; **52**: 302–310.

Drugs and driving

Epidemiology

The use of both illegal and legal drugs presents a significant risk to traffic safety. After alcohol, cannabis, and benzodiazepines are the drugs found most frequently in impaired drivers, with opiates and stimulants found less often. Drivers using drugs are a heterogeneous group who range from individuals taking therapeutic doses of benzodiazepines to those using cocktails of illicit drugs. Generally, drugs with a sedative action taken in high doses have the greatest potential for impairment. Factors that influence drug effects are:

- **Drug type**: e.g. stimulants or sedatives
- **Dose**: e.g. benzodiazepines are more dangerous when taken above recommended doses
- **Mode of administration**: e.g. drugs by injection or inhalation result in lower peak blood levels
- **Time after intake**: e.g. after taking cannabis driving skills are impaired for 2–4 h
- **Half-life of the drug**: e.g. long acting benzodiazepines may impair more than short acting ones
- **Development of tolerance.**

The development of tolerance is particularly important for prescribed drugs where impairment may be greater when a dose changes or a new treatment is commenced; patient factors such as co-morbid liver disease may also be relevant.

Benzodiazepines

Benzodiazepines cause sedation, loss of motor co-ordination, memory impairment and, in high doses, behavioural disinhibition, and paradoxical agitation. All these factors can impair driving, and studies comparing culpable and non-culpable drivers have found increased risks for drivers taking benzodiazepines. Duration of impairment varies with half-life, with 5 mg diazepam causing impairment for 5 h.

Opioids

Long-term treatment with opioids for pain does not significantly impair driving skills, although there is a lack of consensus regarding the responsibility of opiates in road accidents. Acute methadone administration in naïve subjects induces a dose-dependent reduction in reaction times, but once the dose is stable there is little evidence of driving impairment. However, many methadone users take other psychotropic medication which may increase accident risk.

Amphetamines, cocaine and other stimulants

During intoxication with these drugs, reaction time and vigilance may actually be improved, although increased risk taking may be found. Any effects after drug consumption, such as exhaustion and depression may impair driving performance.

Cannabis

THC impairs perception, psychomotor performance, cognitive, and affective functions. The effects of cannabis are dose-related and higher doses are associated with increased accident rates.

Risk level by drug type

- **High risk**: benzodiazepines, cannabis and alcohol
- **High-moderate risk**: cocaine
- **Moderate risk**: cannabis, amphetamines
- **Low moderate risk**: opiates, methadone
- **Low risk** antidepressants.

Testing for drugs

Unlike alcohol, there is no clear dose relationship with driving impairment for drugs that provide the link between dose taken and an unacceptable level of impairment. In the UK, driving impairment is tested by various roadside tests of function, supported by positive tests for drugs. Testing is usually done in blood for evidential purposes.

Driving in illicit drug users

In the UK, The Driver and Vehicle Licensing Agency (DVLA) regularly publishes new editions of its At a Glance Guide (DVLA, 2007), which sets out the medical standards required for the holding of driving licences.

Drug misuse is regarded as a disability in this context. However, the focus and emphasis is on dependent and persistent misuse that is likely to impair driving. If dependent, then the use of prescribed medication to treat drug misuse constitutes a relevant disability and is subject to specific rules in order to obtain permission to continue to retain a licence.

The responsibility to inform the licensing agency of their current medical status lies with the licence holder, not the prescribing clinician or drug service. 'Consultant supervised oral methadone maintenance' or 'an oral buprenorphine programme' are, at the time of writing, the only drug treatments under which a patient may be licensed, subject to specified conditions.

Further reading

Driver and Vehicle Licensing Agency (2007). *At a Glance Guide to Medical Aspects of Fitness to Drive*. Swansea: DVLA.

Tunbridge R, Clark A, Ward BN, Dye L, Berghaus G. *Prioritising Drugs and Medicines for Development of Roadside Impairment Testing*. Project Deliverable DR1, CERTIFIED EU Research Project (Contract No RO-98-3054). Leeds: School of Psychology, University of Leeds, 2000.

Seizures and driving

Alcohol withdrawal seizures occur in 2–5% of alcohol dependent individuals, approximately 6–48 h after cessation of drinking. The seizures are generalized, grand mal (tonic-clonic) and associated with a loss of consciousness. A patient might experience only one seizure during a discrete withdrawal episode or there may be a number of seizures over a period of 3–4 days. Rarely status epilepticus will supervene. Once individuals have experienced a withdrawal seizure they are at increased risk of developing seizures during subsequent episodes of withdrawal.

A number of factors can predispose to withdrawal seizures including hypokalaemia, hypomagnesaemia, hypoglycaemia, a history of previous withdrawal seizures, and concurrent epilepsy. The risk of seizures increases with the duration of alcohol misuse and with repeated withdrawal episodes.

Following a single alcohol-related seizure an individual's licence will be revoked or refused for a minimum of 1 year. Where more than one seizure has occurred consideration under the Epilepsy Regulations is necessary (DVLA, 2007).

Anyone who has experienced an alcohol withdrawal seizure is required to undergo medical assessment with blood analysis prior to having their licence restored. They should be free from alcohol misuse/dependence and seizure free for the appropriate period. In the UK the appropriate periods for drivers of cars and motorcycles are as follows:

• Following a single seizure the licence is restored to individuals who have been seizure free for 1 year. It is restored until 70 years if there are no further attacks and they are otherwise well
• Individuals having had more than one seizure and those with epilepsy must refrain from driving for 1 year. If they have been seizure free for 1 year and pass the medical assessment, a 3-year licence is restored. Those who have been seizure free for 7 years with medication qualify for a licence until 70 years.

Child protection issues

Introduction

Substance misuse does not just affect individuals but their families too. Children's health, safety and emotional wellbeing can be seriously negatively affected when their parents, guardians or siblings have substance misuse problems. Substance misuse in the family can harm children from conception onwards and lead to problems that persist into adult life. The needs of these children or even their presence have all too often been overlooked by treatment agencies commissioned to provide services for adults. Whilst it is true that substance misuse does not always impair parenting, the effects when it does so can cause significant and lasting harm to children and young people.

The scale of the problem

It is estimated that in the United Kingdom there are up to 350,000 children of problem drug users and up to 1.3 million children living with parents who misuse alcohol. This represents up to 3 and 9%, respectively, of children under 16 years. In a sample of substance misusers in treatment in the UK, one-third of mothers and two-thirds of fathers reported that their children were living elsewhere, with around 5% of the sample reporting that their children were living in the care of the local authority. Data from child protection studies show that an increasing level of social work intervention is linked with an increasing rate of parental substance misuse.

Potential harms experienced by children living with adult substance misusers include:

- Intra-uterine exposure to substances ingested by the mother leading to growth impairment, premature birth and in some cases specific foetal damage (for example alcohol)
- Vertical transmission of blood-borne viruses (which may be acquired by the mother through injecting or sexual behaviour)
- Diminished antenatal care through poor attendance and higher incidence of birth complications
- Neonatal abstinence syndrome
- Neglect: parents may be preoccupied with substance acquisition and use, or may be intoxicated with substances
- Poverty: parents may use money for drug use
- Poor nutritional status, poor medical care, lack of immunizations
- Unpredictable adult behaviour (intoxication and withdrawal) and mood swings
- Separations from parents (incarceration, illness)
- Bereavement: parents may die from overdose, complications of alcohol and drug use, and suicide
- Episodes of alternative care provision (grandparents, statutory accommodation)
- Accidental and non-accidental injury
- Exposure to dangerous substances including drugs and drug use paraphernalia. Children have died from ingestion of parental methadone

- Domestic violence: there is an association with substance use, such as alcohol
- Poor school attendance and little support with educational endeavours such as homework and projects
- Separation from extended family
- Stigma from local community: for example, parents known to be using substances, mentally unwell, or seen to be intoxicated, begging, or involved with criminal behaviours
- Children having to parent adults, other children, and themselves
- Inappropriate adults visiting home with attendant child protection risks
- Exposure to violence associated with drug acquisition and drug use
- Exposure to inappropriate adult behaviours such as sex for money or drugs, injecting behaviour
- Drug- or alcohol-impaired driving accidents.

Likely indicators of potential harm from assessment of the parent

All adults presenting for treatment of a substance misuse problem should be assessed with regard to the likely impact of their substance misuse on their children. The following features may suggest greater harm to the children, but this list is not exhaustive and in any situation there are a number of factors that need to be considered. All cases should be assessed on an individual basis and any concerns should be reported to the relevant child protection services so that a full assessment of the children's needs can be undertaken.

- Dependence on large amounts of substance(s) necessitating significant time to fund, obtain and use the substance(s) and mode of use, for example injecting frequently
- Evidence of mood swings and unpredictability
- Presence of significant withdrawal symptoms such as delirium tremens
- Multiple drug and alcohol use with chaotic use, and episodes of intoxication and withdrawal
- Methods of procuring funding for substances such as sex work and criminal activity
- Presence of co-morbid mental illness
- Financial problems, housing problems, legal problems
- No non-substance-using adults in household.

Factors which affect the impact of substance use on parenting ability and the experience of children

Substance misuse is one of many factors that can impact on parenting ability and there are many other factors that can mitigate or exacerbate any problems caused. The following factors need to be considered:

- Severity and type of parental drug and alcohol problems: one or both parents receiving effective treatment is likely to be associated with better outcomes for the children
- Co-morbid mental illness: parental mental illness has associated child protection risks in addition to those associated with substance misuse
- School experience: positive school experiences have been shown to be associated with better outcomes for childhood adversity

- Age of the child and child's needs: for example, younger children are more vulnerable to physical neglect.
- Presence of at least one supportive parent or parental figure is associated with better outcome.
- Level of social support to family: strong social support networks are associated with better outcomes for childhood adversity as is the presence of a committed mentor or other person outside the family .
- Financial status of family: a stable home with adequate financial resources is likely to be associated with better outcomes .
- Parents' ability to prioritise children's needs and general parenting skills (parents may have poor baseline parenting skills).
- Family routines: families report that routines are often difficult to establish where there are substance misuse problems. It is likely that there is a better outcome for children where routines and activities are preserved.

Adverse consequences for children from parental substance misuse

The potential effects of parental problem drug use on children are serious and can cause potentially life long difficulties. They include the following:
- Poor physical and dental health during childhood.
- Incomplete immunizations.
- Acquisition of blood borne viruses.
- Poor educational attainment and difficulty in relationships with peers.
- Emotional and behavioural disorders, such as antisocial acts, truanting, impulsivity, hyperactivity, inattention, aggression, conduct disorders, depression and anxiety.
- Early initiation of smoking, alcohol, and drug use.
- Increased risk of problem alcohol and drug use.
- Increased risk of offending and criminality.
- Increased risk of teenage pregnancy and sexually transmitted infections.

Interventions

A prerequisite for intervention is the identification of children living with adults with substance misuse problems by the relevant agencies.
    Potential interventions include:
- Effective substance misuse treatment for parents.
- Individual specific support for children—depends on age and needs— nursery, after school, counselling, peer support groups, educational support.
- Specific programmes for families with substance misusing parents— research in this area is in its infancy but has shown that it is possible to recruit and retain high risk families and that there may be value in combining clinic-based substance misuse treatment with home visits .
- Social support for family—housing, financial, legal, social.
- Work with children to prevent early initiation of drug and alcohol use.
- Suitable alternative accommodation for children if necessary—where parents are in hospital/prison/unable to provide adequate care. Residential care outside family should be 'last resort'—consider day fostering, family fostering.

Further reading

Advisory Council on the Misuse of Drugs. *Hidden Harm. Responding to the Needs of Children of Problem Drug Users.* London: Home Office, 2003.

Barnard, M. *Drug Addiction and Families.* London: Jessica Kingsley Publishers, 2007.

Barnard MA, McKeganey NP. The impact of parental drug problem use on children: what is the problem and what can be done to help? *Addiction* 2004; **99**: 552–559.

Cleaver H, Unell I, Aldgate J. *Children's Needs—Parenting Capacity. The Impact of Parental Mental Illness, Problem Alcohol and Drug Use, and Domestic Violence on Children's Development.* London: Department of Health, 1999.

Prime Minister's Strategy Unit. *Alcohol Harm Reduction Strategy for England.* London: Cabinet Office, 2004.

Workplace safety/responsibility

There has been increasing focus in recent years on the issue of use of alcohol and other drugs in the workplace. The concern has arisen from four separate considerations:

- A concern about the negative impact on productivity of employees (at various levels) who are impaired as a result of their alcohol or other drug use
- Concern about the legal and ethical implications of employees affected by psychoactive substances particularly in transportation and other industries where public safety is paramount
- The increasing expectation that employees will have a safe workplace, as enshrined by the development of health and safety legislation
- The acknowledgement that the workplace potentially offers a setting in which people with substance use disorders can seek advice and treatment through self referral or employer-initiated mechanisms.

Effects of alcohol on work-related problems

- Volume of alcohol
- Absenteeism due to illness or disciplinary suspension
- Reduced performance and productivity
- Increased turnover of staff
- Inappropriate behaviour
- Theft and other crime
- Poor relationships between workers and low morale
- Work accidents
- Moderate drinking: thought to cause some negative effects
- Patterns of drinking: intoxication and heavy drinking lead to problems, as well as alcohol dependence.

Work accidents

It is estimated that 20–25% of all workplace accidents involve alcohol in some way. Alcohol consumption impairs concentration, judgement, and co-ordination, and accidents can affect the drinker and those around them. Employers have legal responsibilities regarding the safety of employees and, where relevant, the general public. Drinking even small amounts of alcohol before or while carrying out work that is 'safety sensitive' will increase the risk of an accident.

Surveys of many industries have shown a high prevalence of alcohol and other drug use in workforces. In part, this reflects community patterns of substance use. However, other key influences are the socio-demographic make-up of the workforce, and also the nature of the product or service provided. For example, workers in hospitality and catering industries, and in particular those involved in the production or sale of alcohol, have a high rate of alcohol misuse. Workgroups who have ready access to prescribed medications, such as health care professionals have higher rates of dependence on prescribed sedative hypnotics and opioids. In the financial industry there is reportedly a high prevalence of psychostimulant use; whether this involves methamphetamine or cocaine depends on geographical area.

In the music industry and other creative arts there is a high prevalence of multiple substance use, including cannabis, alcohol, heroin, and psychostimulants. In some industries (e.g. trucking) stimulants are sometimes used to increase wakefulness or stamina but pose major safety hazards. Stimulant use has also been associated with the modelling industry, where weight loss is often a desired outcome.

Workplace alcohol policies

Alcohol problems in the workplace should be considered as a health issue, and an alcohol policy should be located in or linked to one or more of an organization's procedures on managing health and safety, as well as personnel and/or general management issues.

An alcohol policy will be more successful if supported by a programme of training that raises alcohol awareness and supports managers in its application. Employers often have a parallel or combined policy to address drug misuse.

Current approaches to the prevention of substance misuse in the workplace include the following:

- A policy covering the use of alcohol or other drugs prior to or during the working day, which is agreed through negotiation with employee groups, unions and management representatives
- Provision through an employee assistance scheme of assessment and referral on a confidential basis of employees who are affected by psychoactive substances. Typically, this would include an employer-initiated process where impairment of work performance or the detection of psychoactive substances has occurred. Secondly, self-initiated referral also occurs where an employee recognizes that their alcohol or drug use is causing problems
- Routine and random testing for alcohol and other drugs has been introduced progressively in recent years into many industries particularly those where there are safety critical working conditions, e.g. using machinery or where there is a responsibility for public safety, as in the transportation industries. Such policies may require employees to provide a urine or saliva sample, which will be tested for drugs or a breath or urine sample for testing for alcohol. The consequences of a positive test will depend on the organization's policy, but may include a warning, a requirement to participate in an employee assistance programme or particularly with repeated infractions, loss of employment (also see p. 413)
- Sometimes the workplace can offer supervision of medication, such as disulfiram to increase adherence to treatment regimes.

Testing

Testing employees or potential employees for alcohol use or related problems remains controversial, raising both industrial relations and civil liberty issues.

Under UK law, employers have a responsibility to demonstrate 'due diligence' (take reasonable care) to prevent an accident if an employee's ability to work safely is impaired. This need to prevent alcohol or drug-related accidents has led companies in the transport sector to introduce testing to prevent employees' substance use in the workplace.

Methods of testing

Alcohol testing indicates whether an individual is under the influence at that time. Drug testing differs, sometimes showing traces of drugs used in the past, but not confirming impairment at the time of testing. Alcohol use can be determined by breath or blood testing. Breath tests are convenient and inexpensive. Blood testing is the most accurate measure of alcohol in the body, but is more invasive than a breath test and not routinely carried out, except in safety critical jobs, e.g. after a positive breath test is returned.

Screening or testing to detect alcohol problems can be used in a variety of ways.

- **Recruitment screening** usually involves testing as part of assessing the health of potential employees during the recruitment process
- **Routine testing** is done at specified times and gives a clear message that it is not acceptable to be affected by alcohol when working. It might be used in situations where employees are in 'safety critical' posts, such as operating public transport or machinery
- **Random testing** is used as a deterrent to identify previously undetected alcohol misuse. Again, this is more likely to be used in safety critical settings
- **'With cause' and post-incident testing** might be used if a manager has reason to believe that an employee has been drinking, by their behaviour or is smelling of alcohol, for instance. After an incident at work, such as an accident, it can be a part of the post-incident investigation.

Getting specialist help

Workforce programmes and interventions tend to be offered by specific organizations which specialize in this area. On occasion, however, an employee may be referred to a public sector or private facility to undergo treatment. In such circumstances it is vital for the clinician to understand clearly the nature of the referral request and any reporting requirements. This is essential to ensure the integrity of the treatment is maintained and that there is a clear understanding by all parties on whether the treatment and response is subject to usual medical confidentiality provisions or whether the clinician or agency is required to provide periodic reports on progress. This is especially important where a person's professional registration or business operating licence is at threat if adherence to treatment is inadequate.

Some larger employers will have an occupational health department or employee assistance programme that may include an in-house counselling service with expertise in alcohol problems. Alternatively, individuals might be encouraged to approach their GP, seek to be referred to a community alcohol service, or attend Alcoholics Anonymous. In-patient detoxification and residential treatment facilities may sometimes also be available, although normally these would be through referral following a full assessment.

Further reading

Babor T, Caetano R, Casswell S *et al*. *Alcohol: No Ordinary Commodity*. Oxford: Oxford University Press, 2003.

Institute of Alcohol Studies. *Fact Sheet on Alcohol in the Workplace*. 2007. Available at: www.ias.org.uk

London Drug Policy Forum. *Tackling Drugs and Alcohol in the Workplace*. 2007. Available at: www.cityof london.gov.uk/ldpf

Mental Health Act, Guardianship Board, Inebriates Act, Diversion into Treatment

Legal provisions for treatment

Although the focus of this handbook is on the management of substance use disorders in standard clinical settings, i.e. with the patients who are voluntarily being treated, occasions exist where patients undergo legally-mandated treatment for their own protection or that of others. The role of the law in coerced or compulsory treatment has undergone significant reassessment in recent years. In some countries patients with serious mental complications, such as a substance-induced psychosis may be detained compulsorily and be treated (with sedation, anti-psychotic drugs and seclusion) without their consent. Typically, such treatment occurs under the provisions of the relevant mental health act.

As an example, in Australia the Mental Health Act of most States & Territories includes provision for the compulsory detention of people with (i) mental illness or who are (ii) mentally disordered. The latter provision is enacted when a person with a substance-related psychosis or delirium is unable to give consent to treatment and when they or others are considered to be at risk of serious harm through their actions. Detention under the mental disorder provisions can take place for a maximum of 3 days, whereupon it lapses.

Legislation to mandate treatment solely on the basis of an alcohol or drug problem (without any mental illness) is uncommonly available and where laws exist, they are rarely used. In New South Wales, Australia the Inebriates Act exists, which was proclaimed in 1912 and has existed practically unchanged in the statute books ever since. It enables a person who has serious recurrent alcohol and other drug-induced disorders to be committed for treatment, typically to a mental hospital, for up to 1 year. No particular form of treatment is specified, this being left to the discretion of the psychiatrist in charge of the case. The Inebriates Act is typically used for people who have a progressive downhill course characterized by significant neuropsychiatric complications and dangerous episodes of extreme intoxication. The decision on whether a person can be committed is that of the magistrate. Committal is more likely if a person's relatives initiate the order and it is backed up by the treating professionals. Individual cases of good outcomes are recognized, but there is no long-term evaluation available of the results of this legislation.

Another uncommonly enacted form of legislation is where a person with a substance use disorder poses, through their actions, a risk to public health and safety. This occurs for example where an HIV+ person engages in sharing of injecting equipment. Treatment such as hospitalization can in these circumstances be imposed. Another instance where this can occur is where a person has multi-drug resistant tuberculosis.

Diversion into treatment, which occurs when the person is apprehended by the police, but not arrested, typically involves the possession of cannabis (in amounts considered only for personal use) and usually entails referral to an education session or a short-term intervention. There may or may not be contingencies if the person fails to abide by the instructions.

Concern is sometimes expressed at the discretionary nature of this form of diversion.

More commonly, diversion into treatment occurs when the person has been arrested and faces Court. As an alternative to the normal penalties, magistrates may decide that diversion into treatment should be offered as an alternative. Typically, this involves referring to a specialist agency for assessment and intervention. This type of diversionary treatment has become common practice in several countries, most notably the USA, and increasingly in Australia and some European countries. In some jurisdictions specially developed 'drug courts' have been established.

Pre-sentence diversion into treatment offers the opportunity for a lesser penalty, if the person found guilty of a drug-related offence accepts the offer of treatment. This may, for example, convert a custodial sentence into a community service order, a fine, or a bond. Again, this form of diversion is undergoing considerable evaluation at present.

Appendix

Detailed list of appendices

Brief alcohol screening instruments
- AUDIT, AUDIT-C
- TWEAK.
- FAST
- Paddington Alcohol Test

ICD-10 and DSM IV TR diagnoses

Withdrawal monitoring scales
- **AWS**: alcohol withdrawal
- **CIWA-AR**: alcohol withdrawal
- **CIWA-B**: benzodiazepine withdrawal
- Opioid withdrawal scale
- Neonatal Abstinence Syndrome.

Mini mental state examination

12-steps of AA

Brief Alcohol Use Screening Questionnaires

AUDIT- The Alcohol Use Disorders Identification Test

1. How often do you have a drink containing alcohol?

| Never | Monthly or less | 2–4 times a month | 2–3 times a week | 4 or more times a week |

2. How many standard drinks containing alcohol do you have on a typical day when you are drinking?

| 1 or 2 | 3 or 4 | 5 or 6 | 7–9 | 10 or more |

3. How often do you have six or more drinks on one occasion?

| Never | Less than monthly | Monthly | Weekly | Daily or almost daily |

4. During the past year, how often have you found that you were not able to stop drinking once you had started?

| Never | Less than monthly | Monthly | Weekly | Daily or almost daily |

5. During the past year, how often have you failed to do what was normally expected of you because of drinking?

| Never | Less than monthly | Monthly | Weekly | Daily or almost daily |

6. During the past year, how often have you needed a drink in the morning to get yourself going after a heavy drinking session?

| Never | Less than monthly | Monthly | Weekly | Daily or almost daily |

7. During the past year, how often have you had a feeling of guilt or remorse after drinking?

| Never | Less than monthly | Monthly | Weekly | Daily or almost daily |

8. During the past year, have you been unable to remember what happened the night before because you had been drinking?

| Never | Less than monthly | Monthly | Weekly | Daily or almost daily |

9. Have you or someone else been injured as a result of your drinking?

| No | Yes, but not in the past year | Yes, during the past year |

10. Has a relative or friend, doctor or other health worker been concerned about your drinking or suggested you cut down?

| No | Yes, but not in the past year | Yes, during the past year |

Scoring the AUDIT

Scores for each question range from 0 to 4, for Questions 1–8 the first response for each question (e.g. never) scoring 0, the second (e.g. less than monthly) scoring 1, the third (e.g. monthly) scoring 2, the fourth (e.g. weekly) scoring 3, and the last response (e.g. daily or almost daily) scoring 4.

For questions 9 and 10, which only have three responses, the scoring is 0, 2 and 4 (from left to right).

A score of 8 or more is associated with harmful or hazardous drinking, a score of 13 or more is likely to indicate alcohol dependence.

AUDIT-C

Consists of the first 3 questions of AUDIT and is scored in the same fashion. Cut-off scores are usually 3 for women and 4 for men, although for expediency in large-scale screening programmes, sometimes a cut-off of 4 is used for both.

Further reading

Babor TF, Higgins-Biddle JC, Saunders JB, Monteiro MG. AUDIT. The *Alcohol Use Disorders Identification Test—Guidelines for Use in Primary Care*, 2nd edn. Geneva: World Health Organization, Department of Mental Health and Substance Dependence 2001. Available at: http://whqlibdoc. who.int/hq/2001/WHO_MSD_MSB_01.6a.pdf

Saunders JB, Aasland OG, Babor TF, de la Fuente JR, Grant M. Development of the Alcohol Use Disorders Identification Test (AUDIT): WHO Collaborative Project on Early Detection of Persons with Harmful Alcohol Consumption—II. *Addiction* 1993; **88**: 791–804.

TWEAK questionnaire

TWEAK is a five-item scale developed originally to screen for risk drinking during pregnancy. It is an acronym for the questions below (Russell, 1994):

T **Tolerance***: How many drinks can you hold?

W **Worried**: Have close friends or relatives worried or complained about your drinking in the past year?

E **Eye-opener**: Do you sometimes take a drink in the morning when you first get up?

A **Amnesia**: stands for blackouts—Has a friend or family member ever told you about things you said or did while you were drinking that you could not remember?

K **K/Cut Down**: Do you sometimes feel the need to cut down on your drinking?

Copies of the TWEAK and scoring instructions are available from Marcia Russell, Prevention Research Center, 1995 University Avenue, Suite 450, Berkeley, CA 94704, USA (email: russell@prev.org).

The Paddington Alcohol Test

Circle number(s)—for specific trigger(s); consider for All the top 10

1. FALL (*inc. trip*) 2. COLLAPSE (*inc. fits*) 3. HEAD INJURY (*inc. facial*) 4. ASSAULT

5. ACCIDENT (*inc. Burn, RTA*) 6. UNWELL (*inc. Request detox/help, self neglect*) 7. NON SPECIFIC GI

8. PSYCHIATRIC 9. CARDIAC (*inc. Chest pain*) 10. REPEAT ATTENDER Other (specify)_____

After dealing with patient's 'agenda,' i.e. patient's reason for attendance: –

1 "We routinely ask all patients in A & E if they drink alcohol—do you drink?" YES – Go to Q2 (No)

2 "Quite a number of people have times when they drink more than usual; what is the most you will drink in any one day?" (*Pub measures in brackets; home measures often x3!*)

Beer/lager/cider	___ Pints (2)	___ Cans (1.5)	**Total units/day**
Strong beer/lager/cider	___ Pints (5)	___ Cans (4)	
Wine	___ Glasses (1.5)	___ Bottles (9)	
Fortified Wine (Sherry, Martini)	___ Glasses (1)	___ Bottles (12)	
Spirits (Gin, Whisky, Vodka)	___ Singles (1)	___ Bottles (30)	

3 If this <u>more than</u> 8 units/day for a man or 6 units/day for a woman, does this happen …..

Once a week or more? = *PAT* +ve (*every day: ? Pabrinex*®)

or if less frequently

At least once a month = *PAT* +ve <1/12 = PAT –ve (trumped by 4.)

4 "Do you fell your current attendance is related to alcohol?" *YES* = *PAT* +ve

No = PAT–ve

Note: the drinking containers and suggested limits in Q3 are for the UK. These can be adapted to drink containers and recommendations from other countries.

Abbreviations: *inc.* – including; RTA – Road traffic accident; GI – gastrointestinal disorders; A & E – Accident and Emergency department.

Further reading

Patton R, Hilton C, Crawford MJ, Touquet R. The Paddington Alcohol Test: a short report. *Alcohol & Alcoholism* 2004; **39**(3): 266–268.

FAST

For the following questions please circle the answer which best applies.

1 drink = ½ pint of beer or 1 glass of wine or 1 single spirits

1. MEN: How often do you have EIGHT or more drinks on one occasion?
   WOMEN: How often do you have SIX or more drinks on one occasion?

   | Never | Less than Monthly | Monthly | Weekly | Daily or almost daily |

2. How often during the last year have you been unable to remember what happened the night before because you had been drinking?

   | Never | Less than Monthly | Monthly | Weekly | Daily or almost daily |

3. How often during the last year have you failed to do what was normally expected of you because of drinking?

   | Never | Less than Monthly | Monthly | Weekly | Daily or almost daily |

4. In the last year has a relative or friend, or a doctor or other health worker been concerned about your drinking or suggested you cut down?

   | No | Yes, on one occasion | Yes, on more than one occasion |

Score questions 1–3: 0, 1, 2, 3, 4. Score question 4: 0, 2, 4.
A score ≥3 indicates probable hazardous drinking

Further reading

Hodgson R, Alwyn T, John B, Thom B, Smith A. The FAST alcohol screening test. *Alcohol and Alcoholism* 2002; **37**(1): 61–66.

ICD and DSM diagnoses

ICD-10 clinical descriptions and diagnostic guidelines

The following are extracts from:

The International Classification of Diseases, 10th Revision, Geneva: World Health Organization.

The ICD-10 Classification of Mental and Behavioural Disorders. Clinical Descriptions and Diagnostic Guidelines. Geneva: World Health Organization 1992. Available at http://www.who.int/substance_abuse/terminology/ICD10ClinicalDiagnosis.pdf F10 - F19.

Mental and behavioural disorders due to psychoactive substance use
Overview of this block

F10 Mental and behavioural disorders due to use of alcohol
F11 Mental and behavioural disorders due to use of opioids
F12 Mental and behavioural disorders due to use of cannabinoids
F13 Mental and behavioural disorders due to use of sedative hypnotics
F14 Mental and behavioural disorders due to use of cocaine
F15 Mental and behavioural disorders due to use of other stimulants, including caffeine
F16 Mental and behavioural disorders due to use of hallucinogens
F17 Mental and behavioural disorders due to use of tobacco
F18 Mental and behavioural disorders due to use of volatile solvents
F19 Mental and behavioural disorders due to multiple drug use and use of other psychoactive substances

Four- and five-character codes may be used to specify the clinical conditions, as follows:

- **F1x.0**: Acute intoxication:
  - .00 Uncomplicated
  - .01 With trauma or other bodily injury
  - .02 With other medical complications
  - .03 With delirium
  - .04 With perceptual distortions
  - .05 With coma
  - .06 With convulsions
  - .07 Pathological intoxication
- **F1x.1**: Harmful use
- **F1x.2**: Dependence syndrome
  - .20 Currently abstinent
  - .21 Currently abstinent, but in a protected environment
  - .22 Currently on a clinically supervised maintenance or replacement regime [controlled dependence]
  - .23 Currently abstinent, but receiving treatment with aversive or blocking drugs
  - .24 Currently using the substance [active dependence]
  - .25 Continuous use
  - .26 Episodic use [dipsomania]
- **F1x.3**: Withdrawal state
  - .30 Uncomplicated
  - .31 With convulsions

- **F1x.4**: Withdrawal state with delirium
  - .40 Without convulsions
  - .41 With convulsions
- **F1x.5**: Psychotic disorder
  - .50 Schizophrenia-like
  - .51 Predominantly delusional
  - .52 Predominantly hallucinatory
  - .53 Predominantly polymorphic
  - .54 Predominantly depressive symptoms
  - .55 Predominantly manic symptoms
  - .56 Mixed
- **F1x.6**: Amnesic syndrome
- **F1x.7**: Residual and late-onset psychotic disorder
  - .70 Flashbacks
  - .71 Personality or behaviour disorder
  - .72 Residual affective behaviour
  - .73 Dementia
  - .74 Other persisting cognitive behaviour
  - .75 Late-onset psychotic disorder
- **F1x.8**: Other mental and behavioural disorders
- **F1x.9**: Unspecified mental and behavioural disorder.

F1x.0. Acute intoxication

A transient condition following the administration of alcohol or other psychoactive substance, resulting in disturbances in level of consciousness, cognition, perception, affect or behaviour, or other psychophysiological functions and responses. This should be a main diagnosis only in cases where intoxication occurs without more persistent alcohol- or drug-related problems being concomitantly present. Where there are such problems, precedence should be given to diagnoses of harmful use (F1x.1), dependence syndrome (F1x.2), or psychotic disorder (F1x.5).

Acute intoxication is usually closely related to dose levels (see ICD-10). Exceptions to this may occur in individuals with certain underlying organic conditions (e.g. renal or hepatic insufficiency) in whom small doses of a substance may produce a disproportionately severe intoxicating effect. Disinhibition due to social context should also be taken into account (e.g. behavioural disinhibition at parties or carnivals). Acute intoxication is a transient phenomenon. Intensity of intoxication lessens with time and effects eventually disappear in the absence of further use of the substance. Recovery is therefore complete except where tissue damage or another complication has arisen.

Symptoms of intoxication need not always reflect primary actions of the substance. For instance, depressant drugs may lead to symptoms of agitation or hyperactivity, and stimulant drugs may lead to socially withdrawn and introverted behaviour. Effects of substances, such as cannabis and hallucinogens may be particularly unpredictable.

Moreover, many psychoactive substances are capable of producing different types of effect at different levels. For example, alcohol may have apparently stimulant effects on behaviour at lower dose levels, lead to agitation and aggression with increasing dose levels, and produce clear sedation at very high levels.

F1x.1. Harmful use

A pattern of psychoactive substance use that is causing damage to health. The damage may be physical (as in cases of hepatitis from the self-administration of injected drugs) or mental (e.g. episodes of depressive disorder secondary to heavy consumption of alcohol).

Diagnostic guidelines

The diagnosis requires that actual damage should have been caused to the mental or physical health of the user.

Harmful patterns of use are often criticized by others and frequently associated with adverse social consequences of various kinds. The fact that a pattern of use or a particular substance is disapproved of by another person or by the culture, or may have led to socially negative consequences such as arrest or marital arguments is not in itself evidence of harmful use.

Acute intoxication (see F1x.0), or 'hangover' is not itself sufficient evidence of the damage to health required for coding harmful use.

Harmful use should not be diagnosed if dependence syndrome (F1x.2), a psychotic disorder (F1x.5), or another specific form of drug- or alcohol-related disorder is present.

F1x.2. Dependence syndrome

A cluster of physiological, behavioural, and cognitive phenomena in which the use of a substance or a class of substances takes on a much higher priority for a given individual than other behaviours that once had greater value. A central descriptive characteristic of the dependence syndrome is the desire (often strong, sometimes overpowering) to take psychoactive drugs (which may or may not have been medically prescribed), alcohol, or tobacco. There may be evidence that return to substance use after a period of abstinence leads to a more rapid reappearance of other features of the syndrome than occurs with nondependent individuals.

Diagnostic guidelines

A definite diagnosis of dependence should usually be made only if three or more of the following have been present together at some time during the previous year:

- A strong desire or sense of compulsion to take the substance
- Difficulties in controlling substance-taking behaviour in terms of its onset, termination, or levels of use
- A physiological withdrawal state (see F1x.3 and F1x.4) when substance use has ceased or been reduced, as evidenced by: the characteristic withdrawal syndrome for the substance; or use of the same (or a closely related) substance with the intention of relieving or avoiding withdrawal symptoms
- Evidence of tolerance, such that increased doses of the psychoactive substances are required in order to achieve effects originally produced by lower doses (clear examples of this are found in alcohol- and opiate-dependent individuals who may take daily doses sufficient to incapacitate or kill non-tolerant users)
- Progressive neglect of alternative pleasures or interests because of psychoactive substance use, increased amount of time necessary to obtain or take the substance or to recover from its effects

- Persisting with substance use despite clear evidence of overtly harmful consequences, such as harm to the liver through excessive drinking, depressive mood states consequent to periods of heavy substance use, or drug-related impairment of cognitive functioning; efforts should be made to determine that the user was actually, or could be expected to be, aware of the nature and extent of the harm.

Narrowing of the personal repertoire of patterns of psychoactive substance use has also been described as a characteristic feature (e.g. a tendency to drink alcoholic drinks in the same way on weekdays and weekends, regardless of social constraints that determine appropriate drinking behaviour).

It is an essential characteristic of the dependence syndrome that either psychoactive substance taking or a desire to take a particular substance should be present; the subjective awareness of compulsion to use drugs is most commonly seen during attempts to stop or control substance use. This diagnostic requirement would exclude, for instance, surgical patients given opioid drugs for the relief of pain, who may show signs of an opioid withdrawal state when drugs are not given, but who have no desire to continue taking drugs.

The dependence syndrome may be present for a specific substance (e.g. tobacco or diazepam), for a class of substances (e.g. opioid drugs), or for a wider range of different substances (as for those individuals who feel a sense of compulsion regularly to use whatever drugs are available, and who show distress, agitation, and/or physical signs of a withdrawal state upon abstinence).

F1x.3. Withdrawal state

A group of symptoms of variable clustering and severity occurring on absolute or relative withdrawal of a substance after repeated, and usually prolonged and/or high dose, use of that substance. Onset and course of the withdrawal state are time-limited and are related to the type of substance and the dose being used immediately before abstinence. The withdrawal state may be complicated by convulsions.

Diagnostic guidelines

Withdrawal state is one of the indicators of dependence syndrome (see F1x.2) and this latter diagnosis should also be considered. Withdrawal state should be coded as the main diagnosis if it is the reason for referral and sufficiently severe to require medical attention in its own right.

Physical symptoms vary according to the substance being used. Psychological disturbances (e.g. anxiety, depression, and sleep disorders) are also common features of withdrawal. Typically, the patient is likely to report that withdrawal symptoms are relieved by further substance use. It should be remembered that withdrawal symptoms can be induced by conditioned/learned stimuli in the absence of immediately preceding substance use. In such cases a diagnosis of withdrawal state should be made only if it is warranted in terms of severity.

F1x.4. Withdrawal state with delirium

A condition in which the withdrawal state (see F1x.3) is complicated by delirium (see criteria for F05. -).

Alcohol-induced delirium tremens should be coded here. Delirium tremens is a short-lived, but occasionally life-threatening, toxic-confusional state with accompanying somatic disturbances. It is usually a consequence of absolute or relative withdrawal of alcohol in severely dependent users with a long history of use. Onset usually occurs after withdrawal of alcohol. In some cases, the disorder appears during an episode of heavy drinking, in which case it should be coded here. Prodromal symptoms typically include insomnia, tremulousness, and fear. Onset may also be preceded by withdrawal convulsions. The classical triad of symptoms includes clouding of consciousness and confusion, vivid hallucinations and illusions affecting any sensory modality, and marked tremor. Delusions, agitation, insomnia or sleep-cycle reversal, and autonomic over activity are usually also present.

Excludes: delirium, not induced by drugs and alcohol (F05. -)

F1x.5. Psychotic disorder

A cluster of psychotic phenomena that occur during or immediately after psychoactive substance use and are characterized by vivid hallucinations (typically auditory, but often in more than one sensory modality), mis-identifications, delusions and/or ideas of reference (often of a paranoid or persecutory nature), psychomotor disturbances (excitement of stupor), and an abnormal affect, which may range from intense fear to ecstasy. The sensorium is usually clear, but some degree of clouding of consciousness, though not severe confusion, may be present. The disorder typically resolves at least partially within 1 month and fully within 6 months.

Diagnostic guidelines

A psychotic disorder occurring during or immediately after drug use (usually within 48 h) should be recorded here provided that it is not a manifestation of drug withdrawal state with delirium (see F1x.4) or of late onset. Late-onset psychotic disorders (with onset more than 2 weeks after substance use) may occur, but should be coded as F1x.75.

Psychoactive substance-induced psychotic disorders may present with varying patterns of symptoms. These variations will be influenced by the type of substance involved and the personality of the user. For stimulant drugs such as cocaine and amphetamines, drug-induced psychotic disorders are generally closely related to high dose levels and/or prolonged use of the substance.

A diagnosis of psychotic disorder should not be made merely on the basis of perceptual distortions or hallucinatory experiences when substances having primary hallucinogenic effects (e.g. lysergic acid (LSD), mescaline, cannabis at high doses) have been taken. In such cases and also for confusional states, a possible diagnoses of acute intoxication (F1x.0) should be considered.

Particular care should also be taken to avoid mistakenly diagnosing a more serious condition (e.g. schizophrenia) when a diagnosis of psychoactive substance-induced psychosis is appropriate. Many psychoactive substance-induced psychotic states are of short duration provided that no further amounts of the drug are taken (as in the case of amphetamine and cocaine psychoses). False diagnosis in such cases may have distressing and costly implications for the patient and for the health services.

F1x.6. Amnesic syndrome

A syndrome associated with chronic prominent impairment of recent memory; remote memory is sometimes impaired, while immediate recall is preserved. Disturbances of time sense and ordering of events are usually evident, as are difficulties in learning new material. Confabulation may be marked but is not invariably present. Other cognitive functions are usually relatively well preserved and amnesic defects are out of proportion to other disturbances.

Diagnostic guidelines

Amnesic syndrome induced by alcohol or other psychoactive substances coded here should meet the general criteria for organic amnesic syndrome (see F04). The primary requirements for this diagnosis are:

- Memory impairment as shown in impairment of recent memory (learning of new material); disturbances of time sense (rearrangements of chronological sequence, telescoping of repeated events into one, etc.)
- Absence of defect in immediate recall, impairment of consciousness, and of generalized cognitive impairment
- History or objective evidence of chronic (and particularly high-dose) use of alcohol or drugs.

Personality changes, often with apparent apathy and loss of initiative, and a tendency towards self-neglect may also be present, but should not be regarded as necessary conditions for diagnosis.

Although confabulation may be marked it should not be regarded as a necessary prerequisite for diagnosis.

Includes: Korsakov's psychosis or syndrome, alcohol- or other psychoactive substance-induced.

F1x.7 Residual and late-onset psychotic disorder

A disorder in which alcohol- or psychoactive substance-induced changes of cognition, affect, personality, or behaviour persist beyond the period during which a direct psychoactive substance-related effect might reasonably be assumed to be operating.

Diagnostic guidelines

Onset of the disorder should be directly related to the use of alcohol or a psychoactive substance. Cases in which initial onset occurs later than episode(s) of substance use should be coded here only where clear and strong evidence is available to attribute the state to the residual effect of the substance. The disorder should represent a change from or marked exaggeration of prior and normal state of functioning.

The disorder should persist beyond any period of time during which direct effects of the psychoactive substance might be assumed to be operative (see F1x.0, acute intoxication). Alcohol- or psychoactive substance-induced dementia is not always irreversible; after an extended period of total abstinence, intellectual functions and memory may improve.

The disorder should be carefully distinguished from withdrawal-related conditions (see F1x.3 and F1x.4). It should be remembered that, under certain conditions and for certain substances, withdrawal state phenomena may be present for a period of many days or weeks after discontinuation of the substance.

Conditions induced by a psychoactive substance, persisting after its use, and meeting the criteria for diagnosis of psychotic disorder should not be diagnosed here (use F1x.5, psychotic disorder). Patients who show the chronic end-state of Korsakov's syndrome should be coded under F1x.6.

DSM IV-TR

The diagnostic guidelines for substance use disorders in DSM IV-TR are available from American Psychiatric Association. Diagnostic and Statistical Manual of Mental Disorders, 4th Edition, Text Revision (DSM-IV-TR). Washington, DC: American Pyschiatric Association 2000.

Below is a summary of the key criteria for a diagnosis of substance abuse and dependence:

Substance abuse

A pattern of recurrent substance use leading to significant impairment or distress, as evidenced by one (or more) of the following, occurring within a 12-month period:

- Recurrent substance use which results in failure to fulfil major obligations at work, school, or home
- Recurrent substance use in situations in which it is physically hazardous (e.g. drink driving)
- Recurrent legal problems related to substance use
- Continued use despite having persistent or recurrent social or interpersonal problems caused or exacerbated by the effects of the substance (e.g. arguments with spouse, physical fights).

A person can only be diagnosed as having substance abuse if they have never met the criteria for Substance Dependence for that class of substance.

Substance dependence

A pattern of recurrent substance use, which leads to significant impairment or distress. Three or more of the following criteria are required for a diagnosis, occurring in the same 12-month period:

- Tolerance, which can be exhibited by either needing more of the substance to achieve the desired effect OR achieving a diminished effect with use of the same amount of the substance
- Withdrawal or use of the substance (or a closely related substance) to relieve or avoid withdrawal
- The substance is often taken in larger amounts or over a longer period than was intended
- A persistent desire or unsuccessful efforts to cut down or control substance use
- A great deal of time spent in obtaining the substance, using the substance, or getting over its effects
- Important social, occupational, or recreational activities are given up or reduced because of substance use
- Continued use despite knowledge of having a persistent or recurrent physical or psychological problem that is likely to have been caused or exacerbated by the substance.

The diagnosis is then further clarified, by specifying whether or not there is physiological dependence (i.e. evidence of tolerance or withdrawal).

Withdrawal monitoring scales

Alcohol withdrawal scale (AWS)

As shown in New South Wales Drug & Alcohol withdrawal Clinical Practice Guidelines. NSW Health Department 2007. http://www.health.nsw.gov.au

Scoring
- Perspiration (0–4)
- Tremor (0–3)
- Anxiety (0–4)
- Agitation (0–4)
- Axilla temperature (0–4)
- Hallucinations (0–4)
- Orientation (0–4)
- **Total (maximum possible is 27).**

Perspiration
0 No abnormal sweating
1 Moist skin
2 Localized beads of sweat, e.g. on face, chest
3 Whole body wet from perspiration
4 Profuse maximal sweating—clothes, linen are wet.

Tremor
0 No tremor
1 Slight tremor
2 Constant slight tremor of upper extremities
3 Constant marked tremor of extremities.

Anxiety
0 No apprehension or anxiety
1 Slight apprehension
2 Apprehension or understandable fear, e.g. of withdrawal symptoms
3 Anxiety occasionally accentuated to a state of panic
4 Constant panic-like anxiety.

Agitation
0 Rests normally during day, no signs of agitation
1 Slight restlessness, cannot sit or lie still. Awake when others asleep
2 Moves constantly, looks tense. Wants to get out of bed but obeys requests to stay in bed
3 Constantly restless. Gets out of bed for no obvious reason
4 Maximally restless, aggressive. Ignores requests to stay in bed.

Axilla temperature
0 Temperature of 37.0°C
1 Temperature of 37.1°C
2 Temperature of 37.6–38.0°C
3 Temperature of 38.1–38.5°C
4 Temperature above 38.5°C.

Hallucinations (sight, sound, taste or touch)

0 No evidence of hallucinations
1 Distortions of real objects, aware that these are not real if this is pointed out
2 Appearance of totally new objects or perceptions, aware that these are not real if this is pointed out
3 Believes the hallucinations are real, but still orientated in place and person
4 Believes him/herself to be in a totally non-existent environment, preoccupied and cannot be diverted or reassured.

Orientation

0 The patient is fully orientated in time, place, and person
1 The patient is fully orientated in person, but is not sure where s/he is or what time it is
2 Orientated in person, but disorientated in time and place
3 Doubtful personal orientation, disorientated in time and place; there may be short periods of lucidity
4 Disorientated in time, place, and person. No meaningful contact can be obtained.

Withdrawal severity:

1–4	Mild
5–9	Mild to moderate
10–14	Moderate to severe
15+	Severe

CIWA-AR

Clinical Institute Withdrawal Assessment for Alcohol—Revised

Sullivan J, Sykora M, Schneiderman J, *et al.* Assessment of alcohol withdrawal: the revised. Clinical Institute withdrawal for alcohol scale (CIWA–AR). *Br J Addict* 1989; **84**: 1353–1357.

Patient .... Date .... Time ....

Pulse or heart rate, taken for one minute: ....

Blood pressure: .... / .... Rater's initials ....

Key to scoring

- Nausea and vomiting (0–7)
- Tremor (0–7)
- Paroxysmal sweats (0–7)
- Anxiety (0–7)
- Agitation (0–7)
- Tactile disturbances (0–7)
- Auditory disturbances (0–7)
- Visual disturbances (0–7)
- Headaches, fullness in head (0–7)
- Orientation and clouding of sensorium (0–4)

Total (maximum possible is 67)

Nausea and vomiting

Ask "Do you feel sick to your stomach? Have you vomited?" and observe.

Score

0 No nausea and no vomiting
1 Mild nausea with no vomiting
2
3
4 Intermittent nausea with dry heaves
5
6
7 Constant nausea, frequent dry heaves and vomiting

Tremor

Observe patient's arms extended and fingers spread apart.

Score

0 No tremor
1 Not visible, but can be felt fingertip to fingertip
2
3
4 Moderate, with patient's arms extended
5
6
7 Severe, even with arms not extended

Paroxysmal sweats
Score
0 No sweat visible
1 Barely perceptible sweating, palms moist
2
3
4 Beads of sweat obvious on forehead
5
6
7 Drenching sweats

Anxiety
Observe, and ask "Do you feel nervous?"

Score
0 No anxiety, at ease
1 Mildly anxious
2
3
4 Moderately anxious, or guarded, so anxiety is inferred
5
6
7 Equivalent to acute panic states as seen in severe delirium or acute schizophrenic reactions

Agitation
Score
0 Normal activity
1 Somewhat more than normal activity
2
3
4 Moderately fidgety and restless
5
6
7 Paces back and forth during most of the interview, or constantly thrashes about

Tactile disturbances
Ask "Have you any itching, pins and needles sensations, any burning, any numbness or do you feel bugs crawling on or under your skin?"

Score
0 None
1 Very mild itching, pins and needles, burning or numbness
2 Mild itching, pins and needles, burning or numbness
3 Moderate itching, pins and needles, burning or numbness
4 Moderately severe hallucinations
5 Severe hallucinations
6 Extremely severe hallucinations
7 Continuous hallucinations

Auditory disturbances

Ask "Are you more aware of sounds around you? Are they harsh? Do they frighten you? Are you hearing anything that is disturbing to you? Are you hearing things you know are not there?", and observe.

Score

0 Not present
1 Very mild harshness or ability to frighten
2 Mild harshness or ability to frighten
3 Moderate harshness or ability to frighten
4 Moderately severe hallucinations
5 Severe hallucinations
6 Extremely severe hallucinations
7 Continuous hallucinations

Visual disturbances

Ask "Does the light appear to be too bright? Is its colour different? Does it hurt your eyes? Are you seeing anything that is disturbing to you? Are you seeing things you know are not there?", and observe.

Score:

0 Not present
1 Very mild sensitivity
2 Mild sensitivity
3 Moderate sensitivity
4 Moderately severe hallucinations
5 Severe hallucinations
6 Extremely severe hallucinations
7 Continuous hallucinations

Headaches, fullness in head

Ask "Does your head feel different? Does it feel like there is a band around your head?"

Do not rate for dizziness or lightheadedness. Otherwise, rate severity.

Score

0 Not present
1 Very mild
2 Mild
3 Moderate
4 Moderately severe
5 Severe
6 Very severe
7 Extremely severe

Orientation and clouding of sensorium

Ask "What day is this? Where are you? Who am 1?"

Score:
0 Orientated and can do serial additions
1 Cannot do serial additions or is uncertain about date
2 Disorientated for date by no more than 2 calendar days
3 Disorientated for date by more than 2 calendar days
4 Disorientated for place and/or person

Withdrawal severity:
Mild withdrawal: Score < 10
Moderate withdrawal: Score 10–20
Severe withdrawal: Score > 20

CIWA-B*: Clinical institute Withdrawal Assessment for Benzodiazepines

Clinician observation

For each of the following items, please circle the number which best describes the severity of each symptom or sign.

Patient self-report

For each of the following items, ask the patient to circle the number which best describes how he/she feels.

		0	1	2	3	4
1.	Observe behaviour for restlessness and agitation	Home, normal activity		Restless		Paces back and forth, unable to sit still
2.	Ask patient to extend arms with fingers apart, observe tremor	No tremor	Not visible, can be felt in fingers	Visible but mild	Moderate with areas extended	Severe, with arms not extended
3.	Observe for sweating, feel palms	No sweating visible	Barely perceptible, palms moist	Palms and forehead moist, reports armpits sweating	Beads of sweat on forehead	Severe drenching sweats
4.	Do you feel irritable?	Not at all				Very much so
5.	Do you feel fatigued?	Not at all				Severely
6.	Do you feel tense?	Not at all				Very much so
7.	Do you have difficulties concentrating?	No difficulty				Can't concentrate
8.	Do you have any loss of appetite?	No loss				No appetite
9.	Have you any numbness or burning sensation on your face, hands or feet?	No				Severe
10.	Do you feel your heart racing?	No				Constantly
11.	Does your head feel full or achy?	No				Severe
12.	Do you feel muscle aches or stiffness?	Not at all				Severe

13. Do you feel anxious, nervous or jittery?	0 Not at all	1	2	3	4 Very much so
14. Do you feel upset?	0 Not at all	1	2	3	4 Very much so
15. How restful was your sleep last night?	0 Very restful	1	2	3	4 Not at all
16. Do you feel weak?	0 Not at all	1	2	3	4 Very much so
17. Do you think you didn't have enough sleep last night?	0 No	1	2	3	4 Not nearly enough
18. Do you have any visual disturbances? (sensitivity to light, blurred vision)	0 Not at all	1	2	3	4 Yes, extreme
19. Are you fearful?	0 Not at all	1	2	3	4 Very much so
20. Have you been worrying about possible misfortunes lately?	0 Not at all	1	2	3	4 Very much so

Total score (Total of Items 1 to 20) . . . .
Rater's initials . . . .

1–20 = mild withdrawal

21–40 = moderate withdrawal

41–60 = severe withdrawal

61–80 = very severe withdrawal

Adapted from: Clinical Institute Withdrawal Assessment for Benzodiazepines.

Further reading

Busto UE, Sykora K, Sellers EM, *et al*. A clinical scale to assess benzodiazepine withdrawal. *Journal of Clinical Psychopharmacology* 1989; **9**: 412–416.

The Subjective Opiate Withdrawal Scale (SOWS)

Date .... Time ....

	Symptom	Not at all	A little	Moderately	Quite a bit	Extremely
1	I feel anxious	0	1	2	3	4
2	I feel like yawning	0	1	2	3	4
3	I am perspiring	0	1	2	3	4
4	My eyes are teary	0	1	2	3	4
5	My nose is running	0	1	2	3	4
6	I have goosebumps	0	1	2	3	4
7	I am shaking	0	1	2	3	4
8	I have hot flushes	0	1	2	3	4
9	I have cold flushes	0	1	2	3	4
10	My bones and muscles ache	0	1	2	3	4
11	I feel restless	0	1	2	3	4
12	I feel nauseous	0	1	2	3	4
13	I feel like vomiting	0	1	2	3	4
14	My muscles twitch	0	1	2	3	4
15	I have stomach cramps	0	1	2	3	4
16	I feel like using now	0	1	2	3	4

Please score each of the 16 items below according to how you feel now (circle one number)

Range 0–64. Handelsman, L., Cochrane, K. J., Aronson, M. J. et al. (1987) Two New Rating Scales for Opiate Withdrawal, *American Journal of Alcohol Abuse*, **13**, 293–308.

Objective Opioid Withdrawal Scale (OOWS)

Date .... Time ....

Observe the patient during a 5 minute observation period

Then indicate a score for each of the opioid withdrawal signs listed below (items 1–13). Add the scores for each item to obtain the total score

	Sign	Measures	Score
1	Yawning	0 = no yawns	1 = ≥ 1 yawn
2	Rhinorrhoea	0 = < 3 sniffs	1 = ≥ 3 sniffs
3	Piloerection (observe arm)	0 = absent	1 = present
4	Perspiration	0 = absent	1 = present
5	Lacrimation	0 = absent	1 = present
6	Tremor (hands)	0 = absent	1 = present
7	Mydriasis	0 = absent	1 = ≥ 3 mm
8	Hot and Cold flushes	0 = absent	1 = shivering/ huddling for warmth
9	Restlessness	0 = absent	1 = frequent shifts of position
10	Vomiting	0 = absent	1 = present
11	Muscle twitches	0 = absent	1 = present
12	Abdominal cramps	0 = absent	1 = Holding stomach
13	Anxiety	0 = absent	1 = mild - severe

Range 0–13 Handelsman, L., Cochrane, K. J., Aronson, M. J. *et al.* (1987) Two New Rating Scales for Opiate Withdrawal, *American Journal of Alcohol Abuse*, **13**, 293–308.

Neonatal Abstinence Syndrome (Modified Finnegan's Scale)

NAS Scoring Chart

For infants at risk of opioid withdrawal—Assess four hourly [½ to 1 hour after each feed]

Name: _____   Frequency: _____   Date and time in hours

System	Signs & Symptoms	Score									
Central nervous system disturbance	High-pitched cry	2									
	Continuous high-pitched cry	3									
	Sleeps <1 h between feeds	3									
	Sleeps < 2 h between feeds	2									
	Sleeps < 3 h between feeds	1									
	Mild tremors disturbed	1									
	Moderate-severe tremors disturbed	2									
	Mild tremors undisturbed	3									
	Moderate-severe tremors undisturbed	4									
	Increased muscle tone	2									
	Excoriation (specify area)	1									
	Myoclonic jerks	3									
	Generalized convulsions	5									

Metabolic/vasomotor respiratory disturbances	Fever (37.3–38.3°C)	1											
	Fever (38.4°C and higher)	2											
	Frequent yawning >3–4 times	1											
	Nasal stuffiness	1											
	Sneezing >3–4 times	1											
	Nasal flaring	2											
	Respiratory rate >60 min	1											
	Respiratory rate >60 min with retractions	2											
Gastro-intestinal disturbance	Excessive sucking	1											
	Poor feeding	2											
	Regurgitation	2											
	Projectile vomiting	3											
	Loose stools	2											
	Watery stools	3											
	Total score												
	Scorer's initials												

Adapted from: Finnegan LP. Neonatal abstinence syndrome: assessment and pharmacotherapy. In: Rubaltelli FF, Granati B (Eds). Neonatal Therapy: an Update. Amsterdam: Elsevier Science 1986: 122–146.
Finnegan LP, Connaughton JR, Kron RE, Emich JP. Neonatal abstinence syndrome: assessment and management. Addictive Diseases 1975; 2: 141–158.

Guidelines for NAS scoring

- High-pitched cry: score 2 if a cry is high-pitched at its peak, score 3 if a cry is high-pitched throughout
- Sleep: consider total amount of time baby was asleep between feeds
- Tremors: this is a scale of increasing severity and only one score should be made from the four categories. Undisturbed sleep means when the baby is asleep or at rest in a cot
- Increased muscle tone: score if the baby has a generalized muscle tone greater than the upper limit of normal
- Excoriation: score if excoriation occurs more than 3–4 times in 30 min
- Nasal flaring: score if nasal flaring is present without other evidence of airways disease
- Respiratory rate: score if respiratory rate of >60/min is present without other evidence of airways disease
- Excessive sucking: score if the baby sucks more than average
- Poor feeding: score if the baby is very slow to feed or takes inadequate amounts
- Regurgitation: score only if the baby regurgitates more frequently than usual in newborn infants.

- A: infants scoring 3 consecutive abstinence scores averaging more than 8 (e.g. 9–7–9) or >12 for 2 scores require treatment. The scoring interval should be 4-hourly until the infant has been stabilized. Infants withdrawing from non-opiates frequently display similar behaviours to those withdrawing from opiates
- B: modifications for prematurity are mainly necessary in the sections on sleeping; e.g. a baby who needs 3-hourly feeds can only sleep at most 2.5 h between them. Scoring should be:
  - if baby sleeps less than 2 h
  - if sleeps less than 1 hour, and
  - if the baby does not sleep between feeds.
  - many premature babies require tube feeding. Babies should not be scored for poor feeding if tube feeding is customary for their period of gestation.
- C: exclude other causes of fever, tachypnoea, and seizures, e.g. infection.

Mini mental state examination

	Patient score	Maximum score
Orientation		
1. What is the (year) (season) (month) (date) (day)?		5
2. Where are we: (State) (country) (city) (suburb) (street or hospital) (house number or ward)? (Accept exact answer only)		5
Registration		
3. I am going to name three objects, after I have said all three objects, I want you to repeat them. Remember what they are because I am going to ask you to name them in a few minutes (say them slowly at 1-s intervals)		3
Please repeat the three items for me. (Score 1 point for each correct reply on the first attempt; allow 20 s for reply, if subject did not repeat all three, repeat until they are learned or up to a maximum of 5 s)		
Attention and calculation		
4. Subtract 7 from 100 and keep subtracting seven from what is left until I tell you to stop. (May repeat three times if patient pauses, just the same instruction—allow 1 min, stop after 5 answers)		5
If unable to subtract, ask him/her to recite the days of the week backwards or spell 'world' backwards		
Recall		
5. Now what were the three objects that I asked you to remember?		3
Please repeat the three items for me. (Score 1 point for each correct reply on the first attempt. Allow 10, allow 1 point for each correct response regardless of order)		

Language

6. Show 2 objects (watch—take off wrist). 'What is this called?' Then pencil. 'What is this called?' (Allow 10 s, use watch, not clock, 0, accept pencil only not pen) — 2

7. I'd like you to repeat a phrase after me. 'No ifs, ands or buts' (Allow 10 s —repetition must be exact) — 1

8. Follow a 3-stage command—ask if the patient is left- or right-handed. 'take this paper in your (right/left) hand, fold it in half once with both hands, and put the paper down on the floor'. (Allow 10 s—repetition must be exact) — 3

9. Read the words on this page and then do what it says (show a sheet of paper with close your eyes typed on it) — 1

(If subject reads and does not close their eyes—may repeat instruction a maximum of 3 times. Allow 10 s; score 1 point only if subject closes eyes. Subject does not have to read aloud)

10. Ask the patient to write any complete sentence on a piece of paper. (Allow 30 s. The sentence should make sense. Ignore spelling errors) — 1

11. Give patient pencil, rubber and paper and the design (see over). Ask him/her to copy the design (two intersecting pen-tangles). (Allow multiple tries until patient is finished and hands it back. Maximum time 1 min. Check if all sides and angles are preserved and if the intersecting sides form a quadrangle) — 1

Total score			30
Interpreting score	0–17	18–23	24–30
	Marked cognitive impairment, very likely to be dementia	Moderate cognitive impairment, quite possibly dementia	Normal range. Interpretation depends on previous level of education, language/culture.

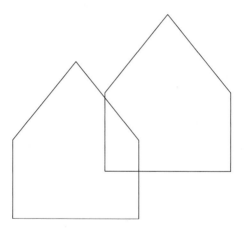

12 Steps of AA

- We admitted we were powerless over alcohol and that our lives had become unmanageable
- We came to believe that a Power greater than ourselves could restore us to sanity
- We made a decision to turn our will and our lives over to the care of God, as we understand him
- We made a searching and fearless moral inventory of ourselves
- We admitted to God, to ourselves, and to another human being the exact nature of our wrongs
- We were entirely ready to have God remove all these defects of character
- We humbly asked Him to remove these shortcomings
- We made a list of all the persons we had harmed and became willing to make amends to them all
- We made direct amends to such people wherever possible, except when to do so would injure them or others
- We continued to take personal inventory and when we were wrong promptly admitted it
- We sought through prayer and meditation to improve our conscious contact with God as we understand him, praying only for knowledge of His will and the power to carry that out
- Having had a spiritual awakening as a result of these steps, we tried to carry this message to others, and to practice these principles in all our affairs.

From Alcoholics Anonymous, USA.

Index

V

varenicline tartrate 159–60
vascular complications of injecting 208–9, 367
venlafaxine 133, 305
ventricular arrhythmias 207
see also tacharrythmias
violent patients 266–7, 392–4
viral hepatitis serology 102
viral infections 208, 220–1, 368
vitamin
  deficiencies 85–6
  B12 102
  thiamine 114–15, 119, 123, 178, 390
volatile solvents 16, 292–4

W

Wernicke's encephalopathy 50, 84, 98, 109, 112, 114, 119–20, 132, 390
withdrawal syndrome 19
  alcohol 110–17, 120–1, 384–91
  anabolic steroids 282
  benzodiazepine withdrawal 172–3, 175, 179–83
  cannabis withdrawal 192, 196
  ICD/DSM diagnosis 78, 426–7
  monitoring scales 430–42
  nicotine withdrawal 149–50
  opioid 206, 360–1
  psychostimulant 247–8

see also alcohol withdrawal, benzodiazepine withdrawal, nicotine withdrawal, opioid withdrawal
workplace safety/responsibility 411–14
work-related stress 349
work place drug testing 413

X

X-ray abdominal 106
X-ray chest 106

Z

zaleplon 184
'Z' drugs 25, 184–5
zidovudine 226
zolpidem 28, 184
zopiclone 28, 184, 355